D0029578

WHY DO I STILL HAVE THYROID SYMPTOMS?

WHEN MY LAB TESTS ARE NORMAL

*A revolutionary breakthrough in understanding
Hashimoto's disease and hypothyroidism*

By Datis Kharrazian, DHSc, DC, MS

Why Do I Still Have Thyroid Symptoms?
When My Lab Tests Are Normal

Copyright © 2010 Datis Kharrazian. All rights reserved.

No part of this publication may be reproduced, stored in a retrieval system, or transmitted in any form or by any means, electronic, mechanical, photocopying, recording, scanning or otherwise, except as permitted under Sections 107 or 108 of the 1976 United States Copyright Act, without either the prior written permission of the Publisher.

LIMIT OF LIABILITY/DISCLAIMER OF WARRANTY: WHILE THE PUBLISHER AND AUTHOR HAVE USED THEIR BEST EFFORTS IN PREPARING THIS BOOK, THEY MAKE NO REPRESENTATIONS OR WARRANTIES WITH RESPECT TO THE ACCURACY OR COMPLETENESS OF THE CONTENTS OF THIS BOOK AND SPECIFICALLY DISCLAIM ANY IMPLIED WARRANTIES OF MERCHANTABILITY OR FITNESS FOR A PARTICULAR PURPOSE. NO WARRANTY MAY BE CREATED OR EXTENDED BY SALES REPRESENTATIVES, WRITTEN SALES OR PROMOTIONAL MATERIALS. THE ADVICE AND STRATEGIES CONTAINED HEREIN MAY NOT BE SUITABLE FOR YOUR SITUATION. THIS BOOK IS SOLD WITH THE UNDERSTANDING THAT THE PUBLISHER IS NOT ENGAGED IN RENDERING MEDICAL, LEGAL, ACCOUNTING, OR OTHER PROFESSIONAL SERVICES. YOU SHOULD CONSULT WITH A PROFESSIONAL WHERE APPROPRIATE. NEITHER THE PUBLISHER NOR AUTHOR SHALL BE LIABLE FOR ANY LOSS OF PROFIT OR ANY OTHER COMMERCIAL DAMAGES, INCLUDING BUT NOT LIMITED TO SPECIAL, INCIDENTAL, CONSEQUENTIAL, OR OTHER DAMAGES.

ISBN 978-0-9856904-0-3

Library of Congress Control Number: 2012948480

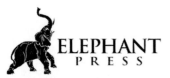

ELEPHANT
P R E S S

Elephant Press LP
7040 Avenida Encinas, Suite 104
Carlsbad, CA 92011 USA
www.ElephantPressBooks.com

ABOUT THE AUTHOR

Datis Kharrazian, DC, DHS, MS, MNeuroSci, FAACP, DACBN, DABCN, DIBAK, CNS

Dr. Datis Kharrazian is considered one of the leading experts in non-pharmaceutical applications to chronic illnesses, autoimmune disorders, and complex neurological disorders. Patients from all over the world fly into his practice located in San Diego, California to understand his perspective regarding their condition and to apply natural medicine alternatives to help them improve their quality of life. Dr. Kharrazian has become the referral source for many doctors nationally and internationally when their cases becomes too complex to evaluate and diagnose.

Dr. Kharrazian is one of the most sought after educators in natural medicine, laboratory analysis, and nutrition. His seminar schedule is booked two years in advance. He lectures both nationally and internationally at various medical and scientific conferences worldwide. He conducts more than 80 professional and scientific presentations a year in addition to giving radio and television interviews. He is also scheduled to appear in upcoming movie documentaries. Dr. Kharrazian has personally trained several thousand health care professionals and currently has educated a group of more than a dozen exceptional doctors to lecture nationally in order to meet the demands for education in his patient management model.

Dr. Kharrazian's first book, Why Do I Still Have Thyroid Symptoms When My Lab Tests Are Normal? quickly became the best-selling thyroid book. It has been listed as the number-one selling thyroid book on Amazon since its release in October of 2009. His book created an international explosion of interest from his detailed review of the scientific literature regarding thyroid disease and his clinical model of patient management. Thousands of positive testimonials have been received globally from the model he created.

Dr. Kharrazian has published numerous professional papers, post-graduate course manuals, and professional journal articles about functional medicine, nutrition, laboratory analysis, and case studies. He has also recorded more than 30 educational audio CDs that cover the latest research and clinical applications related to the topics of autoimmunity, hormone imbalances, and neurological disorders. Dr. Kharrazian is on the editorial board of the Journal of Functional Neurology.

Dr. Kharrazian earned his Bachelor of Science degree from the University of the State of New York with honors and his Doctor of Chiropractic degree graduating

Dr. Kharrazian's material is way beyond the stuff they teach in medical school.
Ron Manzanero, MD
Austin Integrative Medicine
Austin, TX

"This information is critical to all practicing healthcare professionals and their suffering patients, which often includes the doctors themselves. It is eye-opening, relevant to any disease or pathology, and immediately applicable for all your patients. I highly recommend it."
—Kari Vernon, DC, Scottsdale, AZ

What I learned about identifying thyroid disorders from Dr. Kharrazian has been invaluable to my practice. I recently had a woman with all the typical thyroid symptoms but after blood tests and scans, doctors found nothing wrong. Using Dr. Kharrazian's method I was able to identify an autoimmune thyroid condition, which caused her thyroid-stimulating hormone to fluctuate. I was also able to restore thyroid balance to some people whose doctors recommended natural methods to help the thyroid; these natural methods only exacerbated the problem. With so many people suffering with thyroid issues, Dr. Kharrazian's book is a timely lifesaver.
Donna DiMarco, CN, LNC
Pompano Beach, FL

What I have learned from Dr. Kharrazian has changed my entire practice. I am seeing many more chronic patients, and I am getting amazing results. It is astounding how many people have undiagnosed Hashimoto's. People with this condition are the largest part of my practice. I love working with them because they are so responsive to support. When you help them, they tell everyone what you did for them. I would never have been able to understand how to properly care for these patients without the incredible knowledge from Dr. Kharrazian. I am eternally grateful for his vast knowledge of auto-immune disease.
Mark Flannery, DC
HealthWise Chiropractic and Nutrition
Simi Valley, CA

D0004091

I have been attending Dr. Kharrazian's seminars for two years, and each one is better than the last. Much of what he teaches is leaps ahead of what is being done with conventional medicine. Kharrazian's approach is the latest in medical research and as cutting edge as it gets.

Jim Chialtas, LAc
San Diego, CA

Since I met Dr. Kharrazian in 2006, my practice has evolved into one I could not have imagined. His work in evaluating thyroid disorders has given me the tools necessary to affect a person who has all the low thyroid symptoms but normal test results. Thank you, Dr. Kharrazian, for your passion in research and education in developing a clinical approach outside of the traditional, theoretical model we all have been following in our practices.

David G. Arthur, DC, DACNB
Mountain Health Chiropractic and Neurology Center
Englewood, CO

Wow, as practitioners we want to get to the cause of our patients' ailments. This information is leading edge and gets to the cause of the problem.

Paulette Coates, ND
Lakewood, CO

Prior to attending Dr. Kharrazian's classes, I was not seeing consistent results in my health or the health of my patients using the traditional alternative approach to thyroid problems. I was unable to understand or explain what was occurring in our bodies. Each class I attend is a giant step up in understanding science-based thyroid care, functional endocrinology, and blood nutrition analysis. Dr. Kharrazian's classes will change the face of alternative healthcare.

David Peterson, DC
Wellness Alternatives
Town and Country, MO

I have attended all of Dr. Kharrazian's seminars. His approach has caused me to rethink how I approach thyroid treatment. This is excellent material.

Robert Mathis, MD, ABHM, CNS, MCP
Baselinehealth.net
Santa Barbara, CA

www.thyroidbook.com

with honors from Southern California University of Health Sciences, where he was distinguished with the Mindlin Honors at Entrance Award, the Dean's List, and the Delta Sigma Award for Academic Excellence. He has earned a Master of Science degree in Human Nutrition from the University of Bridgeport, a Master of Neurological Sciences from the Carrick Institute of Graduate Studies, and a Doctor of Health Science from Nova Southeastern University. He is currently completing his Ph.D. in health sciences with doctoral research in immunology at Nova Southeastern University.

Dr. Kharrazian has completed many postgraduate specialty programs and has been board certified in numerous specialties that include Diplomate of the Board of Nutrition Specialists, Diplomate of the American Board of Clinical Nutrition, Diplomate of the Chiropractic Board of Clinical Nutrition, Diplomate of the American Board of Chiropractic Neurology, and Diplomate of the International Board of Applied Kinesiology.

His contributions and devotions to clinical practice and educations have earned him several fellowships including Fellow of the American Board of Vestibular Rehabilitation, Fellow of the American Academy of Chiropractic Physicians, Fellow of the International Academy of Functional Neurology and Rehabilitation, and Fellow of the American College of Functional Neurology.

Dr. Kharrazian has been a consultant to several nutritional companies and has formulated more than 60 nutritional products, including topical creams, protein powders, liquid supplements, sublingual hormones, and sublingual nutrients. His formulations are used by thousands of health care professionals nationally for various health disorders.

Dr. Kharrazian was recently recognized by his peers and awarded the Clinician Trailblazer award at the 2010 Annual Conference of Functional Neurology. This award was given to him in recognition for his cutting edge research and for defining the future of clinical practice.

Several institutes and universities have asked Dr. Kharrazian to develop advanced academic programs for graduate and post-graduate programs outlining the latest information in natural approaches to various medical disorders. He is currently teaching postgraduate courses sponsored by the University of Bridgeport and is an associate professor of clinical neurology for the Carrick Institute.

www.thyroidbook.com

INTENDED USE STATEMENT

The content of this book is intended for information purposes only. The medical information in this book is intended as general information only and should not be used in any way to diagnose, treat, cure, or prevent any disease. The goal of this book is to present and highlight nutritionally significant information and offer suggestions and protocols for nutritional support and health maintenance.

It is the sole responsibility of the user of this information to comply with all local and federal laws regarding the use of such information, as it relates to the scope and type of the user's practice.

DISCLAIMER AND NOTICES

The information and recommendations outlined in this book are not intended as a substitute for personalized medical advice; the reader of this book should see a qualified health care provider. This book proposes certain theoretical methods of nutrition not necessarily mainstream. It is left to the discretion and it is the sole responsibility of the user of the information indicated in this book to determine if procedures and recommendations described are appropriate. The author of this information cannot be held responsible for the information or any inadvertent errors or omissions of the information.

The information in this presentation should not be construed as a claim or representation that any procedure or product mentioned constitutes a specific cure, palliative or ameliorative. Procedures and nutritional compounds described should be considered as adjunctive to other accepted conventional procedures deemed necessary by the attending licensed doctor.

It is the concern of the Department of Health and Human Services that no homeopathic or nutritional supplements be used to replace established, conventional medical approaches, especially in cases of emergencies, serious or life-threatening diseases, or conditions.

I share in this concern, as replacing conventional treatment with such remedies, especially in serious cases, may deprive the patient of necessary treatment and thereby cause harm as well as potentially pose a major legal liability for the health professional involved. The nutritional compounds mentioned in this book should not be used as replacements for conventional medical treatment.

The Food and Drug Administration has not evaluated the information detailed in this document. The nutritional supplements mentioned in this manual are not intended to diagnose, treat, cure, or prevent disease.

FOREWORD

By Aristo Vojdani, PhD, MSc, MT

An estimated 27 million Americans suffer from thyroid-related illnesses, the majority of them women. Yet thyroid-related diseases are often ill diagnosed, and there is much about their treatment that bears greater clarification and study. Dr. Datis Kharrazian's *Why Do I Still Have Thyroid Symptoms When My Lab Tests Are Normal?* presents a revolutionary breakthrough in understanding Hashimoto's and hypothyroidism and supporting people who have these conditions.

Using a fascinating approach, Dr. Kharrazian tackles the confusing science of Hashimoto's by emphasizing the root cause of thyroid-related illnesses. After reviewing each of the ten chapters, I was in awe at Dr. Kharrazian's line of reasoning and amazed at its similarity to an article I recently published, "Antibodies as predictors of autoimmune diseases and cancer," in *Expert Opinion on Medical Diagnostics*, (June 2008 593-605). The idea that environmental factors, in particular infectious agents, may cause severe thyroid disorder has been in the literature since the 1940s. This book marks the concept's full reemergence. Dr.

Kharrazian is to be congratulated for bringing together much of the current research and combining it with his vast clinical experience to achieve a greater understanding of clinical and subclinical thyroid disorders. By connecting the dots, Dr. Kharrazian is pioneering the future approach to supporting thyroid disorders.

It is generally accepted that the thyroid autoantibodies thyroglobulin and thyroid peroxidase reflect disease activity and progression and are valuable in disease prediction and the classification of Hashimoto's and Graves' diseases. While clinicians rely on antibody levels and elevations in thyroid stimulating hormone, they give little attention to the factors involved in thyroid autoimmunity, as Dr. Kharrazian indicates. Researchers and clinicians should be asking the question, "Why does the human body react to its own antigens, resulting in the production of potentially harmful autoantibodies?" This event may be caused by environmental factors, such as bacterial or viral infections, or toxic haptenic chemicals binding to human tissue, causing modification of self-antigens and the subsequent production of autoantibodies.

The book begins, in simple terms, with the basics of the thyroid gland and the thyroid metabolic pathway. Since the thyroid gland is connected to many dots including gastrointestinal function, adrenal hormone metabolism, stomach acid production, brain chemistry changes, and liver detoxification, its dysfunction can contribute to clinical manifestations throughout the body. Dr. Kharrazian uses case histories to illustrate the thyroid connection to suboptimal health. For him, a basic understanding of immune function is the first step in managing thyroid disorders. According to Dr. Kharrazian, the immune system must be addressed and supported along with the thyroid to successfully manage Hashimoto's, prevent future autoimmune diseases, and enjoy a better quality of life.

Given its complexity, especially when it comes to autoimmunity, it is no wonder that the immune system is uncharted territory for many medical professionals. Dr. Kharrazian likens this intricate system of checks and balances to a crime movie that involves the mafia, good cops, bad cops, and double-crossers. And, as in a typical crime drama, plans go awry when any of the players deviates from his job. Dr. Kharrazian describes the role of TH-1 and TH-2 cytokine dominance in autoimmune diseases and explains how a new helper T-cell, called the regulatory T-cell, can regulate TH-1 and TH-2 imbalance. Using natural medicine, he guides the reader through the delicate helper T-cell balancing act.

Dr. Kharrazian outlines how to identify the six patterns of low thyroid function, using blood tests. By understanding these functional blood chemistry panels, a physician can assess and support countless people with thyroid disorders early. Dr. Kharrazian draws on his years of clinical experience for specific recommendations to help nutritionally address abnormal chemistries.

For me, the highlight of the book is the final chapter in which Dr. Kharrazian scientifically connects 22 dots to low thyroid function. My favorites are:

- Hypothalamus paraventricular effect promoted by cytokines, leading to low TSH

- Thyroid resistance promoted by elevated cytokines

- Down-regulated 5'deiodinase activity from elevated cytokines

- Down-regulated 5'deiodinase from gastrointestinal dysbiosis and lipopolysaccharides (endotoxins) produced by gram negative bacteria

These four dots link the gut-brain connection to thyroid function, which has been the topic of many recent scientific articles.

By reading this book, practitioners and patients will learn how to connect the dots from environmental factors to Hashimoto's. When these dots are given the proper attention, and are addressed efficiently, then many peoples' lives can be changed for the better. Practitioners must read this book. It will guide them through the intricacies of thyroid disorders, how to identify their causes, and how to tailor the most effective support for each patient. Incorporating the lessons learned from Dr. Datis Kharrazian's *Why Do I Still Have Thyroid Symptoms When My Lab Tests Are Normal?* into clinical practice will make a world of difference in the realm of autoimmune disorders.

References

1. Lipopolysaccharide and a social stressor influence behavior, corticosterone and cytokine levels. Hayley *et al.*, *J. of Neuroimmunology*, 197:29-36, 2008.

2. The gut-brain barrier in major depression: intestinal mucosal dysfunction with an increased translocation of LPS from gram negative enterobacteria (leaky gut) plays a role in the inflammatory pathophysiology of depression. Maes *et al.*, *Neuroendocrinology Letters*, 29:117-124, 2008.

3. Increased serum IgA and IgM against LPS of enterobacteria in chronic fatigue syndrome (CFS): indication for the involvement of gram-negative enterobacteria in the etiology of CFS and for the presence of an increased gut-intestinal permeability. Maes *et al.*, *J. of Affective Disorders*, 99:237-240, 2007.

4. Mechanisms of disease: the role of intestinal barrier function in the pathogenesis of gastrointestinal autoimmune diseases. Fasano and Shea-Donohue, *Nature Clinical Practice Gastroenterology and Hepatology*, 2:416-422, 2005.

5. Bacterial lipopolysaccharide stimulated the thyrotropin-dependent thyroglobulin gene expression at the transcriptional level by involving the transcription factors thyroid transcription factor-1 and paired box domain transcription factor 8. Velez *et al.*, *Endocrinology*, 147:3260-3275, 2006.

DEDICATION

First, I would like to dedicate this book to the millions of thyroid patients who have been ignored and made to feel uncomfortable by their healthcare practitioners.

Second, I would like to dedicate this book to all the healthcare practitioners who are reading this book because they want to better serve their patients.

Third, and most importantly, I would like to dedicate this book to my wife Andrea and to my daughter Maizy for fueling my soul and spirit.

CONTENTS

Introduction

Although she was only in her early forties, Lea feared for her life, convinced she was on the verge of a heart attack. Sometimes her heart pounded so fiercely and quickly she thought it would pop right out of her chest, and she swears she could see it beating under her skin. Her racing heart put such a strain on her lungs that they became sore. When Lea had one of these spells, she could barely walk up a hill or a flight of stairs. Despite feeling exhausted, the nervous energy created by her racing heart made her anxious and kept her up late every night.

And yet at other times, Lea felt as if she were moving underwater — a pressing fatigue, relentless in its grasp, weighed down her limbs and pushed on her head. Her voice grew hoarse as the tissue around her Adam's apple became puffy and tender, and she was always cold. Despite having lost weight easily after the birth of each of her first three children, Lea's body continued to balloon after her fourth child was born. Her puffy eyes and face vexed her deeply and, unsurprisingly, she also battled chronic depression.

Lea visited several medical doctors and had numerous cardiovascular tests done, only to be told she was fine. Natural medicine cardiologists she consulted came to the same conclusion. Finally a friend suggested she get tested for Hashimoto's disease, an autoimmune disease that destroys the thyroid, and sure enough, her blood test came back positive. "Great!" she thought. "Now that I know what's wrong with me, I can finally get some help!" A physician prescribed thyroid hormone, which quickly brought her thyroid hormone levels into a normal range. Lea's symptoms improved for a while, but then slowly returned: The weight wouldn't budge and the chronic fatigue made a come back. So did the terrifying episodes when she thought her heart would jump out of her chest. "What's going on?" Lea asked her doctor. "Why do I still have hypothyroid symptoms when my blood tests are normal?"

Though it weighs less than an ounce, the butterfly-shaped thyroid gland is a formidable figure in the intricate dance of human physiology. The thyroid is the spark plug for energy production — it controls the rate of energy production, maintains body temperature, helps regulate children's growth, and profoundly affects brain chemistry, influencing moods and emotions. When one sees thyroid function within the intelligent matrix of the human body, taking into account the immune system, hormone balance, and even brain function, it becomes easy to see why addressing the entire body — as demonstrated in *Why Do I Still Have Thyroid Symptoms?* — is a very logical way to support the thyroid.

According to the American Association of Clinical Endocrinologists, more than 27 million Americans suffer from thyroid dysfunction, half of which go undiagnosed. Of the detected cases of hypothyroidism, more than half are due to an autoimmune disorder called Hashimoto's disease, in which the immune system attacks and destroys thyroid gland tissue. All too frequently, the question of why the thyroid gland quit working never comes up. Thyroid symptoms are like the person on the airport runway, using giant arm motions and brightly lit orange wands, waving at you in the hopes that you'll steer the right course. Yet standard health care, both conventional and alternative, often treats the thyroid as a car part that simply needs replacing or lubricating. Thyroid replacement hormones are a first line of defense for many doctors, prescribed with the promise of wiping out a number of symptoms in one fell swoop. But taking that approach is turning a blind eye to what caused the thyroid to become depressed in the first place. For example, irregular immune function, poor blood sugar metabolism, gut infections, adrenal problems, and hormonal imbalances can all significantly depress thyroid function. While prescription thyroid hormones might bring their levels in the blood into a normal range, the hormone replacement doesn't address what caused the thyroid to falter in the first place. The drugs may make some people feel better, but for many others the relief is short-lived, if it occurs at all...even when they have normal blood test results

It is far wiser to ask what the faltering thyroid says about the entire body, and proceed from there. I address the conditions that caused the thyroid to slow down in the first place, and find supporting the gland itself either isn't necessary or requires only basic herbal and nutritional therapy for a few months. The conditions creating the hypothyroid symptoms, however, more likely call for lifestyle changes and lasting nutritional support. If the check-engine light on your car lights up, which would be smarter: to investigate the engine or remove the light? Failing to ask what the thyroid symptoms are trying to communicate and prescribing levothyroxine sodium (Synthroid, Armour, or Levoxyl) is like simply removing the engine light. When I started addressing the underlying causes of hypothyroidism in my practice, my patients began to enjoy not only symptom relief but also true health.

In Lea's case, supplementing with thyroid hormone returned her thyroid-stimulating hormone (TSH) level to normal, but her thyroid gland remained swollen and sore, and she still suffered from a racing heart, insomnia, and listless fatigue. That's because taking thyroid medication has no effect on the autoimmune disease that was destroying Lea's thyroid gland. Many years after she was prescribed thyroid hormone, Lea came to me. Our first step was to dampen her immune response and slow its attack on her thyroid gland. When the immune system flares up, it destroys thyroid tissue and releases a flood of metabolism-stimulating thyroid hormone into the bloodstream, which causes a racing, pounding heart and anxiety. When the attack slows, the compromised thyroid gland returns the body to the hypothyroid state of fatigue and depression. Complicating Lea's situation is that, like many working moms, she had long lived a harried and exhausting life, eating a poor diet consisting largely of cheap and easy-to-prepare wheat products. As is the case with most, if not all, Hashimoto's victims, eating wheat and other gluten-containing foods only makes Hashimoto's worse.

With my guidance, Lea was willing and committed to support her thyroid problem by addressing several core lifestyle issues, which will be explained in this book, such as giving up some favorite foods and including nutritional and herbal compounds in her daily routine. Within weeks of following my recommendations, most of Lea's symptoms lifted, and today she is able to maintain normal thyroid hormone levels with no medication.

Some doctors, and patients too, might wish to immediately begin with a thyroid prescription. After all, popping a pill sounds much easier than making major lifestyle changes. My prescriptions for wellness are not always easy, and they are rarely quick, which is why I ask my patients to commit to following my suggestions for at least six months. Although the appropriate thyroid medication is often necessary and important, it does not address the underlying breakdowns that caused thyroid function to fail.

I start by having my patients balance their blood sugar with this handy tip: If you feel sleepy or crave sugar after a meal, you ate more carbohydrates than your system can handle. If they have an advanced case of insulin resistance, I introduce a periodic fasting protocol that I designed, along with blood sugar stabilizing nutritional compounds. I also prescribe a gut-repair regimen, which includes eliminating foods that repeatedly fire up the immune system. Not surprisingly these often happen to be their favorite foods, such as pasta, bread, ice cream, and eggs. In some cases, I order more extensive testing to search out parasitic or bacterial infection. Many people also suffer from some degree of adrenal stress, so I address that as well.

Hypothyroidism is not a one-size-fits-all diagnosis, and while thyroid replacement hormones may be necessary for many, they also produce plenty of misses. For example, if Lea's low thyroid function been the result of adrenal stress or caused by taking birth control pills, thyroid hormone medication would not only have been the wrong call, it may have made her condition worse.

In Chapter One I introduce you to the thyroid gland, how it works, and why proper support is so important. In Chapters Two and Three, I outline the mechanisms behind Hashimoto's, and how to address them, which depends upon understanding and supporting the immune system. When doctors treat Hashimoto's, an immune disorder, with thyroid hormone medication alone, symptoms persist because the underlying problem — the gradual destruction of the thyroid gland — goes ignored.In Chapter Four, I identify six patterns of thyroid dysfunction using blood chemistry panels. Only one of these patterns is helped by thyroid replacement hormone. For the rest the patient is often left on her own and told that something else must underlie her depression, mental fuzziness, constipation, fatigue, or hair loss. Once I determine a person's pattern, I go into the lifestyle strategies necessary to live a thyroid-healthy life, adding the more advanced, brain-related thyroid concepts described in Chapter Nine when necessary. In Chapter Ten, I expand the six patterns of low thyroid function to 22.

For the last ten years I have been teaching thousands of doctors around the country the fundamentals of managing hormone and immune disorders, including hypothyroidism and Hashimoto's. I have been working with patients like Lea for more than ten years, and have increasingly specialized in the nutritional support of autoimmune diseases, including Hashimoto's.

I have tried every lab test available and found the ones that lead to the best patient results. As a consultant for the nutritional manufacturing industry, I helped create a line of herbal and nutritional supplements that I use in my practice. Based on the growth of attendance to my seminars and reactions of doctors who attend, I am clearly offering something new. Here are some samples of what doctors who attend my seminars are saying:

"His research is complete enough that he can trace endocrine problems back to other areas of the body that I have never before seen related to each other in the literature. I can't tell you how impressed I

am, how much help he's given me, and how much he has taught me."
—Betty Ann Childress, CNC, CP, Orange, CA

"Dr. Kharrazian's material is way beyond the stuff they teach in medical school."
—Ron Manzanero, MD, Austin Integrative Medicine, Austin, TX

"To have some of these techniques, which are a new way of evaluating patients, it's been a Godsend. I learned things at this seminar that I never learned at school."
—Barry Sunshine, DC, Knoxville, TN

"I was absolutely amazed at the results that I got."
—Brenda Holcombe, ND, Portland, OR

A variety of thyroid diseases exist, such as Graves' disease, in which the thyroid is over active, and thyroid cancer. However *Why Do I Still Have Thyroid Symptoms?* will address the most common disorder — that is, hypothyroidism, whether it's caused by Hashimoto's disease or physiological stressors in the body. This is a book thyroid patients can use while working with a skilled holistic practitioner (or a progressive MD trained in natural medicine). My goal is to provide the motivated patient and his or her doctor with cutting-edge information backed by peer-reviewed studies, a fresh interpretation of thyroid dysfunction, and clinically proven methods of nutritional support. This book is not about criticizing other approaches, including the use of thyroid hormones. In fact, in my own practice I work with many people whose thyroid dysfunction is so advanced that thyroid hormone replacement is necessary. Nevertheless, it remains critical to address the factors covered in Why Do I Still Have Thyroid Symptoms? to maximize the potential of medication and prevent further damage. For some people, however, thyroid medication is unnecessary.

CHAPTER ONE

GETTING ACQUAINTED WITH THE THYROID GLAND

Maria is running late for work and needs to get to the bus stop on time. It's early winter and yesterday wasn't too cold, so she throws on her sweater (her coat is still packed at the back of the closet), grabs her purse, and rushes out the door. She's barely off her front porch when the cold air sinks into her bones. "I'll warm up," she thinks, picking up the pace. But she doesn't, and soon her hands and feet start to feel as if they're hardening into blocks of ice. The culprit? Faulty thyroid function.

The ancient Greeks named the thyroid gland *thyreos,* which means shield, and it's a fitting description. Not only is the thyroid gland, which stretches over the area of the Adam's apple, shaped like a shield, but it also serves as one, by setting the body's speed limit. If you're cold, the thyroid steps on the gas to create more heat. If you've got a virus, the thyroid revs up the engine of your immune system. If you're overly stressed from too many 18-hour days fueled by coffee and bagels, the thyroid hits the brakes so you don't blow a gasket in the fast lane.

1

Instead, the thyroid slowly but surely steers you into the slow lane (or even onto the shoulder).

The most important thing to remember about the thyroid is that it is highly sensitive to the slightest alterations in the body. It has to be, that's its job. So when the thyroid malfunctions, as it eventually does for an estimated 27 million Americans,[1] the question is not "How can I get 'er up and running as quickly as possible?" but rather "Why on earth is my thyroid mashing the brakes with both feet and yanking on the emergency brake at the same time?" When the thyroid is under active, the condition is called *hypothyroidism.* The causes and remedies of this malfunction guide this book. (Some people with Hashimoto's disease experience episodes of an over active thyroid, too).

Let's look at how the thyroid and the various thyroid hormones work, and why Maria got so cold on her way to the bus stop. The thyroid happens to be one of the most complex hormone-producing, or *endocrine,* glands in the body, which is probably why many people don't fully understand how it functions.

Thyroid Metabolism

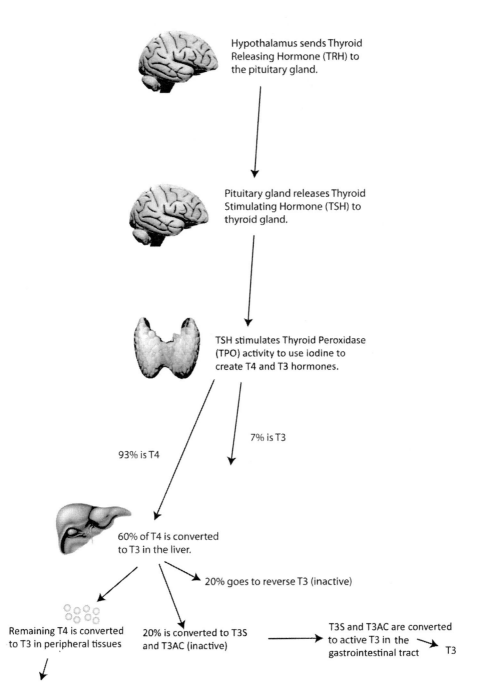

Hypothalamus sends Thyroid Releasing Hormone (TRH) to the pituitary gland.

Pituitary gland releases Thyroid Stimulating Hormone (TSH) to thyroid gland.

TSH stimulates Thyroid Peroxidase (TPO) activity to use iodine to create T4 and T3 hormones.

7% is T3

93% is T4

60% of T4 is converted to T3 in the liver.

20% goes to reverse T3 (inactive)

Remaining T4 is converted to T3 in peripheral tissues

20% is converted to T3S and T3AC (inactive)

T3S and T3AC are converted to active T3 in the gastrointestinal tract

T3

When Maria steps outside on a cold day underdressed, her body becomes cold and sends a message to her *pituitary*, a gland in her brain that is like an air traffic controller for her body, to correct the uncomfortable cold feeling with more body heat. The pituitary pumps out a message to the thyroid called *thyroid stimulating hormone* (TSH) to kick the gland's activity up a notch and create some body heat. The thyroid responds by secreting *thyroxine* (T4), named for its four molecules of iodine, and *triiodothyronine* (T3), named for its three molecules of iodine. The thyroid mostly secretes T4 — only 7 percent is T3. These thyroid hormones then hitch a ride through the bloodstream on thyroid-binding proteins, during which they are referred to as "bound." When they are dropped off at the cells for active duty, they are called "free" hormones.

Although the thyroid gland secretes only a little T3, it happens to be the predominate and most active form the body can use. This means the majority of T4 has to be converted to T3. Most of this happens in the liver, but the conversions also take place in various other cells in the body, such as those of the heart, muscle, and nerves. These cells convert T4 to T3 with an enzyme called *tetraidothyronine 5' deiodinase*, which removes one molecule of iodine. Interestingly, of all the T4 the thyroid secretes, the body uses only about 60 percent of it. Some T4 is converted into *reverse T3* (rT3), a form the body cannot use. Another 20 percent becomes active in the intestines in the presence of a sufficient amount of healthy gut flora, or bacteria. In other words, 20 percent of healthy thyroid hormone activity depends on healthy gut flora. Can you see why something as simple as antibiotic use, which knocks out all gut flora, good and bad, can dampen thyroid function?

In Maria's case, one of the thyroid hormone pathways has broken down so that her body cannot generate enough heat. But assume for a moment that every step in this pathway works: The pituitary, responding to the cold weather, sends TSH to the thyroid gland. The thyroid pumps out T4 and T3, which thyroid-binding proteins carry through the bloodstream to the liver and other cells, where T4 converts to T3. After this conversion, T3 enters the nucleus of each cell, where it turns genes on or off, directing the cells' activities. For Maria, that activity includes generating energy to warm the body.

Are you still with me? It's a logical procession you don't need to memorize since I will review relevant parts of this pathway in discussing the many breakdowns that can happen along the way.

Back to Maria, who is shivering as she walks to the bus stop, silently cursing herself for not taking her winter coat from the back of her closet. What she's not aware of is that the birth control pills she has been taking for a couple of years are creating too much estrogen. Not only will the estrogen dominance in her body fatigue our air-traffic controller, the pituitary gland, but it will also create too many thyroid-binding proteins. Remember those are the proteins that transport thyroid hormones through the bloodstream. Too many of them result in not enough thyroid hormones free to do their jobs. It's like New York City with more than enough cabs, but the drivers won't let their passengers out.

Suppose Maria goes to a doctor complaining of constipation, low energy, and feeling cold most of the time, and her thyroid tests come back normal. She is now relegated to staying bundled in a scarf, mittens, and wool socks even on mildly cool days. Or suppose her blood tests indicate low thyroid function and her doctor prescribes thyroid replacement hormones. She immediately feels great, but as the months go on her symptoms gradually return, even though her blood tests show normal hormone levels. Or, perhaps she doesn't feel any better despite taking thyroid hormone. In fact, her symptoms worsen, and her doctor urges her to exercise more and consider taking an antidepressant. What if her thyroid symptoms are caused by an autoimmune attack on the thyroid gland? Will thyroid hormones and antidepressants address her immune function? The fundamental question has been overlooked: What caused Maria's thyroid to stop working normally? The answer is the premise of this book. Since thyroid function has so many facets, let's explore more of them.

THYROID SYMPTOMS AND SIGNS

How do you know if your thyroid medication is working, or if you have undiagnosed hypothyroidism? Although I use blood chemistry panels and other tests, a person's symptoms and health history are invaluable in accurately assessing a condition. After all, what good are perfect test results if you feel lousy? Below are the most common symptoms of low thyroid function:

- Fatigue
- Weight gain despite adhering to a low-calorie diet
- Morning headaches that wear off as the day progresses
- Depression
- Constipation
- Hypersensitivity to cold weather
- Poor circulation and numbness in hands and feet
- Muscle cramps while at rest
- Increased susceptibility to colds and other viral or bacterial infections and difficulty recovering from them
- Slow wound healing
- Excessive amount of sleep required to function properly
- Chronic digestive problems, such as lack of stomach acid (*hypochlorhydria*)
- Itchy, dry skin
- Dry or brittle hair
- Hair falls out easily
- Dry skin
- Low auxiliary (body-heat) temperature, although this may also be caused by any hormonal imbalance
- Edema, especially facial swelling (*myxedema*)
- Loss of outermost portion of eyebrows

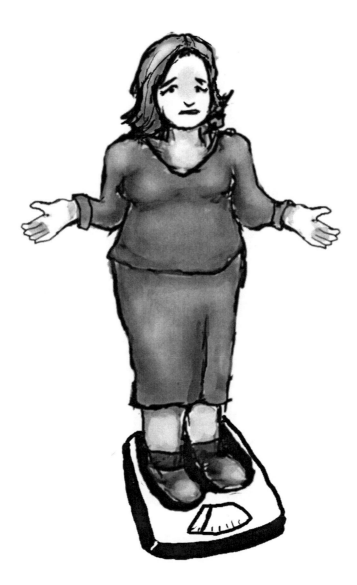

Weight loss can seem impossible for the sufferer of low thyroid function.

OTHER SIGNS THAT CAN INDICATE AUTOIMMUNE HASHIMOTO'S DISEASE:

- Heart palpitations
- Inward trembling
- Increased pulse rate, even at rest
- Feelings of nervousness and emotional distress
- Insomnia
- Night sweats
- Difficulty gaining weight

A BRIEF OVERVIEW OF THYROID HORMONES

Thyroid function is like a relay race, with hormones passing the baton from the brain to the pituitary gland, to the thyroid gland, to the liver, and finally to cells throughout the body. At certain points along the way, these hormones shed some weight by dropping a molecule of iodine before they finish the race. Here is how various hormones perform in the relay race:

Thyrotropin releasing hormone (TRH) To activate the thyroid, the body sends a message to the brain that it needs to speed up metabolism. That's what should have happened to keep Maria warm on a cool day. However, when she was a working, single mother of three, Maria's thyroid often slowed down her metabolism so she wouldn't crash and burn from the chronic stress. The part of the brain that receives the message to either step on the gas or hit the brakes is the *hypothalamus*. This tiny, cone-shaped structure, located in the lower center of the brain, communicates between the nervous and endocrine systems. The hypothalamus delivers messages to the pituitary gland beneath it via the chemical messenger, *thyrotropin releasing hormone* (TRH).

Thyroid stimulating hormone (TSH) or thyrotropin Once TRH delivers its message to the pituitary gland, it releases *thyroid stimulating hormone* (TSH). TSH runs straight to the thyroid gland where it will "pass the baton," ushering in iodine, which stimulates an enzyme called *thyroid peroxidase* (TPO). Enzymes are the body's spark plugs that ignite chemical reactions. In this case, TPO, which is made in the thyroid gland, combines iodine with hydrogen peroxide to create the thyroid hormones T4 and T3.

Why Only Testing TSH is a Model for Failure

Measuring TSH is the most common way to assess thyroid function, and many doctors will prescribe thyroid medications based on TSH alone. When they see that a person's TSH level is high, most physicians assume that the pituitary is producing extra hormone because the thyroid gland isn't doing its job. The solution? Giving medication to boost thyroid performance. But numerous other factors come into play. For instance, measuring TSH alone does not convey pituitary function, whether thyroid hormones are working normally throughout the body, or whether an autoimmune disorder is the culprit.

Thyroxine (T4) Once TSH gets to the thyroid gland, it produces a protein called *thyroglobulin*. The thyroglobulin joins up with four molecules of iodine to produce the thyroid hormone T4, or *thyroxine*. (T4 is identified by four molecules of iodine attached to one molecule of thyroglobulin.) The T4 is then released into the bloodstream, where, as mentioned before, it catches a ride on the taxi known as thyroid-binding protein. About 94 percent of the hormone made in the thyroid gland is T4. The remaining 6 percent is T3, in which only three molecules of iodine are attached to thyroglobulin.

What Happens to T4 Once it Leaves the Thyroid Gland

T4 from the thyroid must be converted to T3 before the body can use it. In the end, however, only about 60 percent of T4 is converted into a usable form of T3. Twenty percent becomes *reverse T3* (rT3), which is permanently inactive. Levels of rT3 can become too high in times of major trauma, surgery, or severe chronic illness. Another 20 percent of T4 becomes *T3 sulfate* and *T3 acetic acid*, which have the potential to become useful if acted upon by healthy bacteria in the digestive tract. The remaining T4 is converted to T3 in the liver and in muscle, heart, and nerve cells.

***Triiodothyronine* (T3).** T3, containing three molecules of iodine, is the predominate thyroid hormone the body uses. The thyroid gland itself secretes only 7 percent, so to get more the liver converts T4 to T3 through conjugation pathways (glucoronidation and sulfation). You can see why a properly functioning liver is essential to healthy thyroid activity. Also, various cells in the body have enzymes that act as spark plugs to make the conversion. These enzymes, called *tetraidothyronine 5' deiodinase enzymes*, remove one molecule of iodine from T4 to make T3. The cells take the usable T3 into the nuclei, where T3 switches on or off the genetic controls. The intestines also convert about 20 percent of T4 into T3, but only in the presence of enough healthy gut bacteria.

Maria's inability to warm up, although it might seem like small potatoes, is actually a distress signal from the body that something, probably more than one thing, is seriously amiss. She may have other symptoms that she thought were a normal part of being in her forties, like chronic constipation, irregular periods, or stubborn weight gain. Instead these changes are clues that some of her body's systems are starting to malfunction. If she pays attention to what her body is communicating, she has the chance to resolve the problem before becoming dependent on a prescription for the rest of her life.

WHY GOOD THYROID HEALTH IS SO IMPORTANT

Because the thyroid has its fingers in so many pots, when its function drags, so does that of many other systems (digestive, hormonal, etc.). It can seem like a vicious cycle. The conventional approach has long been to treat the thyroid so that the other systems it affects will normalize, too. That may work if thyroid hormones are truly needed, but frequently they are inappropriately prescribed, possibly causing more harm than good in the long run. More on that in Chapter Eight. In this section, I will review the many jobs the thyroid performs, and why undiagnosed hypothyroidism can have so many repercussions. Here are some of the functions that come under the gland's influence:

Bone metabolism Although the parathyroid gland (similar name, totally different gland) controls calcium levels in the blood, the thyroid can also affect one's calcium status. That's partly because the thyroid gland manufactures and stores *calcitonin*, a calcium-regulating hormone. Also, hypothyroidism prevents the ends of the long bones from forming fully or correctly. This won't show up as a calcium deficiency on a blood test unless you are looking at the ranges from a "functional" perspective. By that I mean the level that indicates good health.

Gastrointestinal function Chronic constipation is a common complaint of people with an under active thyroid gland. Poor thyroid function slows down the amount of time it takes for food to move through the intestines.[2] This in turn increases the potential of gut infections from harmful yeast and bacteria, leading to inflammation, poor nutrient absorption, and an increased risk of developing food intolerances.

Male reproduction Hypothyroidism in men has been shown to diminish sex drive and cause impotence and a poor sperm count. Although hypothyroidism is rare in men, it must be ruled out when they have testosterone and estrogen imbalances.[3]

Gallbladder and liver The liver has several channels through which it metabolizes hormones, filters toxins, and cleans the blood. Byproducts from these processes are dumped into the gallbladder for final removal. Low thyroid function bogs down this whole process, making the liver and gallbladder sluggish and congested and contributing to gallstones. Gallbladder X-rays in hypothyroid individuals often show a distended gallbladder that contracts sluggishly.[4] And since thyroid hormones are converted into a usable form in the liver, you can see how hypothyroidism creates a vicious cycle — hypothyroidism stymies liver function so that fewer thyroid hormones become active.

Growth hormones Just because you're an adult doesn't mean you don't need *growth hormone* (GH) for regenerating cells and tissues. The pituitary gland releases these "anti-aging" hormones to be dispatched where cell creation and growth are needed. GH then stimulates the synthesis of *insulin-like growth factor* (IGF-1) in the liver in order to complete the job. During this conversion process, an inadequate amount of thyroid hormones hypothyroidism can muck things up, since a healthy amount of thyroid hormones are needed to make IGF-1.

Fat burning One of the most frustrating symptoms of hypothyroidism is the inability to lose weight, even when calories are low and hours logged on the treadmill are high. Hypothyroidism simply slows down the body's overall metabolism and fat burning. For instance, the adrenal hormones epinephrine and norepinephrine that enhance fat burning lose power when the thyroid is under active. What's more, low thyroid function makes it harder for the body to burn fat by shutting down the sites on the cells that respond to lipase, an enzyme that metabolizes fat. So not only does stored fat refuse to budge, but the inability to burn fat for energy also contributes to fatigue and chronic cravings for sweet and starchy foods. Lastly, since hypothyroidism hinders human growth hormone, building muscle through exercise is difficult if not impossible and muscle loss can occur.[5]

Insulin and glucose metabolism Glucose (sugar) metabolism is the rate at which the body uses glucose to make energy. That fuzzy, foggy brain and poor memory so common with hypothyroidism? The brain is the most voracious consumer of glucose, so when glucose metabolism is poor, so is brain function. People with low thyroid function absorb glucose more slowly than normal and their cells don't use it energy as readily. Furthermore, once glucose is absorbed, the body falls behind in eliminating it. Put together, this creates hypoglycemia, or too little sugar available for energy, with symptoms of fatigue, irritability, and light-headedness. The problem is not too little glucose in the blood, but rather that that the glucose can't get into the cells. In fact, glucose blood tests may be normal while symptoms of hypoglycemia rage on. To compensate for low energy, the adrenal glands pump out stress hormones, which activate the liver to release stored glucose into the bloodstream for energy. Eventually this repeating scenario exhausts the adrenal glands, as well as the brain's hypothalamus and pituitary gland, which are responsible for orchestrating so many body functions. Interestingly, hypothyroidism also makes it harder to break down insulin medication, so that diabetics need to take less than they normally might.[6]

Thyroid hormones and cholesterol When I see high triglycerides, high cholesterol, and high LDL ("bad") cholesterol on a blood panel, I always want to rule out thyroid dysfunction before doing anything else. When a person's thyroid is functioning below normal, he or she makes fat much more quickly than it's burned, which drives up triglycerides, cholesterol, and LDL cholesterol. As mentioned earlier, hypothyroidism makes the liver and gallbladder sluggish, so that fat is not easily metabolized and cleared from the body. Cells may be less receptive to taking up LDL, so that too much accumulates.[7] When a person with healthy thyroid function becomes hungry and needs energy, the body is able to readily burn fat for fuel. Not so with low thyroid function. When one of my patients with abnormal lipid panels (cholesterol and triglycerides) has hypothyroidism, I address the thyroid disorder first, after which the lipids in circulation often reach normal levels.

(continued)

Hypothyroidism and Cholesterol

I had a 72-year old female patient come in with triglycerides at 500 mg/dL (the functional range is 75-100 mg/dL). Her other lipid markers were normal. Because I know low thyroid function can cause elevated lipids when other measures are normal, I suggested she take some nutritional compounds Dr. Kharrazian formulated. After one month her triglycerides came down to 327 mg/dL. After another month they were down to 180 mg/dL. At about that time she visited her medical doctor who discontinued the nutritional compounds because he was unfamiliar with them. Unfortunately she did not return so I was unable to see the continuing effects of thyroid support on her lipid levels.

Kari Vernon, DC
Karisma for Life
Scottsdale, AZ

Brain chemistry The adrenal glands, located on top of the kidneys, are our stress-management glands. With hypothyroidism, they do not exert the same energizing effect on the brain as they normally would. This can lead to depression, mood disorders, lethargy, and weight gain.[8]

Estrogen metabolism and breast cancer Estrogen must first be made water soluble in the liver in order to be eliminated from the body. During this process some of the hormone forms a secondary type of estrogen, such as estradiol. Hypothyroidism appears to hinder pathways in the liver that make this possible. The result is the production of too much so-called "proliferative" estrogen, which may lead to breast cancer, uterine fibroids, and ovarian cysts.[9]

Adrenal hormone metabolism I don't like to use urinary adrenal tests for this reason: In people with hypothyroidism, urinary excretion of several adrenal hormones decreases. Instead I prefer salivary adrenal tests. In other words, with a urine test, someone could appear to have an advanced case of adrenal fatigue when in fact they are simply doing a poor job of clearing the hormones through the kidneys.[10]

Liver detoxification Thyroid hormones affect the liver cells responsible for detoxification most of all. The liver has two phases of detoxification. In Phase I, fat-soluble hormones are made water-soluble so the body can eliminate them. This process is finalized in Phase II, and the end products are excreted via the feces, sweat, or urine. It is in Phase II where good thyroid health is most important. When thyroid function is low, the enzymes, or "spark plugs," that carry out the detoxifying tasks, simply don't mature, hindering detoxification.[11] I often see people who do poorly at any attempts at detoxification until thyroid function is restored. Again, this is one of those vicious cycles, as healthy liver function is integral to converting thyroid hormones into a form the body can use.

Stomach acid production Most people think of stomach acid as bad, the sort of thing that causes heartburn. In fact, sufficient stomach acid prevents heartburn by thoroughly digesting your food. (The burning sensation from heartburn is actually from the poorly digested food rotting in your gut and shooting up into your esophagus, not from excess stomach acid). Sufficient stomach acid, or hydrochloric acid (HCl), prevents food poisoning, parasites, and other bad bugs from gaining a foothold in your digestive tract. Lastly, plenty of HCl stimulates the gallbladder and pancreas to complete digestion and preserve the integrity of the whole gastrointestinal tract. The production of HCl depends on the hormone gastrin, which diminishes with hypothyroidism. This can cause such digestive complaints as heartburn, bloating, and gas; hinder the absorption of such vital nutrients as B12, iron, and calcium; and lead to inflammation, lesions, and infections of the intestines. Hypothyroidism and low HCl often go hand in hand.

Protein metabolism Another crucial job stomach acid performs is digesting proteins. In people with hypothyroidism and low stomach acid (hypochlorhydria), protein deficiency may occur. In most cases, simply restoring thyroid function resolves the problem.

Body heat and hot flashes Since the thyroid maintains body temperature, a person with hypothyroidism may develop abnormalities related to body temperature, such as hot flashes and night sweats. These symptoms may be confusing because they are usually associated with perimenopause. Therefore testing the female hormone levels insures addressing the right disorder. Although the thyroid is most commonly associated with regulating body temperature, the ovaries and adrenals affect it, too. A female hormone panel helps determine whether hot flashes and night sweats are caused by estrogen fluctuations or not. If a thyroid disorder causes these symptoms, it's likely other signs of thyroid malfunction are present as well. When the adrenal glands are to blame, the person does not suddenly feel hot, but the adrenal hormone shifts do prompt a sweating attack.[12]

Progesterone production Progesterone and thyroid hormones are intimately connected. Remember that when the pituitary sends TSH to the thyroid, the gland makes T4 and T3 out of thyroglobulin and iodine? The catalyst for this is the enzyme, thyroid peroxidase (TPO), which resides in the follicles of the thyroid gland. (Thyroid *follicles* are small spheres of hormone-producing cells within the gland.) Progesterone appears to both improve the signaling mechanisms of thyroid receptors[13] as well as stimulate TPO production. One reason why a woman's body temperature rises when she ovulates is that the normal progesterone surge that occurs at this point in her cycle ramps up TPO activity, which stimulates overall thyroid activity and metabolism. Progesterone's affect on TPO — too little progesterone depresses TPO activity, lowering T4 production — also explains why a woman with a progesterone deficiency may have mostly normal thyroid levels but a low T4 level. Symptoms of progesterone deficiency include heavy menstrual bleeding, an inability to lose weight, depression, headaches, and other symptoms in the middle of her cycle.

The answer for these women, particularly menstruating women, is not to prescribe progesterone creams. This approach does not take into account the reason for the deficiency, which most often stems from a sluggish pituitary gland (remember, the pituitary is the air traffic control tower that orchestrates the hormones). And factors that lead to poor pituitary function include adrenal fatigue, taking oral contraceptives, or even post-partum hormonal changes. For menopausal women for whom pituitary function may never rebound, sublingual progesterone may be in order. (Progesterone creams almost always guarantee a buildup of excessive levels of progesterone in the fat tissue). For both menstruating and menopausal women, however, supporting the adrenals is integral.

Severe hypothyroidism can lead to loss of ovulation and insufficient progesterone, the buildup of too much tissue lining of the uterus, and excessive and irregular bleeding. Ultimately hypothyroidism raises the risk of infertility and miscarriage.

Lastly, thyroid hormones sensitize the body's cells to progesterone, so that they are able to readily take it up when needed. When the cell's progesterone receptor sites are not exposed to enough thyroid hormones, they lose the ability to allow progesterone into the cells. So even though plenty of progesterone is circulating through the bloodstream, a woman will have symptoms of progesterone deficiency and on progesterone levels will show abnormal surges and dips.

Thyroid hormones and anemia Hypothyroidism can lead to anemia in three different ways. For instance, anemia resulting from a B12 and folic acid deficiency usually stems from low stomach acid, one possible consequence of hypothyroidism. Secondly, about 12 percent of people with hypothyroidism have pernicious anemia, an autoimmune disorder in which the body's immune system destroys a compound in the stomach lining necessary for the absorption of B12. Given that the vast majority of hypothyroid cases are also an autoimmune disorder in which the body destroys its own thyroid gland, it's not surprising that a hyperactive and malfunctioning immune system can lead to both pernicious anemia and hypothyroidism. Lastly, since hypothyroidism leads to a deficiency in stomach acid, iron absorption (among other things) is poor. And remember how hypothyroidism makes it hard for progesterone to get into the cells? That effect causes excessive bleeding during menstruation, and poor iron absorption from low stomach acid coupled with excessive bleeding brings on anemia of iron deficiency.

Protein binding Earlier I mentioned that when the thyroid hormone is traveling to the liver or to various cells, it catches a ride with binding proteins that serve as taxi cabs. The same is true for the reproductive hormones, whose taxis are called *sex hormone-binding globulins* (SHBG). When these "bound" hormones arrive at their destination, they are "free." Research shows that an under active thyroid reduces SHBG levels. In addition to contributing to hormonal imbalances, low SHBG levels can also skew hormone test results.[14]

Heart. Too much *homocysteine*, an amino acid made in the body, seriously increases the risk of heart disease, as well as dementia and neurodegenerative diseases. Hypothyroidism appears to contribute to high homocysteine levels by compromising the liver's ability to manage the amino acid.[15]

CHAPTER HIGHLIGHTS

- The thyroid is a gland that stretches over the Adam's apple of the throat and regulates metabolism.

- Hypothyroidism occurs when the thyroid is consistently under active for a variety of reasons. Prescription thyroid hormones rarely address the true cause of poor thyroid function.

- Hashimoto's disease, an autoimmune disorder that destroys thyroid tissue, is the most common cause of hypothyroidism.

- The brain secretes *thyroid stimulating hormone* (TSH), which tells the thyroid gland to make and secrete the thyroid hormones T4 and T3. T4 and T3 are named for the number of iodine molecules of iodine — four and three respectively.

- The body can only use T3, even though only 7 percent of it is secreted by the thyroid gland. The body must convert T4 to T3 by removing one molecule of iodine with an enzyme called *tetraidothyronine 5'deiodinase*. This happens in the liver, the gastrointestinal tract, and various other cells in the body, such as muscle, heart, and nerve cells T3 goes into the nucleus of these cells to activate the genetic thyroid controls.

- Many things contribute to hypothyroidism. They include poor liver or gut function, a sluggish pituitary gland, too many thyroid-binding proteins in the bloodstream (as a consequence of excess estrogen), and immune dysfunction.

- Twenty percent of T4 is converted to T3 in the intestines, but only in the presence of healthy gut flora.

- Nutritionally supporting hypothyroidism is important as many important functions in the body can become impaired due to faulty thyroid function.

CHAPTER TWO

THE SCOOP ON HASHIMOTO'S DISEASE

After the birth of her second son, Patricia's health seemed to nosedive. Her postpartum blues went on for months, she felt tired all the time, and her hands and feet were always freezing cold. At night, she needed multiple blankets to stay warm, compared to her husband, who was fine with just one. After a visit to her doctor and a blood test, she was diagnosed with hypothyroidism and prescribed Synthroid.

"Even on Synthroid, I felt cold all the time," Patricia says. "I also started to get other symptoms of being hyperthyroid. At night I would lay down and my heart would race and have an irregular heartbeat. All the doctor could do was adjust the dosage of my medication so that my lab tests would look good."

Patricia went on like this for almost 20 years, before a natural medicine doctor diagnosed her with Hashimoto's disease.

"I don't know if my first doctor didn't know I had an autoimmune condition, or just forgot to tell me," Patricia says.

Perhaps no disease is more overlooked in the healthcare system than Hashimoto's, an autoimmune condition in which the body attacks and destroys its own thyroid gland. Although the disorder is the most common cause of hypothyroidism in the United States, many doctors don't test for it since a diagnosis doesn't change the standard treatment, which is to prescribe thyroid hormone. Instead, because they expect the thyroid to continually lose function, they just monitor serum hormone levels and adjust medication accordingly. As other hypothyroid symptoms pop up, the standard of care is to prescribe powerful medications, such as Prozac for depression or even drugs to slow the heart or suppress the adrenal glands. Another approach is to remove the thyroid gland, which doesn't always work either, as some tissue is inevitably left behind and can still serve as a site for autoimmune attacks.

It's not that these people's care is being mismanaged or their condition misdiagnosed, it's just that current conventional health care has no model to successfully manage Hashimoto's. Typically the immune suppressant prednisone is a standard treatment for autoimmune disease, but it's too aggressive for Hashimoto's. Instead, doctors wait for the thyroid to "burn out," meaning to lose function due to extensive tissue death. Then they prescribe thyroid replacement hormone.

The alternatives in natural medicine haven't been much better: Neonatal hormones are prescribed, sometimes along with thyroid glandulars said to act as a "decoy" for the immune system. Or steps to improve overall health are taken, which can do tremendous good, but again it ignores the intricate mechanics of an autoimmune disease. After being diagnosed with Hashimoto's by her alternative health doctor, taking a natural T4/T3 hormone, and improving her diet, Patricia does feel better. She says the T3 hormone, which is the form of thyroid hormone the body can use, is keeping her system functioning better. However her immune system has been ignored. Also, Patricia's doctor prescribes iodine, which, as you will learn later, has the potential to actually speed up the inflammation and destruction of the thyroid gland. Only time will tell how Patricia's thyroid will hold up under this treatment.

In both standards of care, the thyroid gland is the star attraction while the immune system is the mysterious, shadowy stranger relegated to the background. The truth is, the immune system is the one running the Hashimoto's show, and that's where we need to turn the spotlight.

Autoimmune Hashimoto's

Hashimoto's disease is named for Hakuro Hashimoto, a Japanese physician who worked in Europe before World War I. He described the disease in a German publication in 1912. It was the first condition to be recognized as an autoimmune disease.

Approximately one in five people suffer from some form of autoimmune disease. Some estimates say that 75 percent of those affected — some 30 million people — are women.[16]

Thyroid autoimmune diseases are the most common of autoimmune disorders, affecting 7-8 percent of the U.S. population.[17] [18] In the United States, autoimmune disease accounts for approximately 90 percent of adult hypothyroidism, mostly due to Hashimoto's.[19]

HOW DO YOU KNOW IF YOU HAVE HASHIMOTO'S DISEASE?

Let's say hypothyroidism symptoms describe you perfectly. How do you know if your hypothyroidism is due to Hashimoto's disease? Although a positive serum antibody test is the definitive test, it's good to be aware of some classic symptoms and scenarios that typically go along with the condition.

The most common is the person who dutifully takes her thyroid replacement hormones, has her thyroid condition monitored regularly, yet continues to feel worse, needing ever increasing doses of thyroid hormone to function. In fact, this is the person who may even forget to take her medication, only to realize after the fact that she noticed no difference in her symptoms. What's going on? Most cases of Hashimoto's unfold as a gradual attack of the immune system against the thyroid, with TSH levels and symptoms of hypothyroidism slowly escalating. While the person may have normal TSH levels thanks to thyroid hormone medication, the underlying problem of immune dysregulation goes untreated, as do her symptoms.

Another common scenario is one in which the thyroid condition fluctuates between being under active and over active. This is the person whose symptoms are all over the map. One week she fits the classic description of hypothyroidism — she feels tired, complains of headaches and constipation, and has low libido and depression. Then the next week she can't fall asleep, her heart races, she gets anxious, and she has tremors. If her doctor runs blood tests during these episodes, they will show her TSH peaking and dipping, and even appearing normal in between bouts of symptoms. These roller coaster fluctuations can happen for seemingly no rhyme or reason, whether it is days, weeks, months or more between swings. Other times they can be linked to a trigger, such as a stressful event, hormonal fluctuations, or eating foods containing gluten.

Hashimoto's Disease and "Normal" Lab Results

Jan	TSH	4.5
Feb	TSH	0.08
Mar	TSH	2.3
April	TSH	3.8
May	TSH	8.7
June	TSH	7.4
July	TSH	1.6

One reason hypothyroidism often goes misdiagnosed is because a person with Hashimoto's can present with normal TSH. This graph illustrates the monthly TSH levels of a person with Hashimoto's who is receiving no treatment. As the autoimmune condition fluctuates, TSH levels vary wildly. Using a standard lab range of 0.45-4.5, this person would fail to be diagnosed. During the month of March the patient's TSH even falls within the functional range of 1.8-3.0. That's why also testing for immune antibodies and evaluating symptoms and history are so vital.

So what's going on? Is the person hypothyroid or hyperthyroid? Indeed, these fluctuations are sometimes misdiagnosed as anxiety disorders. But in reality, this is just the presentation of Hashimoto's. When an autoimmune flare-up destroys thyroid tissue, hormones stored in the gland flow into the bloodstream. Now flooded with excess thyroid hormone, the body's metabolism speeds up, resulting in hyperthyroid symptoms.

If you suspect you have Hashimoto's, ask yourself if you have any of these symptoms:

HYPOTHYROID SYMPTOMS

- Feeling tired or sluggish
- Feeling cold — hands, feet, all over
- Require excessive amounts of sleep to function well
- Weight gain despite adhering to a low-calorie diet
- Gaining weight easily
- Difficult, infrequent bowel movements
- Depression and lack of motivation
- Morning headaches that wear off as the day progresses
- Outer third of eyebrow thins
- Thinning of hair on scalp, face, or genitals, or excessive hair loss
- Dryness of skin and/or scalp
- Mental sluggishness

HYPERTHYROID SYMPTOMS

- Heart palpitations
- Inward trembling
- Increased pulse rate, even at rest
- Feeling nervous and emotional
- Insomnia
- Night sweats
- Difficulty gaining weight

PERNICIOUS ANEMIA AND GLUTEN INTOLERANCE

In addition to classic symptoms, a couple of medical conditions are red flags for Hashimoto's. If you suffer from the symptoms above and have pernicious anemia,[20] a gluten intolerance, or celiac disease,[21] Hashimoto's may be responsible for your thyroid condition. Pernicious anemia is an autoimmune disease in which the person's body attacks its own intrinsic factor, a substance necessary to absorb B12 that is secreted in the stomach. This appears as B12 anemia. Gluten intolerance and celiac disease are an immune response to gluten that numerous studies link to Hashimoto's. I will talk more about gluten later in this chapter.

CONFIRMING HASHIMOTO'S

Symptoms provide valuable information when it comes to determining whether a person's hypothyroid condition can be attributed to Hashimoto's, but a serum antibody test will confirm the condition.

A test for *thyroid peroxidase antibodies* (TPO Ab) is most important, as Hashimoto's most commonly occurs when the immune system attacks TPO, an enzyme in the thyroid responsible for of thyroid hormone production.[22] [23] Sometimes a *thyroglobulin antibodies* (TGB Ab) test is necessary, since Hashimoto's can follow a TGB attack.[24] TGB is produced in the thyroid and is used by the gland to produce thyroid hormones.

A test for *thyroid stimulating hormone antibodies* (TSH Ab) can identify Grave s' disease (hyperthyroidism), although TSH can also be elevated in Hashimoto's. On lab tests, the TSH marker is commonly referred to as *thyroid stimulating immunoglobulin* (TSI). In severe autoimmune thyroid diseases, antibodies to T4 and T3 can develop. This pattern may be found in polyglandular autoimmune syndrome, systemic lupus erythematosus, and other autoimmune diseases that affect multiple organs. Clinically, people with these conditions do worse and experience more inflammation with bio-identical hormones than synthetic hormones.

Because the immune system fluctuates, it's possible for a person with Hashimoto's to have a negative antibodies test result. In other words, when the autoimmune condition is dormant and the immune system is not attacking the thyroid gland, an antibody test will be negative. However, if I see a negative test result yet a person's symptoms and history strongly suggest Hashimoto's, I do another test, perhaps provoking the immune system to create a flare-up. For instance, numerous studies link gluten, the protein found in wheat, spelt, barley, rye and similar grains to Hashimoto's.[25] [26] [27] [28] [29] [30] [31] [32] If the person is already on a gluten-free diet, I will have them consume wheat for two weeks and then repeat the test, providing gluten doesn't cause other severe symptoms. A positive antibody test confirms an autoimmune thyroid condition and indicates that the immune system, not the thyroid gland, is the target for therapy.

IODINE: THROWING GASOLINE ONTO A FIRE

Iodine is a hot supplement these days. Many people and practitioners have come to value iodine's therapeutic potential, especially for breast and uterine fibroids. Iodine is also vital to thyroid function, as it is a major cofactor and stimulator for the enzyme TPO. But for the person with Hashimoto's, supplementing with iodine is like throwing gasoline onto a fire. Because iodine stimulates production of TPO, this in turn increases the levels of TPO antibodies dramatically, indicating an autoimmune flare-up.[33] Some people develop symptoms of an over active thyroid,[34] while others will have no symptoms despite tests showing an elevated level of TPO antibodies. Therefore, I rigorously advise anyone with an autoimmune thyroid condition to avoid supplements containing iodine, as many thyroid supplements do.

This may seem like confusing advice to the person with hypothyroidism who as been told her condition is the result of an iodine deficiency. Although iodine deficiency is the most common cause of hypothyroidism for most of the world's population,[35] in the United States and other westernized countries, Hashimoto's accounts for the majority of cases of hypothyroidism.[36] Also, studies show that when iodine supplementation is used to correct iodine deficiency in countries such as China, Turkey and Sri Lanka,[37] [38] the rates of autoimmune thyroid disease increase. Also, when iodine is added to table salt in some parts of the world, the rates of autoimmune thyroid disease again increase.[39] Iodine supplementation isn't causing Hashimoto's per se, but it does seem to be a triggering factor.[40]

Some popular books on iodine therapy recommend supplementing with large doses of iodine to quench symptoms of Hashimoto's. That's because taking mega-doses of iodine will shut down the production of the TPO and inhibit thyroid hormone formation. As a result, the thyroid becomes less active, suppressing hyperthyroid symptoms.

If you are considering supplementing with iodine but your symptoms strongly suggest Hashimoto's, be tested several times to rule out an autoimmune thyroid condition. An autoimmune condition can fluctuate, and negative tests are not always definitive. In addition to a gluten-free diet and supporting overall health, which is discussed in later chapters, avoiding iodine supplements is another strategy for preserving thyroid tissue.

HEALTH CONSIDERATIONS

Although no hard and fast rules exist in regards to what triggers an autoimmune disease, there do seem to be certain physiological conditions that can set the stage for Hashimoto's. These include gluten intolerance, estrogen surges, insulin resistance, polycystic ovary syndrome (PCOS), vitamin D deficiency, environmental toxicity, chronic infections and inflammation, and genetic susceptibility to the condition.

STRESS

Without a doubt, stress is the biggest factor when looking at the brew that makes up an autoimmune disease. Although the following factors are considered stressors, the person with Hashimoto's would do well to create a less stressful lifestyle or find ways to mitigate stress in order to better modulate the disease. Stress does many things to upset immune regulation: It suppresses immune function, promotes immune imbalances, weakens and atrophies the thymus gland, and thins the barriers of the gut, lungs, and brain.

GLUTEN INTOLERANCE

One of the main functions of the immune system is to protect the body from foreign invaders. Sometimes it begins to recognize a frequently eaten food as a dangerous invader (often as a result of poor intestinal health), keeping the immune system engaged in constant battle. In time, the beleaguered, over active immune system can start to behave erratically and begin attacking body tissue. The most common example of this scenario for people with Hashimoto's involves gluten, the protein found in wheat and wheat-like grains, including spelt, kamut, rye, barley, triticale, and oats. Actually, the word gluten is a misnomer, as it is the *gliadin* portion of gluten that causes the immune reaction. However, since gluten has become a popular term, I will use here.

Numerous studies from several countries show a strong link between gluten intolerance and Hashimoto's disease.[41][42][43][44][45][46] Because the molecular structure of gluten so closely resembles that of the thyroid gland, the problem may be one of mistaken identity.

Every time undigested gluten mistakenly slips into the bloodstream, the immune system responds by destroying it for removal. That's because gluten doesn't belong in the bloodstream but gets there through overly permeable intestinal walls, or a "leaky gut." (See Chapters 3 and 6 for more on this topic). In people with a genetic predisposition to gluten intolerance — estimated by Kenneth Fine, MD, a gluten researcher, to be up to 81 percent of Americans — gluten itself weakens the intestinal tract, increasing permeability. These individuals are at risk for developing gluten intolerance or celiac disease, a form of gluten intolerance that involves an autoimmune response in the small intestine. Celiac disease affects up to one in 100 Americans, although only 1 in 8 are estimated to be aware of their condition, as symptoms are often silent.[47] Gluten intolerance, however, affects about 35 percent of Americans based on Fine's research, with that number jumping to more than 50 percent if they are at high risk or show symptoms. Most people think gluten intolerance is a gut issue, but for many it causes other problems, such as inflammation in the joints, skin, respiratory tract, or brain. It's important to know if you have a genetic predisposition for gluten intolerance, which you can find out from a test offered through EnteroLab (www.enterolab.com). Once these genes are triggered, gluten must be avoided throughout life.

(continued)

	Permanent Gluten Sensitivity	Celiac Disease	Temporary Gluten Sensitivity
HLA DQ genes	+	+	—
Positive gliadin antibodies	+	+	+
Positive transglutaminase antibodies	—	+	—
Endomysial antibodies	—	+	—
Positive biopsy	—	+ or —	—
Potential Autoimmune disease	Potential autoimmune attack against thyroid, but not the gut	Potential autoimmune attack against the gut and thyroid	—

GLUTEN INTOLERANCE AND CELIAC DISEASE

When it comes to gluten intolerance and celiac disease, scientists look at HLA DQ genes (HLA stands for human leukocyte antigen). Gluten intolerance, celiac disease, and several autoimmune conditions, including Hashimoto's, occur more frequently with certain HLA DQ gene types. (EnteroLab offers an HLA DQ gene test using a cotton-tipped swab of the mouth.) For instance, based on Fine's research, 90 percent of people with celiac disease have the DQ2 gene, which is more common among those of Northern European descent. Nine percent of them have the DQ8 gene, which is a more common among those of European/Mediterranean descent." The DQ1 and DQ3 genes are associated more often with gluten intolerance than celiac disease.

All combined, it's estimated 43 percent of Americans are genetically predisposed to celiac disease, and 81 percent are predisposed to gluten intolerance.

When it comes to diagnosing celiac disease, other markers to consider are positive antibodies against:

- Gliadin, a protein in gluten

- Transglutaminase, an enzyme in the intestines

- Endomysium, a muscle sheath

When any or all of these is positive, it indicates a person is not just gluten intolerant, but has celiac disease.

Sometimes a person will produce gluten antibodies but does not have the HLA DQ genes that predispose him or her to gluten sensitivity. Producing gluten antibodies may simply be from a leaky gut, and the person may be able to safely eat gluten again after repairing the digestive system.

Lastly, a negative biopsy of the small intestine does not rule out celiac disease, since false negative results are possible. However a positive biopsy is conclusive.

So you can see how, if a person with a gluten intolerance or celiac disease eats gluten regularly, her immune system is kept on a constant red alert, toiling virtually non-stop. Here's how it sets the stage for Hashimoto's: When immune antibodies tag gluten for removal, they stimulate the production of antibodies against the thyroid gland as well (again, because they are both so similar in structure). In other words, every time gluten is ingested, the immune system launches an attack not only against gluten but also on the thyroid gland. What's worse, the immune response to gluten can last up to six months each time it's ingested.

My own clinical observations have backed up this scenario over and over. All patients with an autoimmune thyroid condition should be screened for gluten intolerance or celiac disease,[48] just as all patients with a gluten intolerance or celiac disease should be screened for an autoimmune thyroid disorder.[49] I advise my patients with Hashimoto's to give up gluten completely if they wish to preserve their thyroid gland. Eating just a little bit is not OK, since even a small amount will cause irreversible thyroid tissue death. I also remind them to avoid cross-contamination in restaurants, packaged foods, and their own kitchens. Lea can attest to this. When I told her to stop eating gluten to better modulate her Hashimoto's disease, she was amazed to find her frightening bouts of heart palpitations stopped on a gluten-free diet. Like most people, however, some of Lea's favorite comfort foods were wheat-based. "At first I thought I could just enjoy the occasional indulgence, but as soon as I did my heart palpitations came back," says Lea. "Now, even when I order a gluten-free meal at a restaurant, I sometimes get palpitations because my food has been contaminated with gluten. I've learned I have to be careful."

A variety of tests exist to identify gluten intolerance and celiac disease, including EnteroLab's. However one should approach these tests with some skepticism. Sometimes the immune system can be so worn out that, even though it is attacking gluten, the total number of antibodies being produced is extremely low. As a result, test results may look negative, when in fact gluten intolerance is raging on. The best test is the elimination/provocation diet, in which gluten is removed from the diet for two weeks, and then reintroduced while the person monitors her reactions. (For more details, see Chapter Six). Given the overwhelming evidence establishing a link between gluten intolerance and Hashimoto's disease, however, it is wisest to simply remove gluten from your diet if you wish to preserve your thyroid gland.

It is not uncommon to see major resolution of hypothyroid symptoms just by following a gluten-free diet. However, avoiding gluten does not *cure* the disease.[50] It simply helps tame the immune system so it stops attacking the thyroid tissue.

Note: Many clinicians find removing casein, the protein molecule in all forms of dairy, is also integral to thyroid health. There is not as much research on casein intolerance as there is on gluten intolerance, however anecdotal evidence strongly suggests a diet that is not only gluten-free, but also dairy-free promises the best results in managing Hashimoto's.

A Gluten-Free Diet and Thyroid Health

Sam is a 50-year-old practitioner who complained of depression, constipation, and lack of energy. His blood chemistry showed an elevated TSH and TPO antibody count, as well as other markers for low thyroid function. His white blood cell count was elevated, and his fasting glucose was low. An Adrenal Stress Index (ASI) showed he had adrenal fatigue. It was obvious he had Hashimoto's.

Because of Sam's financial limitations, my recommendations were only a glutathione and superoxide dismutase liposomal cream and a gluten-free diet. I also suggested that he eat low-carb, high-protein meals and snacks every three hours to help maintain his blood sugar level. He had difficulty avoiding gluten, and was concerned about additional weight loss.

After a month we re-tested Sam's blood. His TSH dropped to almost normal, and his TPO antibodies decreased quite a bit, too. His depression still lingered, though it was not as severe, and he was less constipated. His energy level was significantly higher. These improvements encouraged him to remove gluten completely from his diet and to add more nutritional compounds to address his other issues. His health became a priority.

Seven months later, his TSH was down in the normal range and his TPO antibodies had dropped significantly. The improvement was also evident by fewer symptoms. We repeated an ASI and also saw significant improvement in his adrenal health. Today Sam has no symptoms and enthusiastically applies similar methods to his own patients. He now regularly attends Dr. Kharrazian's seminars along with me.

Donna DiMarco, CN, LNC
Pompano Beach, FL

ESTROGEN FLUCTUATIONS

Fluctuations of estrogen are another potential trigger for Hashimoto's disease when other risk factors such as genetic susceptibility and immune regulating problems are present.[51] [52] Estrogen triggers Hashimoto's in many women after pregnancy, due to the extreme shifts of hormones and the immune system.[53] [54] Perimenopause is another susceptible period, again due to the estrogen surges and dips.[55] This can be misleading as symptoms of Hashimoto's mimic those of perimenopause. When an autoimmune attack destroys thyroid tissue, excess thyroid hormone enters the bloodstream, increasing metabolic rate and producing symptoms such as hot flashes, nervousness, insomnia, and irritability — all of which appear to the woman and her doctor as signs of perimenopause.

INSULIN RESISTANCE AND POLYCYSTIC OVARY SYNDROME

Studies show polycystic ovary syndrome (PCOS) can trigger Hashimoto's disease. PCOS is the most common female hormone disorder in the United States, affecting 4 to 10 percent of menstruating women, and the most common cause of infertility.[56] [57] PCOS symptoms include the inability to lose weight, hair loss, fatigue after meals, hormone imbalances, and sugar cravings. On blood chemistry tests, PCOS can be identified by insulin resistance patterns, which include a fasting glucose over 100, and elevated triglycerides and cholesterol, especially if triglycerides are higher than cholesterol. Insulin resistance — a condition in which the body's cells become resistant to insulin due to a high-carbohydrate diet — leads to excess testosterone production and PCOS. As testosterone levels rise, the cells become further resistant to insulin, which in turn promotes testosterone elevations, thus creating a vicious cycle.[58] In the meantime, insulin resistance also promotes inflammation and immune system problems, both of which predispose the person to an autoimmune disease.[59] It is the combination of all these factors that can trigger Hashimoto's.[60] (See Chapter Five for more on insulin resistance and how to nutritionally support it.)

VITAMIN D DEFICIENCY

It seems every time you turn the corner, there's a new vitamin deficiency to consider. When it comes to Hashimoto's, however, few are as detrimental as a lack of vitamin D, which technically is a steroid hormone. Modern diets are often lacking in vitamin D-rich foods — liver, organ meats, lard, many forms of seafood, butter, and egg yolks. Although sunlight is another important source of vitamin D, I see a vitamin D deficiency in almost all of my patients here in sunny San Diego. The farther north you go, the worse the potential for deficiency becomes. The Vitamin D Council recommends you maintain a serum 25 (OH) vitamin D level of between 50 – 80 ng/mL, and supplement with 4,000 to 5,000 IU a day of cholecalciferol. Avoid ergocalciferol, which has been shown to be ineffective at raising serum vitamin D levels.[61] People using UVB tanning beds or sunbathing weekly in southern locations such as Florida may not need supplemental vitamin D, however the higher north you live or the darker your skin, the greater your vitamin D need.

Why is vitamin D so important? A vitamin D deficiency is associated with numerous autoimmune conditions, including Hashimoto's,[62] [63] and autoimmune rates have been skyrocketing in recent years. Adequate vitamin D helps keep the immune balanced so it does not swing out of control into an autoimmune disease.[64] [65] [66] The Vitamin D Council offers more information and vitamin D test kits at www.vitamindcouncil.org.

When it comes to Hashimoto's, the problem of a vitamin D deficiency is made worse by genetics — studies show more than 90 percent of people with autoimmune thyroid disease have a genetic defect affecting their ability to process vitamin D. Therefore, many people need higher amounts of vitamin D to maintain health even if a blood test shows sufficient vitamin D. (In ancient times, they may have obtained it through their diets.) This is because the defect is in their cells' vitamin D receptors, so that not enough of the nutrient can gain entry into the cells.[67] [68] Therefore, the blood levels of vitamin D in a person with Hashimoto's should be in the high-normal range. I recommend my patients with the disorder take 5,000 to 20,000 IU daily of emulsified vitamin D in addition to its cofactors (see Nutritional Compounds Resources).

Other contributors to a vitamin D deficiency besides inadequate sunlight or a vitamin D-poor diet include gut inflammation, adrenal stress, obesity,[69] [70] [71] and aging.[72] [73]

CHRONIC INFLAMMATION, INFECTIONS, AND VIRUSES

Rare is the American with a well functioning digestive tract. Just consider the many television commercials for digestive aids, and the billions of dollars spent for over-the-counter antacids, laxatives, and anti-diarrhea medications. Intestinal permeability[74], poor digestion, and bacterial and parasitic infections are common digestive ailments that can lead to autoimmune disease.[75] A gut ravaged by inflammation and infection creates chronic immune and stress responses. Just as in the case of gluten intolerance, chronic stressors on the immune system can predispose it to malfunction and consequently cause an autoimmune disease. Other immune stressors include chronic viruses and infections, such as hepatitis C, Epstein-Barr virus, Lyme disease, and mold infections.[76] [77] [78] [79] Tending to these immune stressors should always be a top priority in managing an autoimmune condition.

A Viral Connection

My client hadn't felt well for some time, and she knew she needed to see someone about it. Having good insurance she went to her physician, who promptly ordered a general blood chemistry report. It was a typical panel of tests and not very comprehensive. After glancing at the report, her doctor said her thyroid and other measures were fine, and that she should just try to relax more. She was very frustrated with that diagnosis. She knew she wasn't fine.

I convinced her to do a more expanded and functional blood chemistry panel. On a hunch I also ordered a TPO antibody test. When the results came back, it showed that her thyroid test results were within the normal lab range, but according to the functional range her thyroid was significantly under functioning.

Plus, she was positive for TPO antibodies. In other words, she had Hashimoto's. Also, her T3 uptake marker was excessively low, prompting me to ask her whether she was on birth control medication. "Oh yes," she said. "My doctor prescribed it for my PMS symptoms." She and I discussed the manner in which excess estrogen can suppress thyroid function and even contribute to her autoimmune issues. These, however, were not the most interesting findings.

What her doctor didn't catch, despite obvious symptoms, was that my client had been suffering from a severe chronic viral infection. On her functional blood chemistry panel, she had a marker (albumin) so low it was in the ominous range.

In terms of nutritional therapy, her thyroid was actually the last priority on the list. The first was addressing the viral infection and her immune system with nutritional compounds. She also stopped taking birth control pills and went on a gluten-free diet. Although Hashimoto's doesn't just "go away", my client is now testing negative for TPO antibodies and her thyroid levels have improved. There is no longer any sign of the viral infection.

I am happy to say that, thanks to what I learned from Dr. Kharrazian, my client is feeling and functioning much better.

Nora Gedgaudes, CNS, CNT
Northwest Neurofeedback, Inc.
Portland, OR

(continued)

ENVIRONMENTAL TOXINS

Other sources of chronic immune stress can come from the toxic chemicals and metals in our environment. We all have some degree of heavy metal and environmental pollution toxicity, however some people's immune systems attack these compounds. The stress of environmental toxins can be a factor in developing autoimmune thyroid disease.[80] [81] [82] [83]

A RED FLAG FOR OTHER AUTOIMMUNE DISEASES

When a person develops an autoimmune response to one tissue, it's not uncommon for her to develop autoimmune attacks against others.[84] [85] In my practice I often see a progression of these attacks, which is why it's so important to modulate the immune system in people with Hashimoto's.

As I mentioned earlier, when a person has Hashimoto's for some time, pernicious anemia, a condition in which the immune system attacks the stomach's intrinsic factor so that B12 can't be absorbed, frequently occurs. The islet cells of the pancreas may become the next target of attack, and the person develops Type I diabetes. (If immune damage goes on unchecked, so does the diabetic condition, despite dietary modifications). For instance, this person is often diagnosed with Type II diabetes since the pancreas is able to still manufacture some insulin even though the disease seems resistant to dietary modifications. If the immune attack goes unchecked, the disease may eventually progress to insulin-dependent Type I diabetes. When I get a patient who tests positive for Hashimoto's, I screen for these other conditions; for instance, I always check to see if antibodies against the pancreatic islet cells are high. In more advanced cases of Hashimoto's, the cerebellum is the final victim.[86] This autoimmune condition manifests as problems with balance, motion sickness, nausea from focusing, and nausea or dizziness from flashing motions on a computer, television, or movie screen. A cerebellar autoimmune disease is also likely the cause behind *gluten ataxia*, a disease in which gluten triggers neurological problems.

As you can imagine, these are the patients who go through life feeling worse and worse, despite normal TSH levels with the use of thyroid hormones. Had their immune condition been modulated from the get-go, they could be living fuller, healthier lives instead of losing the autoimmune battle.

CHAPTER HIGHLIGHTS

- Because it is an immune disease, Hashimoto's often goes undiagnosed, and is largely mismanaged by both conventional and alternative health care systems.

- People with Hashimoto's often don't respond well to thyroid replacement hormones, or they experience symptoms of both and under active and over active thyroid.

- A TPO and TGB serum antibody test helps identify Hashimoto's. A negative test is sometimes false as the immune system fluctuates. If symptoms strongly suggest the disease, repeat tests should be done to confirm the diagnosis. Sometimes it is necessary to challenge the patient with gluten before an antibody test.

- Because supplementing with iodine will exacerbate Hashimoto's, strictly avoid iodine if you have the disease.

- Numerous studies have shown a link between gluten intolerance and Hashimoto's. If you have the disease, eat a gluten-free diet, avoiding wheat and wheat-like grains such as barley, rye, spelt, triticale, kamut, and oats. The gluten molecule is very similar to the thyroid gland molecule, which confuses the overzealous immune system in a gluten-intolerant person.

- Risk factors for developing Hashimoto's include gluten intolerance, insulin resistance, PCOS, estrogen fluctuations, vitamin D deficiency, chronic infection, inflammation, or an immune reaction to heavy metals or environmental pollutants.

Hashimoto's and Diabetes

I was diagnosed with diabetes a few years ago. My doctors were unable to figure out why I was diabetic. I did not have any of the risk factors. I was not over weight, nor was I losing weight or overeating. About a year later I was diagnosed with Hashimoto's as well. My doctors wanted to add another medication to help with the thyroid even though they were at a loss to explain my condition.

Dr. Mark was able to figure out that my problem was not my diabetes nor my thyroid but my immune system. It was attacking my thyroid and pancreas causing these diseases. Ever since I have been under Dr. Mark's care my blood sugar is under control. I have been able to cut down on my diabetes medication and I don't need medication for my thyroid. The hypopigmentation condition I have had on my hands for the last 20 years is starting to resolve. It turns out that was autoimmune disorder as well.

I can't thank Dr. Mark enough. He has been able to improve my health through diet and supplementation. Something my medical doctors were unable to do.

—*Phil, a patient of Mark Flannery, DC*
Mark Flannery, DC
HealthWise Chiropractic & Nutrition
Simi Valley, CA

CHAPTER THREE

HASHIMOTO'S IS AN IMMUNE DISEASE

Laura's thyroid condition began eight years ago when she was 53. Normally a dynamic, fast-moving go-getter who never had weight problems, her energy nosedived and she starting putting on weight. She began losing her hair, her mental focus, and her joy in living, while a cascade of other health problems, like bladder issues, rained down on her. She also has periods of being overtaken by a shortness of breath, a racing heart, and panic attacks. A naturally curious person who loves to travel, now Laura struggles just to get to and from work.

For two years, Laura said she "had to fight for a thyroid test and diagnosis." Finally, her primary care physician sent her to an endocrinologist, who diagnosed her with Hashimoto's. He tests the hormone levels in her blood every three months, constantly adjusting the brand or the dosage of her medication, yet he does not check antibodies. He told her the attacks on her thyroid could not be stopped, but that her TSH could be kept within a normal range.

"My life is a constant up and down," says Laura. "I see improvements, like with a change in my thyroid medication, and then the symptoms come back. I'm tired of this hit-and-miss approach."

Laura thought she was alone with her condition and that no one else is going through what she has to endure. Little did she know she is keeping company with millions of Americans.

Laura's story is one I hear over and over in my clinic: A person is diagnosed with Hashimoto's disease, her TSH levels are brought to normal with thyroid drugs, and yet her symptoms worsen. One woman loses her hair and can barely muster the energy to get out of bed, much less care for her children. Another suffers from mental fogginess, poor memory, chronic constipation, and weight gain, which don't help her depression. Often the autoimmune thyroid disease progresses to autoimmune diseases in other parts of a person's body, manifesting as pernicious anemia, Type I diabetes, joint issues, and even neurological problems.[87] [88] Meanwhile her TSH levels are normal and her doctor manages the symptoms with an ever-increasing array of drugs and hormones and tells her she's fine. In my book, good health means having a zest for life and buoyant energy, neither of which describes the poorly managed person with Hashimoto's disease.

Remember, Hashimoto's is not a thyroid disease but an immune disorder, and it is the immune system that must be addressed (even though thyroid replacement hormones may be warranted if enough thyroid tissue has been destroyed).[89] [90] In order to successfully modulate Hashimoto's, prevent future autoimmune diseases, and enjoy a better quality of life, a basic understanding of the immune system is the first step. Given its complexity, especially when it comes to autoimmune disease, it's no wonder the immune system is uncharted territory for most doctors. In fact, with some autoimmune diseases, some doctors simply remove the thymus gland, the seat of immune regulation.

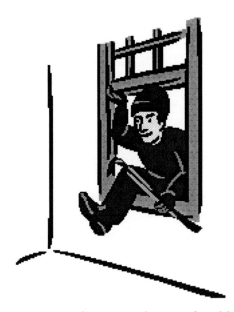

Autoimmune disease can be stimulated by a
"breaking and entering" of the body's immune barriers.

In this chapter I attempt to explain, as simply as possible, the immune system and how it drives Hashimoto's. The cast of characters and the range of duties involved in running the immune system are vast. In order to make it easier to understand, I likened the immune system to crime scene involving a breaking and entering.

Let's say you are a house. Like a house you have barriers that protect you from the outside world, the way windows, walls, a roof and doors protect the inside of a house. Except your windows and walls are your skin and the lining of your intestines, lungs, and brain. You can imagine what it's like to live in a house where the roof leaks, the windows have holes in them, and wind can blow through the slats of the walls. The same thing can happen to your body when holes develop in its protective barriers. A cut in the skin is an obvious example. Less obvious are leaks that develop in the lining of the gut, the lungs, and brain due to stress and an unhealthy diet and lifestyle. After these barriers become leaky, it's not wind or rain that gets in, but instead "antigens" — that is, undigested particles of food, bacteria, parasites, molds, or haptens, environmental toxins.[91] This intrusion triggers a wonderfully orchestrated immune response. The first units on the scene are *macrophages*, a Greek word meaning "big eaters." These cells are stationed in body tissue and constantly on the lookout for intruders, poised to attack and sound the alarm whenever one enters. I like to think of them as overweight security guards carrying clubs but no guns. Although they are the first on the scene, they need help to overcome the antigen.

The macrophage envelops the intruder, creating an *antigen presenting cell* (APC) that acts like a burglar alarm, summoning the rest of the immune system to come help. The first to respond to the alarm are *T-helper cells*, dispatchers who organize the attack. The T-helper cells send messengers to bring the elite police force — *natural killer cells* and *cytotoxic T-cells* to swarm the intruder and destroy it. Back at central headquarters, police sergeants, T-*regulator cells*, monitor the scene to insure there are enough T-helper cells and *T-suppressor cells*, cells that stop the immune reaction once an intruder is disarmed, and that they are doing their jobs.

The immune system takes no chances at another attack, and assumes the intruder is a member of organized crime. T-helper cells fetch the detectives, *B-cell antibodies*, which attach to the intruder and put all his information into a memory bank. This identification process makes the natural killer and cytotoxic T-cells more efficient at recognizing and destroying the intruder if he comes around again. Although the natural killer and cytotoxic T-cells are like an elite S.W.A.T. team, they nevertheless also have poor vision and rely on the B-cells to spot intruders.

TH-1 PATHWAY   **TH-2 PATHWAY**

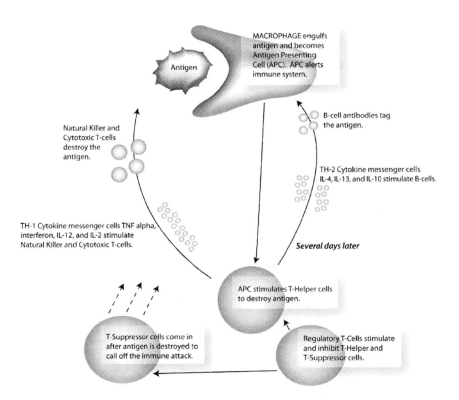

*The immune system's TH-1 and TH-2 pathways at work,
and the sites where things can go wrong in an autoimmune disease.
The TH-1 pathway is the immediate immune response,
whereas the TH-2 pathway is the delayed response.*

THE AUTOIMMUNE CRIME SCENE

Like a movie that involves the mafia, bad cops, and double-crossers, a typical crime scene can go awry when any of the players deviates from his job. This is what happens in the case of autoimmune disease, when some cells of the immune system start destroying the body they were designed to protect. Here are a few possible scenarios:

- Some people don't make enough T-suppressor cells, so the immune system's attack goes on and on. You can see how innocent bystanders, like thyroid tissue, are more likely to be mistaken for the enemy.

- Some people make too much *interleukin 2* (IL-2), a messenger chemical that deploys natural killer and cytotoxic T-cells to destroy the intruder.[92] When there is too much IL-2, an overabundance of natural killer and cytotoxic T-cells are deployed, putting innocent bystanders — that is, healthy tissue — at risk.

- Some people make too much *interleukin 4* (IL-4), a messenger that deploys B-cells.[93][94] An overabundance of B-cells looking for intruders to tag may accidentally mark innocent bystanders.

- People eating high-carbohydrate diets don't handle blood sugar well, causing insulin surges that stimulate overproduction of B-cells.[95]

- A parasitic infection and multiple food intolerances drive up IL-4, causing overproduction of B-cells.[96]

- A chronic virus infection drives up IL-2, causing overproduction of natural killer and cytotoxic T-cells.[97]

Although Hashimoto's is the most common autoimmune disease, it's possible to develop an autoimmune reaction to anything in the body, including organs, joints, hormones, the brain, nerves, muscles, etc. Proper care is based not on the tissue being attacked, but on how the immune system is behaving.[98]Autoimmune diseases are on a precipitous rise in industrialized countries, sending researchers scrambling for explanations and cures. (One example is a whipworm infestation for Crohn's Disease!).[99] According to the American Autoimmune Related Diseases Association, Inc., approximately 50 million Americans, 20 percent of the population or one in five people, suffer from autoimmune diseases.[100] Women are more likely than men to suffer from these disorders. Some experts estimate that 75 percent of some 30 million people affected are women.[101]

It's not always possible to pinpoint what exactly triggers a person's genes to turn on an autoimmune disease. However numerous risk factors exist (See Chapter Two for some examples.) I suspect the weakening of the immune barriers, such as the lining of the digestive tract and respiratory tract, and the blood-brain barrier, plays a big factor.[102] When these barriers are healthy and strong, intruders cannot pass through, so only the occasional emergency and maintenance work such as clearing out dead and dying cells musters the immune system. But as health weakens due to poor diet, unstable blood sugar, gut infections, chronic stress, and adrenal malfunction, these barriers weaken and become porous. The result is intestinal permeability, also known as leaky gut, not to mention leaky lungs and leaky brain.[103] Over time the immune system is working around the clock to battle invaders penetrating the barriers from every direction. These stealthy culprits may be in the foods you eat or the air your breath, and with the immune system so overworked, you have no back up fighters and little relief. An army pushed too far for too long is at risk for mutiny, attacking the very thing it is designed to protect, the human body.

Autism Starts With the Mom

I will no longer address a woman's infertility until she has first restored the integrity and function of her health and immune system. I am finding an autoimmune disorder is often at the root of autism, with the immune system attacking brain or nerve tissue of the child with autism. Children born with an immune system that is a ticking time bomb are vulnerable to anything that can launch a self-attack, whether it is a vaccine, food intolerance, blood sugar imbalance, or heavy metal toxicity. When a woman goes into a pregnancy with a leaky gut, dysglycemia, multiple food intolerances, and adrenal fatigue, I believe she is putting her baby at risk for developing one of the increasingly common, modern health disorders, including autism spectrum disorders, eczema, asthma, food allergies, and food intolerances.[104] [105] [106] [107] [108] [109]

ARE YOU TH–1 OR TH–2 DOMINANT?

Once the gene for an autoimmune disease has been turned on, it can't be turned off. The only thing to be done clinically is to turn down the volume on the immune response by restoring balance.[110] The trick is to discover which side of your immune system is more active — the side that deploys natural killer and cytotoxic T-cells, or the side that deploys B-cell antibodies. Are you producing too many natural killer and cytotoxic T-cells, the ones responsible for killing invaders? If so, you are *TH-1 dominant.* (TH stands for T-helper cell) Or are you producing too many B-cells, the ones in charge of tagging the intruder so it can be readily identified? If so, you are *TH-2 dominant.* If you are dominant in one or the other, your immune system is out of balance and autoimmune disease is either highly likely or already underway.

In our crime scene, T-helper cells communicate and orchestrate an immune attack. They are the dispatchers that send messengers to fetch natural killer, cytotoxic T-cells, and B-cells to the crime scene. By measuring these messengers, or *cytokines*, in blood tests, I can find out whether a patient with an autoimmune disease is TH-1 or TH-2 dominant. Cytokines are like hormones — they are chemical messengers that make things happen. Interestingly, TH-1 and TH-2 cytokines affect thyroid function beyond driving Hashimoto's disease: Elevated TH-1 or TH-2 cytokines also block thyroid receptor sites,[111] [112] [113] [114] preventing thyroid hormone from getting into the cells, thus causing symptoms of low thyroid activity.

Thyroid Cytokines and Hormones

Interestingly, TH-1 and TH-2 cytokines affect thyroid function beyond driving Hashimoto's disease: Elevated TH-1 or TH-2 cytokines also block thyroid receptor sites. This prevents thyroid hormone from getting into the cells, thus causing symptoms of low thyroid activity.

Are You TH–1 OR TH–2 Dominant?

Too much natural killer and cytotoxic T-cell activity:
- **TH-1 DOMINANT**

Too much B-cell activity:
- **TH-2 DOMINANT**

We determine whether someone is TH-1 or TH-2 dominant by measuring cytokines, chemical messengers that stimulate production of natural killer and cytotoxic T-cells or B cells.

The TH-1 cytokines include:
- IL(interleukin) -2
- IL-12
- Tumor necrosis factor alpha (TNFa)
- Interferon

The TH-2 cytokines include:
- IL-4
- IL-13
- IL-10

Although there are exceptions to every rule, I have seen recurring patterns of TH-1 versus TH-2 dominance.[115] For instance, about 90 percent of my patients with Hashimoto's are TH-1 dominant. Their natural killer and cytotoxic T-cells are over active, thus attacking thyroid tissue. Research not only confirms my experience, but studies also show that Type I diabetes, multiple sclerosis, and chronic viral infections are often associated with a TH-1 dominance.[116] [117] On the other hand, lupus, dermatitis, asthma, and multiple chemical sensitivities are often associated with a TH-2 dominance.[118] [119] However, these are generalities, and should not be taken as the rule. Also, it's important to note that not *all* autoimmune diseases can be traced to a TH-1 or TH-2 dominance; other possible causes include immune defects and deficiencies. In other words, no cookbook recipes exist to managing an autoimmune disease. Instead, a basic understanding of immunology is key.

(continued)

Hashimoto's and Pregnancy

Autoimmune diseases are more common in women, and pregnancy is a common trigger, so we know hormones play a big role in turning on autoimmune genes.[120][121] During the third trimester, a pregnant woman becomes TH-2 dominant, and during the postpartum period, she becomes TH-1 dominant. Many women complain their thyroid problems started after they had children. Combined with other risk factors, such as stress, gut infections, insulin surges, gluten intolerance, and environmental toxins, pregnancy can indeed trigger Hashimoto's disease.[122][123] The following story illustrates this point:

A patient asked me to evaluate her thyroid condition, because she had Hashimoto's and wasn't feeling better under her physicians care, which involved monitoring her TSH levels every month and adjusting her medication accordingly. This went on for four years, during which time she became pregnant and had a baby. Looking at the lab tests done over those years, I was fascinated to see how her immune system shifted during and after the pregnancy. In the first half of pregnancy, a woman is TH-1 dominant. My patient's Hashimoto's had gone into remission during those months. Towards the second half of pregnancy women shift into TH-2 dominance, and this woman's TSH peaked at 58 during this stage (normal is 1.8-3). She was obviously TH-2 dominant. While the TH-1 dominance of early pregnancy tamed her autoimmune thyroid condition, the TH-2 dominance of later pregnancy kicked it into high gear. Blood tests of her immune system confirmed that her TH-2 pathway was dominant.

By taking sufficient emulsified vitamin D and fish oil, applying a lipsomal glutathione and superoxide dismutase cream, and sticking to a gluten-free diet, this patient was able to get off her thyroid medication and live a symptom-free life. However when she eats gluten, her symptoms return.

Shane Steadman, DC, DACNB
Mountain Health Chiropractic and Neurology
Englewood, Colorado

HOW TO ADDRESS A TH–1 OR TH–2 DOMINANCE

When addressing autoimmune disease, the goal is to restore balance to the immune system. I approach this in several ways. The foundation of care is to support my patient's overall health, which will be covered in following chapters. Unstable blood sugar, gut infections, and poor adrenal health (all of which are practically universal in this country) worsen an autoimmune condition.[124] Removing gluten from the diet is also vital, given the studied links between Hashimoto's and gluten intolerance.[125] [126]

STEP ONE: SUPPORT THE T–REGULATORY CELLS

Beyond those basics, however, I use natural medicine to balance the immune system. My first step is to support the T-regulatory cells. At our crime scene, these were the sergeants monitoring the situation from headquarters, sending more T-helper or T-suppressor cells as necessary to boost, slow down, or halt an immune attack. In an autoimmune crime scene, these T-regulatory cells start behaving erratically, as if they are drunk or working for the bad guys. As a result, they issue bad commands — dispatching too many or not enough T-helper or T-suppressor cells — that ultimately destroy body tissue. By restoring sanity to their actions, we can restore balance to the immune system and tame an autoimmune response.

Emulsified vitamin D (cholecalciferol) is a powerful immune modulator [127] and best supports the T-regulatory cells [128] [129] [130] when prescribed in therapeutic doses by a licensed healthcare practitioner qualified to work with vitamin D therapy. Emulsification is important so that someone with poor digestion can absorb the nutrient. It also prevents toxicity at higher doses. Cod liver oil, although high in vitamin D and possessing necessary cofactors for its absorption, does not provide enough of the vitamin to modulate an autoimmune disease. The EPA and DHA in fish oil also support the T-regulatory cells. (Taken in large amounts, cod liver oil delivers too much EPA and DHA, which has blood-thinning properties).

Vitamin D supplementation is important for another reason: Studies have found that more than 90 percent of people with autoimmune thyroid disease have a genetic defect affecting their ability to process vitamin D. Therefore, they need higher amounts of vitamin D to maintain health.[131] This can be the case even if a blood test shows sufficient vitamin D: The defect is at the cellular receptor site, so not enough vitamin D can gain entry into the cells. On a lab test, I like to see high-normal vitamin D levels for patients with thyroid disorders.

Other nutrients that modulate the immune system and support the T-regulatory cells are glutathione cream and superoxide dismutase, both powerful antioxidants.[138] [139] [140] [141] Glutathione works best when delivered intravenously or absorbed through the skin (especially the bottom of the feet).[142] Since giving glutathione intravenously is usually not practical, I recommend a cream that delivers these nutrients into the circulatory system via a liposomal delivery method through the skin to act as a powerful immune modulator.

STEP TWO: BALANCE TH-1 AND TH-2

After I establish immune modulation with vitamin D and the glutathione cream, I work directly on taming a dominant TH-1 or TH-2 pathway. I do this is by stimulating the side of the immune system that is *not* dominant. Imagine your immune system is a seesaw, on which TH-1 and TH-2 are sitting. TH-1, which stimulates production of natural killer and cytotoxic T-cells, is sitting on the ground because it is big and heavy, while TH-2, the B-cell pathway, is way up in the air, waving its skinny little legs in an attempt to come down. To restore balance to that seesaw, I use natural compounds to stimulate TH-2, beefing it up so it can level the seesaw. If TH-2 is the dominant one sitting on the ground, then I support TH-1 to achieve the same balance.

Hashimoto's and Vitamin D

If you have Hashimoto's, you may need additional vitamin D for another reason: Studies have found that more than 90 percent of people with autoimmune thyroid disease have a genetic defect affecting their ability to process the nutrient.[132] [133] [134] [135] [136] [137] Therefore, these people need higher amounts of vitamin D to maintain health.

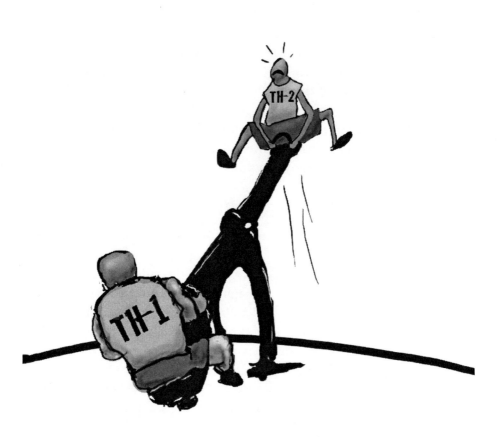

When it comes to managing autoimmune disease, it's important to know whether you are TH-1 or TH-2 dominant.

I have put together a short list of compounds that stimulate TH-1 and TH-2. Sometimes, one or more of these nutrients can be used to determine the dominant state. For instance, coffee stimulates the TH-2 pathway. Drinking coffee will worsen a TH-2 dominant person's autoimmune condition. This is the person who says she can't drink coffee because it makes her autoimmune condition flare up. The TH-1 dominant person, however, may sheepishly admit to drinking coffee because she finds it lessens her symptoms and makes her feel better. Coffee, however, can be a tricky tool for diagnosis. Since it also stimulates the adrenal glands, coffee can cause irritability, insomnia, and other symptoms that resemble an autoimmune thyroid flare-up. I have had cases, however, in which my patients with rheumatoid arthritis have less joint pain when they drink coffee. That's a clue that they have a TH-1 dominance.

Echinacea, a common component of antiviral remedies, stimulates the TH-1 pathway. It can make the person with TH-1 dominance feel worse and exacerbate autoimmune tissue destruction. The person with TH-2 dominance, in contrast, might feel better using echinacea.

Both the scientific literature and my clinical experience have allowed me to put together a list of botanical and nutritional compounds that affect the TH-1 and TH-2 pathways. Although I list these compounds here, it is important for the person with Hashimoto's to see a healthcare practitioner trained and qualified in working with autoimmune disease to use these compounds correctly, safely and in the right combinations.

COMPOUNDS THAT STIMULATE TH-1 [143] [144]
(These dampen a TH-2 dominance and will worsen the autoimmune condition of a TH-1 dominant person):

Astragalus[145]

Echinacea[146]

Beta-glucan mushroom[147]

Maitake mushroom[148]

Glycyrrhiza (from licorice)[149]

Melissa Officinalis (lemon balm)[150]

COMPOUNDS THAT STIMULATE TH-2 [151]
(These dampen a TH-1 dominance and will worsen the autoimmune condition of a TH-2 dominant person):

Caffeine[152]

Green tea extract[153]

Grape seed extract[154]

Pine bark extract[155]

White willow bark[156]

Lycopene[157]

Resveratrol[158]

Pycnogenol[159]

COMPOUNDS THAT MODULATE BOTH TH-1 AND TH-2[160]

Probiotics[161 162 163 164]

Vitamin A[165 166]

Vitamin E[167 168]

Colostrum[169 170 171 172 173]

COMPOUNDS THAT DAMPEN IL-1 ACTIVATING TH-1 OR TH-2:[174]

Boswellia[175 176 177 178]

Pancreatic enzymes

Turmeric/Curcumin[179 180 181]

I always use immunological lab tests to determine whether a person is TH-1 or TH-2 dominant so that I know how to properly tame and support her over active and poorly regulated immune system. So if she is TH-1 dominant, I prescribe compounds that stimulate TH-2, and if she is TH-2 dominant, I recommend compounds that stimulate TH-1. Because unstable blood sugar, adrenal dysfunction, and poor digestive health exacerbate autoimmune disorders, supporting the entire body is also integral to managing Hashimoto's. Also, don't forget that the first priority is to enhance T-regulatory cell function with emulsified vitamin D, fish oil and glutathione cream. It's important to add in the right combination of nutritional compounds, as determined by your healthcare practitioner, one at a time every three days to monitor response.

How do I know if the protocol for immune modulation is working? Monitoring symptoms is important of course, but I also use blood tests to monitor cytokines and T and B cell populations along the way, too. They should begin to reach normal levels and antibody tests should become negative. That doesn't mean the condition is cured, but it is dormant.

Supporting Hashimoto's Disease

A 36-year-old woman with scleroderma was referred to our office by the nanny who cared for her two children. She was being treated by a chiropractor using NAET for food allergies. Her antinuclear antibodies (ANA) were at 1,380. ANAs are found in patients with a number of different autoimmune diseases. Comprehensive blood tests revealed her TSH and T4 were functionally low. She was experiencing extreme fatigue and was not able to get out of bed. The nanny who cared for her two children referred her to our office. Her other symptoms included severe sugar cravings, heartburn, weight gain, and cellulite deposits all over her body.

She began taking nutritional compounds for autoimmune modulation developed by Dr. Kharrazian. After two months, her energy improved to the point where she felt able to start an exercise program.

Her second group of blood tests done sixty days after starting the program, showed her TSH and T4 in normal range. Four months after first coming to our office, she went to her endocrinologist to check her ANA count. It had dropped to 26. When she questioned her doctor about the dramatic ANA drop, he responded that the original test was probably an error. He could not account for why she was feeling better on our autoimmune protocol. By this time she was playing two hours of tennis several times a week. Her weight was dropping, and her cellulite was disappearing. The endocrinologist measures her ANA every two months, and it remains in the 26-28 range.

David Peterson, DC
Wellness Alternatives
Town & Country, MO

USING LAB TESTS TO ASSESS IMMUNE FUNCTION

Advancements in technology and testing have given us wonderful tools to assess health. When used in conjunction with these cutting-edge tests, natural medicine is a very effective model of support.

The first thing to establish is whether the person has an autoimmune condition. I use TPO and TGB serum antibody tests to rule out Hashimoto's. If a test comes back negative but symptoms strongly suggest the disorder, I'll repeat the test since antibody counts can fluctuate. Sometimes I'll ask the person to eat gluten-containing foods for two weeks prior to the test, in order to heighten the autoimmune response.

From there, I delve into the immune system mechanics. I measure TH-1 and TH-2 cytokines to determine if the person is TH-1 or TH-2 dominant. When a person is placed on an immune-modulating protocol, I retest these cytokines to see whether the immune system is coming into better balance. When looking at these test results, it is important to look at the *percentages* of the cytokines and not the totals.

Remember, regardless of whether a person with Hashimoto's has TH-1 or TH-2 dominance, managing his or her condition requires modulating the immune system with emulsified vitamin D, fish oil, glutathione cream, a gluten-free diet, and dietary support.

Hashimoto's and Other Complaints

A patient with Hashimoto's came to see me complaining of double vision. Within two to three weeks of using glutathione cream and therapeutic levels of emulsified vitamin D, her thyroid symptoms began to normalize and her double vision disappeared.

Another patient with the same diagnosis experienced a lot of joint pain. After two to three weeks on the same protocol plus nutrients to dampen the TH-1 pathway, her discomfort was gone and her energy increased so much that she said she had not felt that good in 15 years.

Brian Hickey, DC
Arlington Natural Wellness Center
Arlington, TX

USING A SUPPLEMENT CHALLENGE

About 30 percent of the time, the labs don't clearly show a dominant pathway. When that happens, I may turn to TH-1 and TH-2 stimulators to establish which state is dominant. As I mentioned earlier, I look for clues while talking to my patients: Does she feel better or worse after drinking coffee, or taking something like echinacea? If a person with Hashimoto's complains of irritability and insomnia whenever she takes echinacea, that is a clue she might be TH-1 dominant as echinacea stimulates the TH-1 pathway.

I will send patients home with three days each of a specially formulated combination of nutritional compounds that support TH-1 pathways and TH-2 pathways. I have them take the TH-1 compound first and monitor how they feel. Then I instruct them to take the TH-2 compound and compare the difference in how they feel. (A patient should not take both formulations at the same time for the purpose of assessment.) Sometimes the effects are very noticeable: A person may experience a flare-up of thyroid symptoms on one product and a noticeable improvement with the other. However some people don't notice anything, which requires more sleuthing on my part.

NOTE: This challenge should only be done under the supervision of a licensed healthcare professional. Also, some people develop autoimmune reactions to brain and nerve tissue, such as with muscular dystrophy or autism. It is important *not* to use this protocol when destruction of nerve or brain tissue is at risk.

Hashimoto's is an Immune Disease

My late teens were riddled with reoccurring respiratory infections, skin rashes, fatigue, sharp abdominal pain, extreme menstrual cramping, irregular periods, and weight gain. I was finally diagnosed with hypothyroidism in my early twenties by a nurse practitioner and was told to take Synthroid. I decided to see a chiropractic nutritionist who helped bring my thyroid hormone levels back into normal range. I could tell I was feeling somewhat better and I was losing weight, but I still was suffering from skin rashes, fatigue, severe menstrual cramping, and irregular periods. I went back a year or so later to have my blood work done by an endocrinologist. He diagnosed me with Hashimoto's. I was stunned! My doctor seemed adamant that I would be on thyroid replacement hormone forever. I decided medication was not the answer and worked even harder on my diet. I sought the help of Dr. Mark Flannery, who trained with Dr. Kharrazian. He took the time to educate me that my immune system needed to be regulated in order to help my autoimmune thyroid condition. After a series of blood tests, I started a very simple program that targeted the immune system and not the thyroid. I was concerned that Dr. Flannery did not have me on any specific supplementation for the thyroid. However, the blood test results proved I was headed in the right direction. This baffled the endocrinologist who insisted I must have been taking medication. My energy came back full force, my hair and skin were softer than ever, my menstrual cycle became regular, and I haven't had cramping in over two years. I owe my good health to Dr. Mark Flannery, for his expert knowledge of the immune system and for giving me my life back.

— VJ, *a patient of Mark Flannery, DC*
Mark Flannery, DC
HealthWise Chiropractic & Nutrition
Simi Valley, CA

STEP THREE: REMOVE THE ANTIGEN
PROVOKING THE AUTOIMMUNE ATTACK

Quite often I will find that a specific antigen — a food, mold, bacteria, chronic virus, or parasite — is provoking the autoimmune attack. The perfect example with Hashimoto's is gluten, which provokes at attack on the thyroid gland every time the gluten-intolerant person eats it. People can also develop an immune response to haptens, which are environmental chemicals or heavy metals that provoke an immune response. It's important to note that not everyone will develop an autoimmune response to antigens or haptens. For instance, we all have varying degrees of heavy metal toxicity, but not everyone's immune system will mount an attack against mercury, lead, cadmium, or other metals. (Although antigen refers to organic compounds and hapten refers to inorganic compounds such as heavy metals, I refer to both as antigens for the sake of simplicity.)

The Bacterial Connection

Researchers have found the prevalence of antibodies to *Yersinia enterocolitica*, which indicates evidence of exposure to the bacterium, was 14 times higher in people with Hashimoto's than in those who didn't have the disorder.[182] Being tested for and removing this particular bacterium is an example of how removing the antigen can be an effective tool in managing Hashimoto's disease.

When an antigen is to blame for stimulating an autoimmune attack, an immune panel of tests may show both the TH-1 and TH-2 cytokines are high and T-suppressor cells are low. This indicates the body is currently in a heated battle against something the immune system recognizes as an enemy, which is stoking the autoimmune mechanism. Another essential immune panel measures the ratio of T-helper cells to T-suppressor cells. This is the CD4/CD8 test (CD4 measures T-helper cells and CD8 measures T-suppressor cells). Typically when an autoimmune disease such as Hashimoto's is being driven by an antigen response, the CD4/CD8 ratio is above 2. If follow-up tests of the CD4/CD8 ratio show it lowering, then you know the approach you're using is having an effect.

Identifying the responsible antigen can be tricky but is important. Questioning the person about their health and lifestyle yields essential clues. For instance, does she live in a house with toxic mold? Does she have Hepatitis C? Did he work at a job or have a hobby that regularly exposed him to toxic heavy metals? Immune tests to detect antibodies to particular antigens help, too, once you have narrowed down the possibilities. With Hashimoto's, remove gluten, a common antigen, from the diet immediately. Also, antigens such as molds, viruses, parasites and other organic compounds typically fire up the TH-1 pathway. Haptens, inorganic compounds such as heavy metals, pesticides, and other environmental compounds typically fire up the TH-2 pathway. But this is a generality and not a rule. Another clue that a hapten may be responsible for driving an autoimmune disease is when the person's response to both TH-1 and TH-2 stimulators makes them feel worse. In this case, restoring the immune barriers, discussed later in this chapter, is key.

As with all cases of autoimmune disease, effective modulation begins with support of the regulatory T-cells using emulsified vitamin D, EPA/DHA and a glutathione cream, an effective delivery method for glutathione.

WHEN TO STIMULATE THE *DOMINANT* PATHWAY

What distinguishes the approach to managing an active antigen is that *you support the TH pathway that is dominant* in order to remove the antigen or drive it into remission. By squelching the antigen, you help restore balance and calm to the stressed immune system.

Let's simplify this with some examples. Say a person with hepatitis C, a chronic virus infecting the liver, develops Hashimoto's. An immune panel shows me the Hashimoto's disease is a result of an active antigen response — both TH-1 and TH-2 pathways are elevated, and the CD4/CD8 ratio is higher than 2. Because I know that an active antigen, such as a chronic virus, can sometimes trigger autoimmune attacks, I support the immune system to drive the hepatitis C into a dormant state. Treating viruses is beyond the scope of this book, but managing this person's case would include a viral load test to monitor the liver infection, as well as an immune panel to determine whether the person was more TH-1 or TH-2 dominant. (Even though both TH-1 and TH-2 could be high, I see which is the highest). If the person's TH-1 pathway is more dominant, then I further stimulate TH-1 with compounds to help the body overcome the virus, and vice versa with TH-2 dominance. This is opposite to my standard immune support for Hashimoto's caused by an immune system malfunction in which you support the *depressed* TH pathway. By relieving the immune system of the chronic infection, it can relax and the autoimmune attacks fade into remission.

Again, add in nutritional compounds geared toward modulating immunity one at a time every three days to monitor response.

RESTORING THE IMMUNE BARRIERS

Sometimes the active antigen infection can be due to a heavy metal such as mercury. When the gut, respiratory tract, or brain barriers become permeable (i.e., "leaky gut" "leaky lungs," or "leaky brain"), antigens such as mercury can pass through them, potentially creating a chronic and powerful immune response and possibly triggering the gene for an autoimmune disease. Although most people have some degree of mercury in their bodies, not everyone's immune system will respond to it as if it's an infectious agent.

If mercury or other environmental compounds are creating an autoimmune response, this can be verified by an antibody tests against that particular compound (by running chemical hapten or heavy metal antibody tests). If the test comes back positive, removing the compound is one way to address Hashimoto's.

A recent study, for instance, looked at the impact of dental amalgams on Hashimoto's disease in people having an immune response to mercury. The researchers concluded that the removal of mercury-containing dental amalgams contributed to the successful management of those with the thyroid disorder.[9]

In other cases, however, liberating stored mercury with methods like chelation can exacerbate an autoimmune response. A good example involves autism. Many doctors peg autism on heavy metal toxicity and prescribe chelation. I, on the other hand, think that an *immune response to mercury* can trigger an autoimmune attack on nerve or brain tissue, causing autism. Chelation releases stored mercury into the system and can exacerbate an autoimmune autistic condition, causing more tissue death and a worsening of symptoms.

In this situation, the most important action is to restore integrity to the immune barriers, (See my protocol for repairing leaky gut in Chapter Six), especially if immunoglobulin M (IgM) antibodies are elevated. This prevents mercury from slipping into places it doesn't belong, like brain and nerve tissue. In addition to supplying the right nutrients to restore these barriers, remember that stress significantly weakens these tissues. Since poor blood sugar handling is a top stressor, balancing blood sugar (See Chapter Five) is key. When restoring integrity to the immune barriers has resulted in successful dampening of the autoimmune condition, chelation may be appropriate with careful monitoring, but perhaps not. It is better to live in peace with mercury than permanently destroy brain tissue in an attempt to eliminate it.

Monitoring and Supporting Hashimoto's

- After Hashimoto's is assessed with a positive TPO and/or TGB serum antibody test, establish TH-1 or TH-2 dominance with an immunological serum test. Look at the percentage values, not the total.
- A TH-1 serum profile includes interferon, IL-2, IL-12, interferon-gamma, and TNF alpha.
- A TH-2 serum profile includes IL-4, IL-13 and IL-10.
- If the TH-1 cytokines are high, then modulate the autoimmune condition by supporting the TH-2 pathway with TH-2 stimulators.
- If the TH-2 cytokines are high, then support the TH-1 pathway with TH-1 stimulators.
- A CD4/CD8 (T-suppressor cell/T-helper cell) ratio of 2 or higher is an indication that an active antigen is driving the autoimmune response. This test is also a baseline from which to monitor overall progress.
- If an active antigen or hapten is at work, then stimulate the *dominant* TH pathway to eradicate the antigen or drive it into remission.
- If both TH-1 and TH-2 stimulators make you feel worse, a hapten may be driving the autoimmune condition. In that case, restore the immune barriers.
- In all instances, modulate immune T-helper cell response with therapeutic doses of emulsified vitamin D plus cofactors, fish oil, and liposomal glutathione and superoxide dismutase cream. Have a licensed healthcare practitioner qualified to work with vitamin D therapy prescribe the appropriate dose.
- Add in nutritional compounds individually every three days to monitor response.
- Remove gluten and possibly dairy from the diet and support other systems, organs, and functions in the body. (Managing blood sugar, digestive function, and adrenal health using functional medicine principles is explained in later chapters.)
- Monitor whether support is effective with follow-up TSH, CD4/CD8, and TH-1 and TH-2 cytokine tests.

- The immune system can be likened to a crime scene, with security guards, police officers, dispatchers, and detectives.

- We don't always know what triggers an autoimmune disease, although a compromised immune barrier in the digestive tract is often a factor. When the gut lining loses integrity due to poor diet, infections, blood sugar swings, and adrenal malfunctions, the immune system is called into action on a constant basis. This can lead to an immune system imbalance and the development of an autoimmune disease, such as Hashimoto's.

- Hashimoto's is an immune disease, not a thyroid disease, so the immune system must be supported.

- Determining whether a person is TH-1 dominant or TH-2 dominant is key to managing Hashimoto's.

- Vitamin D, fish oil and glutathione cream modulate the immune system whether one is TH-1 dominant or TH-2 dominant.

- Gluten is a common trigger for Hashimoto's.

- If Hashimoto's is being triggered by an active infection, remove the antigen, support the TH dominant pathway differently, or focus on restoring the immune barrier of the gut and brain (see Chapter Six).

CHAPTER FOUR

SIX PATTERNS OF LOW THYROID FUNCTION AND HOW TO FIND THEM ON A BLOOD TEST

Eileen's gut seemed to be moving slowly, and she was constipated. She also had a hard time staying warm on winter nights and needed to take a very hot shower before hopping into a bed piled high with extra blankets. She noticed feeling depressed more and more frequently. After researching her symptoms on the Internet, she decided to get her thyroid function tested. Her medical doctor told her she was in excellent health and her TSH level, the only marker ordered, was well within normal range. However when Eileen finally got her thyroid checked by a natural medicine doctor who requested several tests and considered the ranges differently than her MD, her TSH was low. After just one month of taking the nutritional compounds her healthcare practitioner recommended, supporting her adrenal health, and making a few dietary changes, Eileen's symptoms resolved and her mood lifted.

She had been spared of potentially months or even years of worsening health just by examining her thyroid blood tests correctly.

THE TROUBLE WITH BLOOD TESTS

Although Hashimoto's is the most common cause of hypothyroidism in the United States, six other factors can lead to low thyroid function. In this chapter I'll introduce you to the six different patterns of low thyroid function, only one of which is successfully served, if at all, with thyroid replacement hormone medication. This is because most people with symptoms of hypothyroidism have "functional hypothyroidism," and not an actual thyroid disease. Some facet of their health is breaking down and producing hypothyroid symptoms, but the condition does not warrant lifelong medication. It's all a matter of learning how to correctly order and interpret a panel of blood chemistry tests.

Perhaps the grossest mismanagement of hypothyroidism begins and ends with the blood test. It is estimated 13 million cases of thyroid dysfunction go undiagnosed each year,[183] and inadequate blood testing is a big factor. Why?

Only one of the six patterns will show up on a blood test to measure TSH, the thyroid hormone test doctors commonly order. Also, many doctors use the lab ranges that come with the test results, instead of the "functional" ranges, which have been carefully researched and formulated as parameters of good thyroid health. By the time someone's thyroid levels are outside of the typical ranges the lab provides, his or her condition is so advanced that taking medication throughout life may be the only treatment option. That is why the standard lab ranges are referred to as pathological or disease ranges. As a result, countless people suffer months or years with hypothyroid conditions that could have been easily reversed with proper diagnoses.

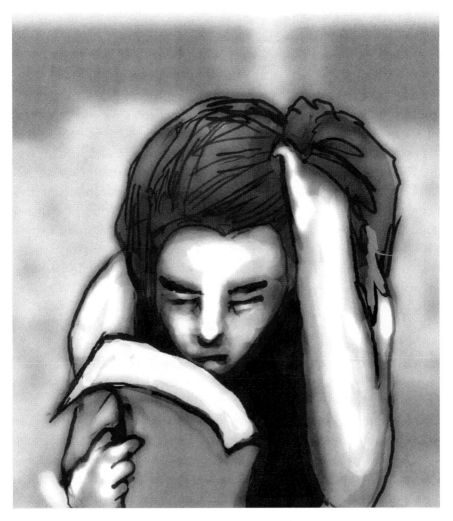

It can be frustrating when your
blood test results are normal but your health isn't.

Although pathological ranges are useful for diagnosing diseases that require medical intervention, they are of little value for gauging what constitutes good health. You may be surprised to know that pathological ranges are simply the averages of all the people who have had blood work analyzed by that lab in the last year. So this means the guidelines for diagnosing a thyroid condition are based on all the people who visited the lab over the previous year, most of whom we can assume are in some degree of poor health. What's worse, many of these folks already take thyroid hormones, which skew the results even more. We can also assume that many of them have undiagnosed thyroid conditions, which are then added into the stew defining what is normal.

Furthermore, pathological ranges have broadened over the past 50 years as the health of the American population has declined. For instance, as Americans hurtle toward a diabetes epidemic, the ranges for what constitute healthy blood sugar have widened. What was considered hypoglycemic or pre-diabetic 30 years ago, before junk foods became dietary staples, is now considered normal on many lab tests.

Do you really want to evaluate your health based on all the sick people in your area? Or do you want to know what constitutes good health? I certainly don't want to treat my patients using disease parameters, so I use functional blood ranges. Functional ranges assess risk for disease before it develops. For instance, the functional range for fasting blood glucose is 85-100 mg/dL. The pathological range may be 65-110 mg/dL. By using the functional range, we can reverse the risk of diabetes with lifestyle, diet, and nutritional compounds, before it's too late. The same holds true for hypothyroidism. A standard TSH lab range is 0.35 – 5.5 uIU/mL, but the functional range is a much narrower 1.8 – 3.0 uIU/mL, allowing the natural medicine doctor to reverse the downward swing of the thyroid before it's too late.

Conventional medicine, however, is geared toward providing care once a disease manifests, and often has little to offer before it occurs. In other words, a person is considered healthy because no disease is present, even if she goes through her days feeling awful. As a functional doctor, I define health as having adequate energy, healthy digestion, ideal physiological function, and other markers of wellbeing.

Functional ranges have been determined over the years by healthcare providers and researchers who embrace the principles of preventative medicine, including guiding a person to make healthy diet and other lifestyle changes.

The Importance of Blood Work

Virginia was a vivacious entrepreneur who started getting sick constantly after she turned 40. She struggled with pneumonia, shingles, respiratory infections, sinus infections, and every virus that came through. Doctors ran tests but they all showed her to be healthy. When she saw Dr. Steadman she learned she had Hashimoto's and a TH-1 dominance. All the echinacea tea she drank was actually making her worse. As Dr. Steadman managed her Hashimoto's Virginia's immune system became stronger and she no longer became sick so frequently and severely.

Shane Steadman, DC, DACNB
Denver, Colorado

USING A BLOOD TEST TO ASSESS THYROID HEALTH

Many people suffer from thyroid imbalances that are not advanced enough to create a pathological range on a blood test. From a functional perspective, however, one can find these imbalances by looking at a combination of markers. In this chapter I will review individual markers to include on blood tests, their functional ranges and explain how to put the markers together to look at the six different patterns of thyroid dysfunction.

(continued)

Getting the Terminology Straight

Throughout this book I use the term *functional hypothyroidism* to define depressed thyroid activity that can be nutritionally supported without the use of medication. I use this term because it is widely recognized in the alternative medicine world. However, what I'm really referring to is *euthyroid*, a condition in which the thyroid gland itself is fine but the thyroid metabolic pathways are impaired. The six patterns in this chapter primarily explain defects in these metabolic pathways.

Technically, in the alternative medicine world, functional hypothyroidism means lab tests are normal but the patient still has symptoms. In conventional medicine, functional hypothyroidism means the opposite — blood tests are abnormal, but the person has symptoms.

Because euthyroid is an unfamiliar word to most people, and because I explain functional blood test ranges and functional medicine, I will stick with the popularly used term *functional hypothyroidism* to describe low thyroid activity that arises from defects in the thyroid metabolic pathways.

UNDERSTANDING INDIVIDUAL THYROID MARKERS

TSH Thyroid Stimulating Hormone (TSH), or thyrotropin, is released by the pituitary gland. This is the most common and sensitive marker of thyroid function. TSH increases when T4 drops, and TSH decreases when T4 rises. This is frequently the only test performed by conventional doctors to screen for thyroid disorders, yet it fails to consider myriad factors.

Functional Range: 1.8-3.0 mU/L

Typical Laboratory Range: 0.5-5.5 mU/L

Total Thyroxine (TT4) The TT4 test measures both bound and un-bound T4 levels. (Remember, thyroid hormones travel through the bloodstream bound to proteins before they are released to enter into cells, becoming unbound.) Therefore, it does not give you an idea of how active T4 is, unless other markers are included, such as T3 uptake. T3 uptake indicates how much thyroid hormone is entering cells. By measuring T4 along with T3 uptake, you can calculate the activity of free T4. Total T4 can be altered by many drugs (See sidebar at the end of the chapter).

Functional Range: 6-12 ug/d

Typical Laboratory Range: 5.4-11.5 ug/d

Free Thyroxine Index (FTI) Total T4 and T3 uptake must be considered together to measure the activity of free or unbound T4. This index is measured by multiplying TT4 levels by the T3 uptake and determines how much active T4 is available. If TT4 is depressed, then T3 uptake is high; if the TT4 is high, then resin uptake is low. (Resin T3 uptake will be discussed in this section.) Even when drugs impact thyroid binding, the Free Thyroxine Index should be within normal range if the thyroid is functioning properly.

Functional Range: 1.2-4.9 mg/dl

Typical Laboratory Range: 4.6-10.9 mg/dl

Free Thyroxine (FT4) The free thyroxine (FT4) test is used to measure the amount of free, or active, T4 in the blood. Factors that affect TT4 will not impact FT4. Free T4 is high with hyperthyroidism and low with hypothyroidism. It's important to note that even a high TSH with normal T4 is enough to identify hypothyroidism. A rare pattern and one indicative of a hereditary thyroid resistance condition is high FT4. High FT4 can also be caused by taking heparin or by an acute illness that causes binding protein levels to suddenly fall. If an illness other than thyroid disease becomes severe or chronic, it may decrease FT4.

Functional Range: 1.0-1.5 ng/ dL

Typical Laboratory Range: 0.7-1.53 ng/dL

Resin T3 Uptake The resin T3 uptake measures the amount of sites for active or unbound T3 to bind with proteins. The more binding sites open on the proteins, the lower the resin uptake result will be, and vice versa. For example, anything that reduces the binding sites, such as elevated testosterone or testosterone replacement therapy, can cause a low T4, because it leaves very few binding sites for thyroid hormone. On the other hand, anything that raises the binding sites, such as estrogen or birth control pills, would cause a pattern of high total T4 and low T3 uptake.

Functional Range: 28-38 md/dl
Typical laboratory Range: 24-39 md/dl

Free Triiodothyroxine (FT3) This test measures free T3 hormone, and is the best marker for measuring active thyroid hormones available to thyroid receptor sites. However it is rarely completed in conventional medicine, but it is typically ordered when a patient has hyperthyroid symptoms and FT4 levels are normal.

Functional Range: 300- 450 pg/mL
Typical Laboratory Range: 260-480 pg/mL

Reverse T3 (rT3) This test measures the amount of reverse T3 that is produced. The production of rT3 typically takes place in cases of extreme stress, such as major trauma, surgery, or severe chronic stress. It appears the increased production of T3 is due to an inability to clear rT3, as well as from elevated levels of cortisol.

Functional Range: 90-350 pg/ml
Typical Laboratory Range: 90-350 pg/ml

Thyroid Binding Globulin (TBG) This test measures the amount of proteins in the blood that transport thyroid hormones to the cells. Elevated testosterone can lower TBG levels, while elevated estrogen can raise TBG, both of which produce hypothyroid symptoms.

Functional Range: 18-27 ug/dl
Typical Laboratory Range: 15-30 ug/dl

Thyroid Antibodies Thyroid autoantibodies indicate the body's immune system is attacking itself and if an autoimmune thyroid condition is present, whether it be hypothyroidism or hyperthyroidism.

Specific antibody tests identify Hashimoto's. A *thyroid peroxidase antibodies* (TPO Ab) test is the most important diagnostic one, since TPO is the enzyme responsible for the production of thyroid hormones, and the most popular target of attack in Hashimoto's. Although sometimes a *thyroglobulin antibodies* (TGB Ab) test is necessary, too. TGB, which is made in the thyroid gland and used to produce thyroid hormones, is another common target for Hashimoto's disease. A *thyroid stimulating hormone antibodies* (TSH Ab) — typically referred to as thyroid stimulating immunoglobulin (TSI) — test is used to identify hyperthyroidism, or Grave's Disease, although TSH can also be elevated in Hashimoto's disease, too.

Because the immune system fluctuates, a person with Hashimoto's may produce a negative antibodies test. If I see negative test results yet suspect the person has the disorder, I will repeat the test. If the person is already on a gluten-free diet, I will have them consume wheat for two weeks and then repeat the test. Once you see a positive antibody test, you have confirmed an autoimmune thyroid condition.

THE SIX PATTERNS OF HYPOTHYROIDISM — WHICH ONE ARE YOU?

The thyroid is extremely sensitive to the slightest changes in body chemistry; that's its job — to detect subtle shifts and compensate for them. When these shifts become chronic, however, the thyroid fatigues and falters. Blood sugar that is always too low or too high, hormone imbalances, adrenal dysfunction, chronic inflammation, nutritional deficiencies, toxicity, liver congestion, poor digestive health, and the use of hormone creams or pills are all triggers for a functional thyroid imbalance.

Low thyroid function falls into one of six patterns, only one of which can be resolved with thyroid hormone medication. Also, two or more patterns may exist simultaneously. While a serum blood test is integral to assessment, a person's symptoms, medical history, and prescription drug use, such as oral contraceptives or estrogen cream, are also important considerations. The following descriptions introduce the patterns. Please see Resources for more information on the products and ingredients I recommend.

1. PRIMARY HYPOTHYROIDISM

If the pituitary gland senses the thyroid isn't doing its job, it will pump out extra TSH, giving the thyroid a kick in the pants to work harder.

Primary hypothyroidism is a true dysfunction of the thyroid gland, and is the only pattern of hypothyroidism that can be effectively managed with thyroid replacement hormone — unless it's autoimmune Hashimoto's. Then it is an immune issue, and needs to be supported as such. If tissue destruction is severe, replacement hormones prevent complications due to deficient thyroid hormones. However, if the health care practitioner detects primary hypothyroidism before the damage is too far-gone and approaches it nutritionally, it may be possible to manage the condition, delaying or even preventing the need for medication. An elevated TSH on a blood test primarily identifies this pattern.

> In standard health care, doctors typically do not screen for Hashimoto's in people with an elevated TSH level because it does not change the treatment. The standard health care system is based largely on doing tests only if it affects treatment.

If the TSH does not come down to normal after a nutritional protocol, testing thyroid antibodies to rule out autoimmune disease is in order. In the event of autoimmunity, the immune system must be managed. If the hypothyroidism is advanced then thyroid medication may also be necessary to support overall health.

Functional blood chemistry pattern
Thyroid Stimulating Hormone (TSH) – Elevated
Total T4 (TT4) – Normal or low
Free T4 (FT4) – Normal or low
Free Thyroxine Index (FTI) – Normal or low
Resin T3 Uptake (T3U) – Normal or low
Free T3 (FT3) – Normal or low
Reverse T3 (rT3) – Normal

Nutritional support
- Nutritional compounds to support healthy thyroid function. Key ingredients include porcine thyroid gland, ashwagandha, vitamin A, vitamin D, selenium, and zinc.

- Nutritional compounds to help support T4 to T3 synthesis. Key ingredients include guggulu, selenium, zinc, and antiperoxidative compounds.

Note: I do not recommend tyrosine and iodine, which are in many thyroid products. Tyrosine can suppress TPO activity. Iodine can exacerbate or potentially trigger an autoimmune thyroid disease.

For treating pathological thyroid condition: Appropriate drug intervention by a physician.

It is vital to retest the TSH 30 days after beginning this protocol to be sure it is working. If the TSH has returned to normal, the patient may decrease dosages of nutritional compounds and repeat the TSH blood test in another 30 days. At some point the clinician should be able to determine proper dosage of supplementation to maintain the TSH. If the patient does not respond to the above protocol, the clinician will need to consider natural thyroid replacement, and, most importantly, rule out an autoimmune thyroid condition. Thyroid support has little effect in people with positive thyroid antibodies. For them, nutritional support is essential.

Non-Autoimmune Hypothyroidism

Sandi consulted me for her thyroid symptoms because I had successfully addressed her daughter's Hashimoto's disease. Sandi was your classic hypothyroid patient with elevated TSH. Since her original TSH level was 16.64, her general practitioner prescribed hormone replacement therapy for several months, and her TSH returned to normal. Sandi began to have symptoms again, but her TSH was normal (4.74).

After assessing her blood tests and salivary hormones, I discovered that Sandi had true hypothyroidism. Her TSH level was within the normal medical range, but it did not satisfy the functional ranges I use. Coupled with her increasing symptoms of low thyroid (constipation, weight gain despite exercising, and elevated cholesterol), I knew right away how to support this person and change her life once and for all.

After a month of nutritional support, her TSH level was 2.25, well within the functional range. Her constipation cleared, and her cholesterol dropped from 214 to 197. She decided she didn't need to go on statins and showed her general practitioner the test results. Sandi is also no longer taking thyroid replacement hormones and her TSH remains in the functional range. She has been able to successfully manage her weight for the last two years with the proper diet and exercise routine we designed for her.

Dr. David G. Arthur, DC, DACNB
Denver, CO

2. HYPOTHYROIDISM SECONDARY TO PITUITARY HYPOFUNCTION

This is a very common pattern of functional hypothyroidism. In this case, TSH will be low (below 1.8), although not as low as with hyperthyroidism, and the person will have symptoms of an under active thyroid. Chronic stressors are at the root of this pattern because they fatigue the pituitary gland at the base of the brain. As a result, the pituitary fails to signal the thyroid to release enough TSH to stimulate its activity. In other words, the thyroid gland may be perfectly fine, but nobody is telling it to go to work because the pituitary is asleep on the job.

Pituitary hypofunction is usually the result of one of four things. The first and most common trigger is an active stress response, which is nearly universal in the United States. A busy lifestyle, poor diet, inadequate sleep, too much caffeine, a high-carbohydrate diet, chronic inflammation, and viral or bacterial infections are just a few of the factors that wear out our adrenal glands and depress thyroid function.[184] [185] [186] [187] [188] [189]

Second is post-partum depression. It's not uncommon for women to dip into a low thyroid state after pregnancy. That's because pregnancy amplifies the demands on all hormonal systems, keeping the pituitary gland busy 24/7.[190] [191] Also, many women enter pregnancy in some state of adrenal stress, and the increased demands of pregnancy overwhelm the pituitary gland.

Third, interestingly, is the inappropriate use of thyroid medications. Many doctors prescribe their symptomatic patients thyroid medication, even if their blood test results are normal. These patients may feel better once they start taking the medication…for a little while. But because they are flooding their system with unnecessary thyroid hormone, their cells develop resistance to it. Weary of being incessantly bombarded by too much thyroid hormone, the cells slam the doors shut so no more can get in.

When thyroid hormones can't get into the cells to regulate metabolism, hypothyroidism symptoms return. The person either quits taking the medication or is prescribed a higher dose, ultimately exacerbating the problem. Also, with an overabundance of thyroid hormones circulating in the bloodstream, the pituitary gets the message it's no longer needed, and eventually stops communicating with the thyroid gland. Sometimes in this scenario, the pituitary/thyroid loop is permanently lost, and the dependence on medication becomes life long.

This scenario can also come into play when a clinician prescribes thyroid medication to a person with Hashimoto's but doesn't address their autoimmune condition.

In summary, there are three criteria for identifying hypothyroidism secondary to hypopituitary function:

- TSH below 1.8

- T4 below 6

- hypothyroid symptoms

Functional blood chemistry pattern

Thyroid Stimulating Hormone (TSH) – Low, below 1.8
Total T4 (TT4) – Normal or low
Free T4 (FT4) – Normal or low
Free Thyroxine Index (FTI) – Normal or low
Resin T3 Uptake (T3U) – Normal
Free T3 (FT3) – Normal or low
Reverse T3 (rT3) – Normal
Thyroid Antibodies – Negative

Nutritional support

Nutritional compounds to support the pituitary-thyroid axis. Key ingredients include porcine thyroid gland, porcine pituitary gland, rubidium sulfate, sage leaf extract, L-arginine, gamma oryzanol, magnesium, zinc and manganese.

Appropriate adrenal support based on the Adrenal Salivary Index test. (See Chapter Seven.)

Postpartum Hypothyroidism

There are a ton of postpartum thyroid stories, more than anyone knows, with TSH levels ranging between 1.5 and 1.7. Everyone is focused on the baby's health and wellbeing, but meanwhile the mother starts suffering from postpartum depression, weight gain, and hair loss. She is often just prescribed antidepressants, and her problems are blamed on the baby not sleeping through the night. I support the adrenals, and use compounds that support the thyroid-pituitary axis. When a new mother's TSH level increases to 2 and 3, she starts losing weight and her hair begins growing. The stress of pregnancy and birth has just overwhelmed the thyroid, especially since most women are in some state adrenal stress before getting pregnant. I also see a lot of Hashimoto's kick in postpartum because of the immune shifts of pregnancy.

Shane Steadman, DC, DACNB
Mountain Health Chiropractic and Neurology
Englewood, CO

3. THYROID UNDER CONVERSION

This is a common pattern associated with chronic adrenal stress and excess production of the adrenal hormone cortisol.[192] [193] In this scenario, the body makes plenty of T4, but too much cortisol prevents the body from being able to convert enough T4 to T3, the form of thyroid hormone the body can use. An elevated cortisol level suppresses the conversion of T4 to the useable form of T3.

Another common cause for thyroid under conversion is deterioration of the body's cell membranes in response to chronic infection or inflammation.[194] [195] [196] Cell membranes are in charge of multiple functions, including the conversion of T4 to T3. Chronic inflammation causes lipid peroxidation, in which harmful free radicals damage cell walls. And damaged cell walls hamper thyroid conversion. In this case, finding the cause of the inflammation and improving antioxidant status are keys to support. Inadequate conversion of T4 to T3 often isn't diagnosed because a low T3 level doesn't affect TSH levels.

Functional blood chemistry pattern
Thyroid Stimulating Hormone (TSH) – Normal
Total T4 (TT4) – Normal
Free T4 (FT4) – Normal
Free Thyroxine Index (FTI) – Normal
Resin T3 Uptake (T3U) – Normal
Total T3 — Low
Free T3 (FT3) – Low
Reverse T3 (rT3) – Low or normal
Thyroid Antibodies – Negative

Nutritional support
- Liposomal cream that delivers nutritional compounds to re-duce inflammation and oxidative stress. Key ingredients include glutathione and superoxide dismutase.

- Nutritional compounds to help support T4 to T3 synthesis. Key ingredients include guggulu, selenium, zinc, and antiper-oxidative compounds.

- Liposomal cream that delivers nutritional compounds to mod-ulate the stress response. Key ingredient includes 2,000 mg a day of phosphatidylserine.

4. THYROID OVER CONVERSION AND DECREASED TBG

Elevated levels of testosterone in women create this pattern of too much T4 being converted into T3, and under production of thyroid binding globulin (TBG).[197] The excess T3 overwhelms the cells so they develop a resistance to the thyroid hormone and it can't get into the cells. As a result, the person with this disorder has hypothyroid symptoms.

This pattern is most often found in women with insulin resistance and polycystic ovary syndrome (PCOS), since excess testosterone production accompanies these conditions.[198] In this pattern, therefore, reversing insulin resistance reverses hypothyroid symptoms.

This pattern may also arise in those who have already developed diabetes and are taking insulin. For them, gaining control over blood sugar and insulin needs with diet, supplementation and exercise is critical.

Using testosterone cream can lead to thyroid over conversion, too. In this situation, the testosterone dose needs to be reduced, and the liver cleared through a liver detoxification program.

Functional blood chemistry pattern
   Thyroid Stimulating Hormone (TSH) – Normal
   Total T4 (TT4) – Normal
   Free T4 (FT4) – High or high end of normal
   Free Thyroxine Index (FTI) – Normal
   Resin T3 Uptake (T3U) – High or high end of normal
   Free T3 (FT3) – High or high end of normal
   Reverse T3 (rT3) – Normal
   Thyroid Antibodies – Negative

Nutritional support
   Address insulin resistance with proper nutritional support (See Chapter Five.) and hormone overload with a liver detoxification (See Chapter Eight.).

5. THYROID BINDING GLOBULIN ELEVATION[199 200 201 202]

This pattern is often associated with oral contraceptives or estrogen replacement therapy. Thyroid hormones hitch a ride through the bloodstream on thyroid binding globulin (TBG). When estrogen levels are too high, as often happens in women taking birth control pills or hormone replacement therapy (such as Premarin or estrogen creams), the body makes too much TBG. Since thyroid hormones in the bloodstream bind to the excess TBGs, not enough free hormone is available to enter the cells. In people with this pattern, clearing the body of excess estrogen (See Chapter Six) addresses hypothyroidism.

Functional blood chemistry pattern

Thyroid Stimulating Hormone (TSH) – Normal

Total T4 (TT4) – Normal

Free T4 (FT4) – Low

Free Thyroxine Index (FTI) – Low or normal

Resin T3 Uptake (T3U) – Low

Free T3 (FT3) – Low

Reverse T3 (rT3) – Normal

Thyroid Antibodies – Negative

Nutritional support

- Nutritional compounds to support healthy methylation re-actions. Key ingredients include choline, trimethylglycine, (methylsulfonylmethane) MSM, beet root, and betaine HCl.

- Nutritional compounds to improve Phase I and II liver de-toxification. Key ingredients include molybdenum chelate, milk thistle extract seed, dandelion root, gotu kola nut, panax ginseng, L-glutathione, glycine, N-acetyl-L-cysteine, and DL-methionine.

- Nutritional compounds to support healthy bile formation, se-cretion, and flow. Key ingredients include dandelion root, milk thistle seed, ginger, taurine, beet concentrate, vitamin C, and phosphatidylcholine.

6. THYROID RESISTANCE

This is another stress-related pattern in which the pituitary and thyroid glands function normally and make the right amount of thyroid hormones, but the hormones are not getting into the cells to take effect. Symptoms of hypothyroidism ensue. Elevated levels of cortisol in response to chronic stress cause the cells to become resistant to thyroid hormones.[203] [204] In this case, managing adrenal health is the ticket to addressing hypothyroidism. Other causes included elevated homocysteine levels[205] and a genetic predisposition to hypothyroidism.

Functional blood chemistry pattern

Thyroid Stimulating Hormone (TSH) – Normal

Total T4 (TT4) – Normal

Free T4 (FT4) – Normal

Free Thyroxine Index (FTI) – Normal

Resin T3 Uptake (T3U) – Normal

Free T3 (FT3) – Normal

Reverse T3 (rT3) – Normal

Thyroid Antibodies – Negative

Nutritional support

Support of this pattern requires addressing adrenal malfunction and excess cortisol (See Chapter Seven). Thyroid resistance is also caused if thyroid replacement hormone therapy is not properly monitored (See Chapter Eight).

Thyroid Symptoms and Insulin Resistance

Amanda came to me with low thyroid symptoms. She had the classic ones: low energy, cold hands and feet, weight gain and the inability to lose weight, and thinning eyebrows. However, blood tests, according to her general practitioner, were normal. It was discouraging to see her suffer from what we have all been taught was low thyroid and not be able to do anything for her with traditional nutritional support.

I had just started utilizing salivary hormone testing in my practice but was unaware of the impact it would have on the support of her thyroid. Her cortisol levels were elevated, and her blood test results indicated that her blood sugar issues were creating inflammation. Amanda had a few other patterns that needed addressing, but we both wanted to work on the thyroid first. As we assessed new salivary and complete thyroid blood tests, we uncovered much of the same information to confirm what I was thinking. Every one of her thyroid hormone levels came back NORMAL. It was not Hashimoto's or classic hypothyroid. However, we did find elevated cortisol and testosterone levels. Not good to say the least.

I immediately began managing her insulin resistance and elevated cortisol levels. After about 35 days, I retested her again to find that her thyroid levels had not changed but her cortisol had returned to a normal. Her circadian rhythm was within the normal range as well. Her follow-up questionnaire and health history revealed that many of her symptoms had begun to improve, mainly over the pervious two weeks. Her tolerance to cold was much better, and she was even able to ski more. She had suddenly lost about two inches from her waist with no additional exercise. Her aesthetician even commented that she was growing new eyebrows.

David G. Arthur, DC, DACNB
Denver, CO

ANEMIA IS A DEAL BREAKER

Most markers of a thyroid problem are on an expanded blood test. Again, by looking at functional ranges instead of pathological ones, these test panels give enormous insight into the person's overall health. For instance, markers can point to a possible gut infection, a chronic or acute viral infection, adrenal stress, poor digestion, liver malfunction, blood sugar regulation problems, abnormal cholesterol levels, and more. One marker that often comes up with my thyroid patients, especially people with Hashimoto's and gluten intolerance, is anemia.

Anemia as is a deal breaker for nutritional support of any kind, including thyroid support, since anemia literally starves your body of oxygen. When your red blood cells are deprived of oxygen, basic functions that maintain, regenerate, and heal the body simply cannot operate adequately, if at all. Therefore, clinicians must always consider anemia and address it in a person with any thyroid condition.

Anemia can be due to a variety of factors, including pernicious anemia (an autoimmune disease). Some forms of anemia do not seem to respond to iron supplements because red blood cell breakdown is the culprit. When this happens, supplementing won't increase iron levels and can, in fact, worsen health. Too much iron in the body is more toxic than mercury, lead, or other heavy metals we commonly associate with heavy metal toxicity.

A qualified health care provider should evaluate a person with anemia.

A Whole-Body Approach

When Ellen came to me, she had suffered from many health problems throughout her adult life, and had had her thyroid removed because it was enlarged. At 49, her health was deteriorating to the point where her memory constantly failed her and she had to quit her job.

Her gynecologist had prescribed bio-identical estrogen twice daily and daily progesterone for two weeks of the month. We started her on a protocol to clear excess hormones in her system. Ellen began to feel better and began questioning taking the bio-identical hormones, especially after I educated her on what these hormones were doing in her body. Her hair was still coming out in clumps but the loss had significantly decreased. We then shifted the focus to repairing her gut, and she said she felt like a new woman.

I then turned my attention to supporting her pituitary. Although she was still losing hair, she noticed new hair growth. Ellen's blood test indicated she was anemic yet she responded poorly to iron supplementation, which is typical with chronic inflammation. An immune tests revealed a chronic viral infection and abnormal immune regulation. The protocol to control inflammation and the immune system made a serious impact with Ellen. Her iron levels moved towards the functional range without iron supplementation. Switching to a gluten-free diet appeared to help alleviate her symptoms.

Endocrine testing showed she was suffering from a disorganized ovarian-pituitary feedback loop. She was placed on a supplement protocol to support this pattern for several months. She now reports normal periods, and she is able to maintain her health with diet and lifestyle changes. There are occasional flare-ups when she is stressed or eats gluten.

David Peterson, DC
Wellness Alternatives
Town & Country, MO

NUTRITIONAL FACTORS

Entire books are dedicated to the subject of foods that support healthy thyroid function, so I won't delve into that subject here. However, a few nutrients are worth mention as their deficiencies can cause poor thyroid function.

Essential fatty acids

Healthy hormone production, including the production of thyroid hormones, depends on essential fatty acids (EFAs) — the wonder nutrients you've heard about touted in fish oil, flax seed, evening primrose oil, borage oil, and black currant seed oil. In our diets, these nutrients can be found in cold-water fish and in many raw, unprocessed nuts and seeds. EFAs not only contribute nutrients for hormones, but also for proper cellular communication, brain function, and more.[206] [207 208]

EFA deficiencies and disorders are common in the United States. It's estimated that up to 80 percent of the U.S. population fail to get enough each day, thanks to our modern, overly processed diets. To make matters worse, hydrogenated and trans fats in so many processed foods skew the body's ability to properly metabolize EFAs so that the body converts anti-inflammatory good fats into inflammatory ones. As a result, one becomes even more deficient in EFAs.

The ideal ratio between omega 6 and omega 3 fats in EFAs is estimated to be 3:1 to 5:1.[209] The average American's ratio is more like 25:1, thanks to diets heavy in processed vegetable oils in our diets.[210]

For my patients with hypoglycemia I recommend a well-rounded EFA supplement that includes flax seed oil and evening primrose oil. For those with insulin resistance, I recommend a fish-oil based EFA supplement. Insulin resistance creates a condition in which the body cannot properly metabolize the EFAs in flax, borage, evening primrose, or black currant seed oils. In fact, it shunts these otherwise beneficial fatty acids into pro-inflammatory compounds.[211 212] Also, because the EPA and DHA in fish oil helps receptor sites on cells become more sensitive to insulin, fish oil is a must-have for people with insulin resistance.

Blood tests are available to determine EFA status. It's important when working to establish the sufficiency and proper metabolism of EFAs to root out and resolve any source of inflammation in the body, including gut infections, food intolerances, and chronic virus infection. EFA status won't improve without resolving the source of inflammation.

THE IMPACT OF NUTRITIONAL DEFICIENCIES ON THYROID FUNCTION

Thyroid peroxidase (TPO) is the enzyme in the thyroid responsible for making thyroid hormones. It liberates iodine to be added to tyrosine for T4 and T3 production. This process involves many cofactors, including selenium, copper, magnesium, niacin, riboflavin, pyridoxal-5-phosphate (the active form of vitamin B6), and zinc.[213]

Vitamin A is another critical nutrient for thyroid activity. When a thyroid hormone binds to a cell's receptor site, it sets off a series of biochemical reactions that carry messages to the cell's nucleus. Once the nucleus has been activated, it responds by producing proteins that carry out such thyroid functions as increasing metabolic rate and producing energy. Vitamin A appears to influence how well the thyroid hormone receptors in the nucleus function.[214] [215]

Tyrosine and iodine If you've ever supported your thyroid naturally, chances are you recognize tyrosine and iodine, as they're in most nutritional thyroid supplements. Here is where I depart from the average natural medicine doctor. Although tyrosine and iodine are vital thyroid nutrients, my research shows that supplementing them may actually make a thyroid condition worse even though they can make a person feel more energetic.

Iodine, which is discussed in more detail in Chapter Two, has been shown to trigger autoimmune thyroid conditions, and will also exacerbate an existing autoimmune thyroid disease, such as Hashimoto's. Because this disorder is so prevalent, I consider it prudent to leave iodine out of a thyroid supplement.

Although tyrosine is an integral part of thyroid hormone production, supplementing with it has the potential to suppress thyroid activity. Not a single study exists showing the ability of tyrosine to increase thyroid hormones, even when they are low.[216] [217] Tyrosine will, however, increase the adrenal hormones (epinephrine and norepinephrine) that create that wired, energetic feeling,[218] which may feel like progress when a person has been plagued with the fatigue and fogginess of hypothyroidism. For the person in an active stress response (See Chapter Seven), however, this stimulating effect on the adrenals will also suppress TPO activity and, consequently, thyroid hormone production, just as caffeine and other adrenal stimulants do.[219] [220] [221] Because the majority of people in the U.S. must cope with some degree of stress and adrenal malfunction, tyrosine supplementation is often inappropriate.

I recommend formulas that have all the nutritional cofactors that support thyroid hormone production and function along with very clean Argentine porcine thyroid glandulars and ashwagandha root. These formulas stimulate TPO and vitamin A for healthy, responsive thyroid receptors.

Thyroid Hormone Replacement Prescription Medicine

Armour Trade name for natural (non-synthetic) thyroid hormone, made with desiccated animal (usually pig) thyroid gland.

Cytomel Trade name for synthetic triiodothyroinine (T3). Used alone or in combination with thyroxine to treat hypothyroidism.

Dessicated Thyroid Generic name for tablets of animal thyroid gland used to treat low thyroid conditions. (Trade names include Armour, Westroid, Naturthroid, and Proloid.) Active ingredients include T3 and T4.

Levothroid Trade name for drug containing synthetic thyroxine (T4), the most common of the synthetic thyroid medications. It is usually in the top five of the most commonly prescribed medications in the United States each year.

Levothyroixine Generic name for synthetic thyroxine (T4).

Levoxyl Trade name drug containing synthetic thyroxine (T4).

Synthroid Trade name for drug containing synthetic thyroxine (T4).

Thyrolar Trade name for drug containing a fixed-ratio mixture of synthetic T3 and T4.

Drugs That Influence Thyroid Metabolism

(New England Journal of Medicine, 333(25) 1688, Table 2, December 1995)

Clinicians need to be familiar with commonly prescribed medications that have adverse impacts on thyroid physiology and can cause symptoms of thyroid imbalances.

Drugs that decrease TSH secretion Dopamine, glucocorticoids, octreotide (Sandostatin)

Drugs that decrease thyroid hormone secretion Lithium, iodide, aminoglutethimide (Citroden)

Drugs that increase thyroid hormone secretion Iodide, amiodarone (Cordarone)

Drugs that decrease T4 absorption Colestipol (Colstid), cholestyramine, aluminum hydroxide, ferrous sulfate, sucralfate (Carafate)

Drugs that alter T4 and T3 transport in the bloodstream by increasing the concentration of thyroid binding globulin Estrogens, Tomoxifen, heroin, methadone, mitotane (Lysodren), fluorouracil

Drugs that alter T4 and T3 transport in the bloodstream by decreasing the concentration of thyroid binding globulins Androgens, anabolic steroids, slow-release nicotinic acid, glucocorticoids

Drugs that alter T4 and T3 transport by displacement from protein-binding sites furosemide (Lasix), fenclofanac, mefanamic Acid, salicylates

Drugs that alter T4 and T3 metabolism by increasing hepatic metabolism Phenobarbital, rifampin (Rifadin), phenytoin (Dilantin), Carbamazapine (Tegretol)

Drugs that decrease T4 5' deiodinase activity Propylthiouracil, amiodarone (Cordorone), beta-adrenergic-antagonistic drugs

CHAPTER HIGHLIGHTS

- The majority of people with hypothyroidism do not need thyroid hormone medication. In fact, medication can make functional hypothyroidism irreversible.

- There are six patterns of functional hypothyroidism, only one of which would respond to medication (even though it is rarely necessary). Most of these patterns are related to poor blood sugar control, stress, poor gut health, a sluggish liver, and hormonal imbalances. Only one of these patterns will appear on standard thyroid blood tests that measure only TSH.

- Incomplete or inaccurately interpreted thyroid blood tests allow countless people with hypothyroidism to go undiagnosed.

- Hypothyroidism can be caught in time to be reversed nutritionally through properly interpreting appropriate thyroid blood tests.

- By the time your hypothyroid condition shows up in blood test, it may be too late to support it nutritionally and you may require prescription medicine.

- Abnormal blood test ranges are based on pathological ranges, the stage at which the condition is a disease requiring medical intervention. Normal functional ranges are based on what constitutes good health and if abnormal can alert a clinician to the person's risk of developing a disease and help him or her support that potential disorder nutritionally.

- Sometimes a person with hypothyroidism has normal blood test results.

- Anemia is a deal breaker to managing hypothyroidism or Hashimoto's, and should always be addressed first. When anemia doesn't respond to iron supplementation, it is often a result of chronic inflammation and managing that problem often resolves the anemia.

- Iodine and tyrosine are not always appropriate if people with thyroid conditions.

CHAPTER FIVE

TAMING THE BLOOD SUGAR BEAST
FOR THYROID HEALTH

Lauren is a mother of two young children who keeps busy tending her vegetable garden, canning, knitting, baking, teaching part-time, and doing volunteer work. However, each day felt like a struggle. Her energy crashed around 3 or 4 p.m., from which point she counted the hours until she could collapse into bed, only to awaken at 3 a.m., besieged with worry and anxiety over nitpicky aspects of her life. She felt completely powerless to combat her relentless sugar cravings and frequently binged on chocolate chips or brownies. She couldn't leave the house for more than 30 minutes unless she packed enough food for an army, since she worried about becoming hungry and crashing. Lauren also found herself becoming intolerant to an increasing number of foods. On the advice of a nutritionist who takes my classes, Lauren finally mustered the courage to remove grains, starchy vegetables, fruits, and all sweeteners from her diet — cold turkey. It wasn't easy, as her husband is Mexican, and her family had been eating meals based on rice, beans, and corn. In their place, however, she ate plenty of produce, and high quality proteins and fats. In only three days her energy was abundant and even, like a clean-burning fuel, she slept soundly through the nights.

"I can't believe what a big difference the change in diet made," Lauren says. "And the weird thing is I don't even miss the sugar or the grains. Eating this way feels easy, and it is so worth the effort."

America's addiction to sugar, fast foods, and a grain-based diet has produced a nation of carbohydrate-addicts riding the highs and lows of blood sugar swings. When you look at all sweeteners combined, Americans consume an average of 200 pounds each of sweet stuff a year. It's no wonder the Centers for Disease Control and Prevention predicts that one in three Caucasian children born after 2000 will become diabetic. For Hispanics and African-Americans, that number jumps to 1 in 2.[222] My experience shows that attempts at successfully managing a person with Hashimoto's or functional hypothyroidism are futile as long as continue he or she indulges in a sugar-laden, high-carbohydrate diet.

The Glycemic Index

When I say high-carbohydrate, I am technically referring to foods with a high glycemic index (GI) or glycemic load (GL), which measure how rapidly carbohydrates turn into sugar in the body. The faster the food is converted to sugar, the higher the insulin spike. The GI of a food is based on 50 grams of a food while the GL is based on an average serving size, and also factors in grams of carbohydrates.[223] Raw carrots, for instance, measure high using the Glycemic Index, but low using Glycemic Load, meaning carrots are acceptable for the person wishing to eat a lower-carbohydrate diet.

For most of human history, our bodies have evolved to weather times of famine when blood sugar levels drop and sweets were scarce. An indulgence in carbohydrates, whether it's mashed potatoes or a caramel latte with whipped cream, causes a blood sugar spike. To bring blood sugar back to normal, the pancreas pumps insulin into the bloodstream. When this mechanism occurs frequently, the pancreas begins to overcompensate, shooting too much insulin into the bloodstream. Now blood sugar drops *too* low, and our adrenal "fight or flight" hormones are called in for backup. The adrenal glands, which recognize low blood sugar as a threat to survival, send out hormones to boost it. The problem is these hormones also cause stress. Every time this happens, and for many people it happens every time they eat, convenient functions like digestive health, immunity, hormone balancing, and, you guessed it, thyroid function, take a back seat.

Dysglycemia is a condition in which the body loses the ability to keep blood sugar stable. As I explain below, the modern person's blood sugar is either chronically low or high, and both are stepping-stones to diabetes, a disease becoming so widespread it is predicted to bankrupt our healthcare system. Dysglycemia and its effects on adrenal function are at the heart of numerous health imbalances that frequently end in hypothyroidism: Dysglycemia weakens and inflames the digestive tract, weakens the immune barriers of the gut,[224] lungs and brain,[225] drives the adrenal glands into exhaustion,[226] [227] sets the stage for hormonal imbalances (premenstrual syndrome, polycystic ovary syndrome, or a miserable transition into menopause),[228] [229] [230] clogs the body's attempts at detoxification, impairs fatty acid metabolism,[231] [232] and fatigues metabolism. All of these significantly weaken thyroid metabolism and set the stage for and exacerbate Hashimoto's. In fact, insulin surges can drive autoimmune tissue destruction of the thyroid gland in Hashimoto's disease.[233] As long as dysglycemia goes unchecked, attempts at supporting hypothyroidism or Hashimoto's are futile.

Low Blood Sugar

When the pancreas pumps out too much insulin due to chronic spikes in blood sugar (cereal, Milky Way lattes, pastries, pasta salad… you get the picture), blood sugar levels swing from high to low. So do one's energy, mood, and mental cognition. This person spaces out easily, has poor short-term memory, is grouchy and explosive if she goes too long without eating, and is prone to crashing, especially around 3 or 4 p.m. This is what your typical person with *reactive hypoglycemia*, or low blood sugar, experiences. It's *reactive* because the drop in blood sugar occurs two to five hours after eating. Reactive hypoglycemia is an early stage of insulin resistance, discussed below, and can lead to diabetes. The person with reactive hypoglycemic typically misses meals, eats foods high in sugar, depends on caffeine to function, craves sweets and salt during the day, and has a hard time waking up in the morning and sleeping through the night. The problem can be reversed with diet.

Some people are simply *hypoglycemic*, meaning a fasting blood glucose test reveals their blood sugar is chronically low. A poor diet, adrenal fatigue, hypothyroidism, drug side effects, and certain tumors are usually at fault. Symptoms include fatigue, mental confusion, lethargy, and headaches. People with hypoglycemia are past the point of regaining normal blood sugar function and need to adapt a lifelong diet that keeps their blood sugar stable.

Hypoglycemia is linked to all forms of hypothyroidism, but the most common type is that caused by a sluggish pituitary function. The pituitary gland is located at the base of the brain and is responsible for directing hormonal traffic. Constant blood sugar swings stress the adrenal glands, which in turn drag down function of the pituitary gland, ultimately affecting thyroid health.[234] [235] [236] [237] [238] [239]

Hypoglycemia symptoms
- Craving for sweets
- Irritability if meals are missed
- Dependency on coffee for energy
- Becoming lightheaded if meals are missed
- Eating to relieve fatigue
- Feeling shaky, jittery, or tremulous
- Feeling agitated and nervous
- Become upset easily
- Poor memory, forgetfulness
- Blurred vision

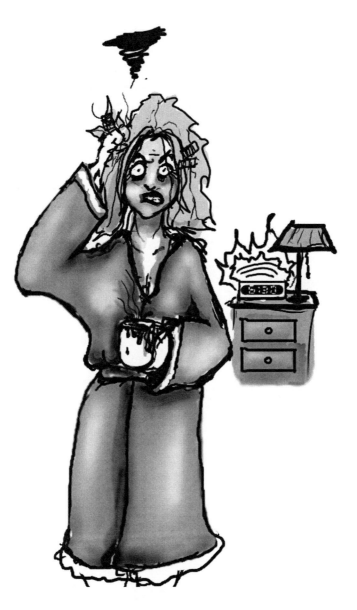

Being grouchy in the morning is a common symptom of reactive hypoglycemia.

High Blood Sugar

Other people slip from hypoglycemia into high blood sugar, or insulin resistance (also knows as Metabolic Syndrome, or Syndrome X). Insulin normally escorts glucose into the cells, where it is made into energy. The chronic release of insulin to battle high blood sugar exhausts the cells until they start refusing entry to insulin. In other words, the cells become insulin resistant. This is the person who feels like she needs a nap after every meal, and if she eats a carbohydrate-rich meal, she may in fact nod off (Let's hope she's not driving.). She may also feel like she will die if she doesn't get some sugar after each meal, and she's hungry all day, even after big meals. This is also the person who carries a lot of fat on her belly and complains of insomnia. Insulin resistance promotes testosterone production in women,[240] so one with the disorder may grow a faint mustache and beard while going bald; men develop more breast tissue and their hips widen. At this point, hypothyroidism is a likely possibility if not already evident. Insulin resistance is also a driving factor of Hashimoto's.

It is conservatively estimated that 25-35 percent of the population in developed countries suffers from degree of insulin resistance.[241] Insulin resistance has also been found to be a contributing factor to diabetes,[242] cardiovascular disease,[243] sleep apnea,[244] hormone metabolism disorders,[245] obesity,[246] and certain types of cancer.[247]

Insulin resistance symptoms

- Fatigue after meals
- General fatigue
- Constant hunger
- Craving for sweets that is not relieved by eating them
- Must have sweets after meals
- Waist girth is equal or larger than hip girth
- Frequent urination
- Increased appetite and thirst
- Difficulty losing weight
- Migrating aches and pains

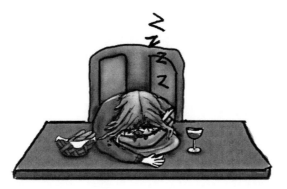

Fatigue after meals is a common symptom of insulin resistance.

The Hypoglycemia/Insulin Resistance Combo

In truth, everyone who is hypoglycemic has some degree of insulin resistance, and everyone who is insulin resistant has some degree of hypoglycemia. The bottom line is if your blood sugar is either chronically low or high, you are subjecting your body to dangerous insulin surges. When blood sugar drops too low with hypoglycemia, the body releases a surge of insulin to carry whatever glucose is left in the bloodstream into the cells for energy. Eventually this creates insulin resistance and glucose can't get into the cells to make energy so the body releases another surge of insulin in a more concerted effort to transport glucose into the cells. As a result, blood sugar drops too low, creating symptoms of hypoglycemia. These insulin surges create a cascade of problems that ultimately drag down thyroid function or set the stage for Hashimoto's.

CHECKING YOUR BLOOD SUGAR

I recommend buying a glucometer at your pharmacy and checking your blood sugar first thing in the morning before eating or drinking anything other than water, and again two to four hours after each meal. A normal blood sugar range falls between 80-100 mgdL. If yours goes under 80, you are in the hypoglycemic range, and if it is over 100, you are in the range of insulin resistance. In functional medicine anything over 110 indicates diabetes, whereas the American Diabetes Association says a person with a fasting blood glucose level above 126 has diabetes.

HOW HYPOTHYROIDISM AFFECTS BLOOD SUGAR CONTROL

I've gone over the basics of blood sugar metabolism. Unfortunately, in the case of hypothyroidism, some of these basics are skewed. For instance, low thyroid function slows the response of insulin to elevated blood sugar, so that glucose is slow to get into the cells to make energy. (Insulin also breaks down more slowly, which is why people with diabetes and hypothyroidism need less insulin.) Because hypothyroidism slows down the absorption of glucose both into the bloodstream and the cells, a blood test will show normal blood sugar levels, but the person will experience symptoms of hypoglycemia. The brain also interprets this as hypoglycemia and calls in the adrenal glands to raise blood sugar, but to no avail. Eventually this pattern wears out communication between the pituitary and adrenal glands.[248]

DIET PLAN FOR DYSGLYCEMIA

Whether you are hypoglycemic or insulin resistant, you must make changes to your diet; there are no exceptions to this. With insulin resistance, you can no longer simply eat what you please when you please; with hypoglycemia, you cannot continue missing meals or snacking on something sugary or starchy. The worst thing a person with insulin resistance can do is to eat more carbohydrates than he or she can tolerate or overeat. (If you feel sleepy or crave sugar after a meal, you just ate too many carbohydrates.) The worst things a hypoglycemic person can do are skip breakfast, eat starchy/sugary snacks, and eat sugar or starchy foods before going to bed. (A person with insulin resistance should avoid these habits, too).

Sticking to a diet that stabilizes blood sugar is challenging, due to intense cravings and the addictive nature of certain foods. Also, unidentified food intolerances stimulate the adrenals so that people actually get an "adrenaline rush" from the foods to which they are sensitive, which creates intense cravings. However, support with the right blood sugar stabilizing nutritional compounds and the determination to weather the hardest period — that is, the first three days after changing the diet — will make following a new healthy way of eating easier and more rewarding.

Dysglycemia and Hair Loss

A 33-year-old woman consulted me, complaining of fatigue and hair loss lasting for several years. An endocrinologist had diagnosed her with Hashimoto's, and her primary care physician prescribed Synthroid. Each time she saw her doctor, he tested her TSH level and adjusted her medications, but her fatigue and hair loss persisted. She cried every night over her hair and her inability to properly take care of her children due to lack of energy. She even bought several wigs to conceal her severe hair loss. She had lost all hope.

A friend of hers referred her to me, but she was skeptical that I could help her. It was difficult convincing her and her husband that they needed to spend several hundred dollars on immune testing that was not covered by insurance, but they eventually came around out of desperation. We ran thorough immune testing, which showed that she had increased levels of TNF alpha, which means her TH-1 was dominant as is common in those with Hashimoto's. In addition, the tests revealed that her immune system was not properly regulated. I recommended daily therapeutic doses of emulsified vitamin D, a liposomal cream containing high dosages of glutathione and superoxide dismutase, and nutritional compounds to support the TH-2 response. Her fatigue resolved after one a half weeks on this protocol. (continued)

Follow up testing showed that her TNF alpha level had returned to normal, thus slowing the immune attack on her thyroid tissue, which was the root cause of her thyroid problems. After one month on the protocol she was still losing hair but at a much slower rate. Further testing revealed that she had dysglycemia, high testosterone levels — which is known to cause hair loss in women, and a leaky gut. Currently she is being supported for blood sugar issues and intestinal barrier repair. Her hair loss has stopped, although at this time, hair growth has not returned to normal. Nevertheless, she is happy to have her energy back, and enjoys doing activities with her children that she had not been able to do. I am personally grateful for all the wisdom that Dr. Kharrazian has shared with me to enable me to help patient after patient. I am so thankful that I am now seeing more and more chronic patients and I have the tools to help them. Thank you Dr. Kharrazian for all the long hours of research and the years of managing chronic patients that has given you this great knowledge. If only you could share this knowledge with every doctor out there, you would revolutionize health care.

Mark Flannery, DC
HealthWise Chiropractic & Nutrition
Simi Valley, CA

Whether you are hypoglycemic or insulin resistant, a few basic rules apply to support your low thyroid condition by addressing unstable blood sugar:

- **Eat a high-quality protein breakfast.** When you wake up in the morning, you have gone a long time without eating. Chances are your adrenal "fight or flight" hormones have been called into action (particularly if you woke up at 3 or 4 a.m. feeling anxious). You need to calm down your system by eating a low-carbohydrate breakfast of high quality proteins and fats. I realize eating breakfast is difficult when you have dyglycemia. Chances are you wake up with no appetite at all, perhaps even feeling nauseous. That is a side effect of your adrenal hormones, and that cup of coffee is only making the problem worse. You simply must force yourself to eat some protein, even if it's a little bit. It will dissipate your nausea, and in just two to three days of stabilizing your blood sugar, you will no longer wake up feeling nauseous. Supporting blood sugar issues is futile unless you eat breakfast. If you like to work out first thing in the morning, just make sure you eat within one hour of waking up.

- **Eat a small amount of protein every two to three hours.** The name of the game is to keep your blood sugar stable and leave the adrenal glands out of the picture. Going for long stretches without eating when you have dysglycemia exacerbates your blood sugar issues, which exacerbates your thyroid problems. Nuts, seeds, a boiled egg, cheese or meat, or a low-carbohydrate protein shake are some examples of protein snacks. As your dysglycemia improves, you will find you can go longer between snacks.

- **Find your carbohydrate tolerance and stick to it.** A high-carbohydrate diet is at the root of dysglycemia, not to mention hormonal imbalances (including hypothyroidism), poor digestion, and weakened immunity. How many grams of carbohydrates should you eat each day? I follow this simple rule: **If you feel sleepy or crave sugar after you eat, you have eaten too many carbohydrates.** Sometimes insulin resistance causes you to feel sleepy even if you haven't eaten anything starchy or sweet. In this case, you need to work with your practitioner to reverse the problem using specific nutritional compounds. What are carbohydrate-rich foods? Grains (remember, corn is a grain), legumes, starchy vegetables like potatoes and peas, and, of course, sweets, including natural sweeteners like agave nectar. The more processed the grain, the more likely it is to trigger a surge of insulin into your bloodstream. I realize carbohydrates are comfort foods. They are ubiquitous in our society and difficult to avoid. However if you weather the first few days, it becomes not only easier to refuse them but rewarding as well. Many symptoms of dysglycemia, such as poor sleep, irritability, and energy crashes, start to diminish on a low-carbohydrate diet.

Also, unidentified food intolerances can create sugar cravings or fatigue after meals, so it's important to find out if that's an issue for you (See Chapter Four.).

- **Never eat high-sugar foods without some fiber, fat or protein.** If and when you do eat high-carbohydrate foods, always eat it with some high quality fiber, fat or protein. This will slow down the rate at which the glucose is absorbed into the bloodstream and help prevent "insulin shock."

- **Do not eat sweets or sugary foods before bed.** This is one of the worst things the hypoglycemic person can do. Your blood sugar will crash during the night, long before your next meal is due. Chances are your adrenals will kick into action, creating restless sleep or that 3 a.m. wake up with anxiety.

- **Avoid all fruit juices and carrot juice.** These can be more sugary than soda, and will quickly have you crashing.

- **Avoid all adrenal stimulants.** For most people, this means caffeine, including decaffeinated coffee. The energy boosting drinks on the market should also be avoided. Dysglycemia is hard enough on the adrenal glands, adding in adrenal stimulants fatigues them further and moves you away from thyroid health. The exception is green tea, which can actually be helpful for people with insulin resistance.

- **Eat a well balanced diet consisting mostly of vegetables, and quality meats and fats.** A diet of junk food, fast foods, and other processed foods works against you. To restore your thyroid health you must find ways to restore your diet closer to what our ancestors ate. A diet dominated by leafy, green vegetables, and adequate in quality protein and fats is enormously restorative.

- **Eliminate food allergens and intolerances.** Whenever a food creates an immune response, such as an allergy or intolerance, it also creates blood sugar instability and insulin surges. Common food intolerances include gluten, dairy, eggs, corn, soy, and yeast. Eating these foods can create sugar cravings and fatigue after meals. To stabilize blood sugar and promote thyroid health, problem foods should be eliminated and the gut repaired. This will be explored further in Chapter Six.

- **Eliminate parasites and toxicities.** Similarly, parasites, pathogens, infections and heavy metal or chemical toxicities can affect the immune system in a way that impacts blood sugar.

- **Important note for people with hypoglycemia when fasting.** Fasting, whether it's a juice fast, vegetable fast, or a simple food-free fast, has long been touted as a way to detoxify and rejuvenate the body. This may have been appropriate before the advent of refined sugars, processed flours, industrialized foods, and stressed-out lifestyles. Today, however, fasts are detrimental to the modern human on a blood-sugar roller coaster. Folks with symptoms of hypoglycemia and reactive hypoglycemia should never undergo a fast, as extended periods without eating will exacerbate the hypoglycemic condition, which in turn will accelerate damage to brain tissue, gastrointestinal function, and adrenal health. A simple blood sugar check with a store-bought glucometer during a fast will quickly bring this fact to light. Fasts can, however, be appropriate for insulin resistance. More on that later in this chapter.

In addition to the dietary protocol outlined above, I also recommend the following:

Nutrients to support a healthy response to insulin resistance Certain nutrients help the cells to regain their sensitivity to insulin so that it can bring glucose into the cells for energy. Key ingredients include chromium, vanadium, alpha-lipoic acid, mixed tocopherols, magnesium, biotin, zinc, inositol, and gymnema sylvestre. Please work with a qualified healthcare practitioner to safely and correctly use these nutrients in the right amounts.

Nutrients to support a healthy response to hypoglycemia Key ingredients include chromium, bovine adrenal gland, choline bitartrate, bovine liver gland, bovine pancreas gland, inositol, L-carnitine, co-enzyme Q10, rubidium chelate, and vanadium aspartate.

Sometimes a person will swing back and forth between insulin resistance and hypoglycemia. In these cases I recommend taking nutritional compounds for insulin resistance with meals, and nutritional compounds for hypoglycemia between meals.

It's important to work with a properly educated, qualified doctor or nutritionist so you take the right nutrients and botanicals in the right amounts. Taking the wrong nutrients for your blood sugar condition has the potential make your condition worse.

SPECIAL CONSIDERATIONS FOR INSULIN RESISTANCE

Insulin resistant folks are those who become drowsy after meals, or even need to lie down and take a nap, especially after a meal heavy in rice, pasta, bread, or other carbohydrates. Women with insulin resistance tend to have excess facial hair and a large belly. The rule of thumb for insulin resistance is that if you feel sleepy after you eat, you just ate too many carbohydrates. What if your meal was virtually carbohydrate-free, say a chicken breast and green beans drizzled in olive oil, and you still feel sleepy after eating? It means your insulin resistance has advanced to such a degree that you may need specialized nutrients to correct insulin resistance.

What exactly causes that symptom? Insulin escorts glucose from the bloodstream into individual cells, where the glucose is made into energy. When cells become insulin resistant, the glucose can't get in, so it circulates round and round the bloodstream, damaging arterial walls and the brain. Because the body wants to normalize blood sugar levels as soon as possible, it converts the excess glucose into triglycerides to be stored as fat. This process demands so much energy that you become sleepy. Furthermore, insulin resistance decreases the body's ability to use stored fat for energy. This process also raises serotonin levels, a brain chemical that can induce drowsiness.

UNWINDING INSULIN RESISTANCE —
A FASTING PROTOCOL

Insulin resistance creates a serious risk for heart disease and diabetes, not to mention low thyroid activity. Successfully managing

Hashimoto's or functional hypothyroidism is dependent upon reversing insulin resistance.

As I mentioned earlier, fasting is harmful to the hypoglycemic person. However, I have developed a fasting protocol that is quite successful for "unwinding" insulin resistance. A person with hypoglycemia will feel crummy on a fast — spacey, dopey, half-dead and hungry. My patients with insulin resistance, on the other hand, report feeling great on this fast — they're more energetic and think more clearly. They start burning fat for energy, their digestive and immune problems calm down, and their blood becomes less acidic.

PHASE 1

First of all, you must do this fast under the supervision of a doctor, preferably a nutritionally oriented chiropractor, naturopath, or medical doctor. I also recommend you do blood tests for, among other things, fasting glucose and lipid levels (cholesterol, triglycerides, and HDL and LDL cholesterol), so that you can compare results with a follow-up test after a sequence of fasts.

I suggest fasting three to five days. A minimum of three days is required for best results. If you are feeling good and following my fasting rules, you may go longer than five days (one of my patients went as long as four weeks). During the fast, do not take any supplements, use hormone creams, or even popular brand skin creams, as many skin creams contain hidden estrogens that will hamper your results.

The fast is limited to the following drink:

DR. KHARRAZIAN'S FAST FOR UNWINDING INSULIN RESISTANCE

- Freshly squeezed lemon or lime juice with pulp
- Water
- Organic maple syrup (Grade B preferred), using just enough to take the edge off the tartness of the lemon or lime
- Brewed green tea (optional). Do not have tea at night

Exact proportions are not important. Although this looks very similar to the Master Cleanse, do not add cayenne pepper — it can be too irritating for some. **YOU MUST TAKE SIPS OF THE DRINK EVERY 10 TO 15 MINUTES THROUGHOUT THE DAY.** This step is critical. If you go too long between sips, your blood sugar drops and you move backwards in progress. I ask my patients to make two gallons in the morning and have plenty of water bottles on hand so they have no excuse to go too long between sips. It's also important to anticipate frequent trips to the bathroom to urinate on this fast. In other words, don't start your fast when traveling or having long meetings at work.

Taking a break from food is important because most people with insulin resistance have multiple food sensitivities and intolerances to the foods they eat most often. The fast gives your digestive tract time to start recovering. If, however, you become truly hungry, you may eat a vegetable that you rarely eat. No spices or dressings are permitted.

Lemon or lime juice alkalinizes blood. Grade B maple syrup is sweeter than other grades, so you need less. Green tea helps fire up the hormone lipase, which in turn helps burn body fat. You may also drink hot green tea separately, as long as you maintain your sips of the fasting liquid every 10-15 minutes.

> Remember, if you do the Fast for Unwinding Insulin Resistance, **YOU MUST TAKE SIPS OF THE DRINK EVERY 10 TO 15 MINUTES THROUGHOUT THE DAY.**

PHASE 2

After fasting for three to five days, I ask my patients to stick to an anti-inflammatory diet that is free of sugars, grains, and processed foods, for three weeks. While on this diet, they consume a nutritional hypoallergenic protein powder that is high in antioxidants, enzymes, pre- and probiotics, and nutrients that aid in detoxification, liver support, and gut repair. Key ingredients include medium chain triglycerides, gamma oryzanol, biotin, glutamine, lactobacilli acidophilus, Jerusalem artichoke and inulin, marshmallow root, quercetin, grape seed extract, rutin and hesperiden, evening primrose, milk thistle seed, and an enzyme blend.

This is also the time to take nutritional compounds for insulin resistance. If detox reactions such as nausea, digestive upset, skin eruptions, or anxiety occur, you are detoxifying too fast and need to reduce the nutritional powder dose. Sometimes you may need to reduce the insulin resistance compounds doses as well. Please work with a qualified healthcare practitioner to safely and correctly use these nutrients in the right amounts.

It is important to notice how you feel in general after your elimination diet and nutritional powder program. You should feel much better, have more energy, and have smoothly functioning digestion. If you don't, there's a possibility you have a gut infection from parasites or bacteria that needs to be addressed by a qualified health care practitioner. It could also mean your immune system is over active, which also needs to be supported by a qualified health care practitioner.

MY ANTI-INFLAMMATORY DIET

All foods may be selected from the food list provided with the program. The basic nutritional requirement of this program is to eat according to your appetite, selecting from the food list provided and eating the most nutritionally dense foods, including those that offer soluble and insoluble dietary fibers. Drink plenty of clean water, and do not overeat. I also suggest a nutritional hypoallergenic protein powder along with the diet.

Two-Week Plan

Days 1 and 2: One serving of protein powder, just before breakfast

Foods to avoid:
- Any food you are allergic to
- Dairy (milk, cheeses, yogurt, butter), margarine, and shortening
- Eggs
- Gluten, such as wheat, oats, rye, barley, spelt or kamut
- Tomatoes and tomato sauces and corn
- Alcohol, and caffeine (coffee, black tea, sodas)

- Soy or products made from soy, such soymilk or tofu
- Peanuts or peanut butter
- Beef that is not grass-fed, pork, cold cuts, bacon, hotdogs, canned meat, sausage, shellfish, and meat analogues made from soy

Foods to eat:
- Drink plenty of water (8-10 glasses), herbal teas, green tea, vegetable juices
- Rice, millet, quinoa, buckwheat, or tapioca (although be mindful of your tolerance level for carbohydrates with hypoglycemia or insulin resistance)
- Fresh fruits, vegetables, beans (again, be mindful of your carbohydrate tolerance with fruits, beans and starchy vegetables)
- Consume mainly fish (not shellfish), and moderate amounts of chicken, turkey, and lamb
- Use mainly olive oil and flax seed oil

Days 3 and 4: Two servings of protein powder daily, one before breakfast, one before dinner, and follow the food directions above

Days 5 to 10: Three servings of protein powder, one before breakfast, one before lunch and one before dinner
During this phase of the plan:
- Avoid all of the foods in the "Foods to avoid" listed above.
- Use all of the foods in the "Foods to eat" list, except eliminate all animal products from the diet (including fish, chicken, turkey, and lamb)

Days 11 and 12: Two servings of protein powder, one before breakfast, one before dinner
During this phase of the plan:
- Avoid all of the foods in the "Foods to avoid" listed above.

- Use all of the foods in the "Foods to eat" in the above list, including all of the animal products (fish, chicken, turkey, and lamb)

Days 13 and 14: One serving of protein powder, just before breakfast, and follow the food directions above

PHASE 3

In Phase 2 you eliminated possible problem foods for two weeks. In this phase you will introduce each of the eliminated foods one at a time, every 72 hours, keeping a journal to note any symptoms that arise when the food is reintroduced. If you have reactions to any foods, eliminate them from your diet so that your entire system may heal. It does not necessarily have to be a life-long elimination if you fully restore your gut integrity. For more information on this Elimination/Provocation Diet, please see Chapter Six.

PHASE 4

Four to eight weeks after your first fast, you undergo another fast that is three to five days or longer, following the directions in PHASE 1. I suggest at least one more round of a nutritional hypoallergenic protein powder for two to three weeks after this second fast.

PHASE 5: REPEATED PHASE 1 FASTS

Continue doing the three- to five-day fasts (or longer), with breaks of four to eight weeks in between. Remember, you must eliminate your problem foods, as well as sugars and high-carbohydrate foods between fasts. Most people need to go through the entire cycle four to six times to reverse their insulin resistance. By working with your practitioner and having blood tests, you can track the progress of your thyroid health, immune health, and other markers.

If your functional thyroid condition is not so advanced that it is beyond nutritional repair, you can restore its function and avoid or delay taking medications. You can also help successfully address Hashimoto's through dietary changes. This route is not as easy as popping a pill, but instead requires making lifestyle changes to care for your whole body. You may need to seek additional help to assist you in modifying your habits and behavior. Committing to a diet low in sugars, starches, and processed foods suddenly has one sitting on the outside of normal American life. But you have to ask yourself, do you want to live your life plagued with normal American diseases?

We will discuss more steps in reversing or managing hypothyroidism in this book, including the use of nutritional compounds, but the first and most important step is to reign in those wild blood sugar swings by cleaning up your diet. This will free up energy so your body can restore itself well being.

CHAPTER HIGHLIGHTS

- Supporting hypothyroidism is futile if your blood sugar is too low or too high. This is called dysglycemia, a stepping-stone to diabetes. Diabetes is becoming so prevalent that authorities predict it will bankrupt our healthcare system.

- Reactive hypoglycemia is a condition in which blood sugar repeatedly drops too low in response to high-carbohydrate foods or going too long without eating, such as skipping breakfast. Eating some protein every two to three hours is critical to reverse this trend.

- Insulin resistance is high blood sugar as a result of the cells becoming resistant to insulin, so that no glucose enters the cells to make energy. Instead, glucose travels the bloodstream until it is turned into triglycerides for fat storage. This process demands considerable energy, causing a person to feel tired after eating.

- How many carbohydrates can you eat and still keep your blood sugar stable? If you feel sleepy or crave sugar after eating, you just ate too many carbohydrates. If you feel sleepy after a low/no-carbohydrate meal, you are most likely insulin resistant.

- It is impossible to support hypoglycemia or insulin resistance unless you eat a breakfast with ample high-quality protein. Even if you feel nauseous in the morning, eating breakfast is critical, and will most likely relieve your nausea.

- If you have hypoglycemia, you should never fast — it will make matters worse.

- My *Fast for Unwinding Insulin Resistance* protocol, however, is helpful for addressing insulin resistance.

Chapter Six

THE DIGESTION CONNECTION:
THYROID HEALTH DEPENDS ON GUT HEALTH

Hashimoto's and the Gut

A mother of three in her late thirties came to see me about her chronic depression. Her depression improved quite a bit with some amino acid supplements.

However, about five months after the birth of her fourth child, she crashed. Her depression and fatigue were so bad she could not get out of bed, and she spent her days crying. This was a normally very engaged, loving mother, who could now no longer care for her family.

She was barely able to muster the energy to come to my office. I suspected her recent pregnancy triggered the expression of an autoimmune thyroid disease, and that anemia was also at play. We ran tests and discovered she was indeed severely anemic, and her TSH was high at 122 (the functional range is 1.8-3). Her adrenal salivary index also revealed that she was in total adrenal fatigue and barely able to make cortisol. Stool tests revealed several serious bacterial and parasitic infections. From her symptoms, we ascertained she had dysglycemia.

Because her TSH was so high, I sent her to an endocrinologist and suggested she have her TPO antibodies tested immediately. The endocrinologist didn't want to test for TPO antibodies, saying it was more important to get her TSH under control first. She came back to me to get her TPO antibodies tested, since I had explained the mechanics of autoimmune disease. Sure enough, her TPO antibody count was high, at 934! This was a serious case of Hashimoto's.

We also had her do a provocation/elimination diet and found she had multiple food intolerances. Further testing showed she had celiac disease. (In fact, her four children tested positive for gluten intolerance.) She was also dairy intolerant, as are about 95 percent of my autoimmune clients. I advise them to remove not only gluten from their diets, but dairy as well, since I see so many problems with it.

We changed her diet to stabilize her blood sugar, cleared up her parasitic and bacterial infections, supported her adrenal glands with liposomal phosphatidylserine, and a liposomal cream that includes licorice, B vitamins and other nutrients that address adrenal health. I also supplemented her with iron and modulated her Hashimoto's with therapeutic doses of emulsified vitamin D and a liposomal glutathione cream.

Within two weeks she completely rebounded, and she is now back to normal. She is no longer depressed and her energy returned. Her whole family follows a gluten-free, dairy-free diet and is enjoying better health, including her baby, who had been suffering from sleep apnea due to a dairy-intolerance.

Linda Clark, MA, CN
Universal Wellness Associates
Fair Oaks, CA

Hippocrates said that all disease begins in the gut, and my clinical experience has shown that is largely the case. Yet gastrointestinal (GI) dysfunctions are the most overlooked and exceedingly common disorders today, affecting about 70 million Americans[249] and accounting for billions of dollars in annual sales of over-the-counter digestive aids. While these drugs can offer immediate relief, the underlying causes of the dysfunction, whether it is acid reflux or constipation, go ignored, and people end up with far worse problems down the road. Since most of the immune system is situated in the digestive tract, a problematic gut leads to a problematic immune system.[250] Because the lining of the digestive tract is an important immune barrier, poor gut health is a significant factor in triggering autoimmune diseases[251] [252] such as Hashimoto's, as well as functional hypothyroidism.

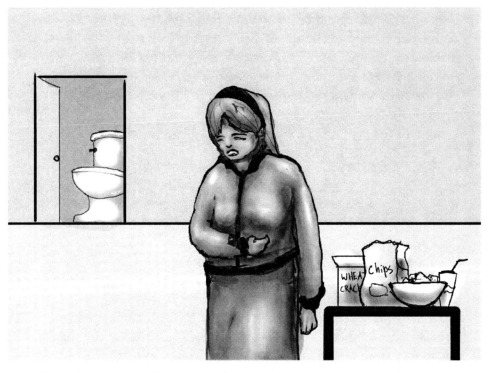

Poor digestive health is extremely common in this country and a major contributor to low thyroid function.

Although stabilizing blood sugar is integral to supporting thyroid health, it is also necessary to restore gut health. A blood sugar that swings wildly from lows to highs compromises the health of your gut tissue and your digestive function. Likewise, poor gut health lends a hand in blood sugar problems, and gut health is integral to stabilizing blood sugar. (The reason why is the adrenal glands, which will be discussed in the next chapter.)

THE THYROID–GUT CONNECTION

One of the first things to go in a poor digestive environment is the balance of healthy gut flora in the intestines, and 20 percent of healthy thyroid activity depends on healthy gut bacteria. Poor digestive function depletes the body of nutrients that support thyroid health, particularly zinc, tyrosine, selenium, and vitamins A and D. Also, faulty digestion is believed to be a leading cause of autoimmune disorders,[253] [254] including Hashimoto's, since at least 60 percent of the immune system is located in the digestive tract. An inflamed GI tract and parasitic infections exhaust the adrenal glands,[255] which in turn drags down thyroid function. Constipation from poor GI health makes it difficult for the body to eliminate unneeded hormones, so estrogen accumulates, which slows down thyroid function. These are just a few reasons why supporting gut health is paramount to successfully managing an autoimmune thyroid condition and supporting functional hypothyroidism.

STOMACH ACID

Hypothyroidism can lead to *hypochlorhydria*, a condition in which the stomach produces too little stomach acid, or hydrochloric acid (HCl). For someone with acid reflux, this may sound like a good thing, but in fact hypochlorhydria often causes that problem. When food is not digested thoroughly by sufficient stomach acid, it putrefies, ferments, and becomes rancid in the stomach. The small intestine naturally tries to refuse entry to this rotting mess, so it backs up into the esophagus, irritating the delicate tissue and causing heartburn. Also, because the food is not sufficiently acidic (although it's certainly acidic enough to burn your esophagus), it does not stimulate the gallbladder to secrete bile to emulsify fats, nor does it signal the pancreas to secrete digestive enzymes for further digestion. The poorly digested, rotting food moves through the intestines, eventually causing inflammation, infection, and intestinal permeability. Whenever a pattern of hypochlorhydria is observed, a thyroid disorder should be ruled out, and any time thyroid malfunction is observed, hypochlorhydria must be considered.[256] [257] In either case, supplemental hydrochloric acid should be used until the patterns resolve.

FAT DIGESTION

Many don't realize it, but the gallbladder is an important digestive organ because it secretes bile to emulsify fats so the body can easily assimilate them. When fats are sufficiently emulsified by bile they transport minerals, and they don't go rancid in the GI tract, which would cause inflammation and infection. Hypothyroidism has been shown to impair gallbladder function, causing the organ to become distended and contract sluggishly, thus not releasing enough bile.[258] [259] A sluggish gallbladder also causes the liver's detoxification pathways to become sluggish and backed up, so that the organ cannot effectively detoxify hormones, toxins, and other metabolites.[260] It is important to support hypothyroidism and cleanse the liver and gallbladder to restore gallbladder function.

CONSTIPATION

Ideally, It takes food 19 to 24 hours to move through a healthy digestive tract. Hypothyroidism has been shown to slow this transit time, as well as impair intestinal absorption rates. This frequently results in constipation, bowel inflammation, malabsorption, and the growth of too much harmful gut bacteria.

HEALTHY GUT BACTERIA

As mentioned earlier, 20 percent of thyroid function depends on a healthy balance of gut flora. We carry approximately four pounds of healthy bacteria in our colons. These bacteria serve many functions, one of which is to facilitate the conversion of T4 to T3. When diets are poor and digestion falters, *dysbiosis*, an overabundance of bad bacteria, occurs crowding out the beneficial bacteria and hampering thyroid function.[261]

Interestingly, some studies have found connections between *Yersinia enterocolitica* and Hashimoto's. Researchers have found that antibodies to this bacteria, which indicates exposure to it, was 14 times higher in people with Hashimoto's than in those without the disease.[262] Being tested for and removing this particular bacterium can be another effective tool in managing Hashimoto's.

Bacterial Infection in the Gut and Thyroid Metabolism

Many people have an overabundance of harmful bacteria in their guts. Studies have shown that the bacteria cell walls, called lipopolysaccharides (LPS) impact thyroid metabolism in numerous ways: They reduce thyroid hormone levels, dull thyroid hormone receptor sites, increase the amount of inactive T3, decrease TSH, and promote autoimmune thyroid disorders.[263] [264] [265] [266] The strain of LPS on the immune system also promotes an abnormal relationship between the thyroid and pituitary glands. When I have a patient complaining of digestive disorders, chronic pain and inflammation, and excessive immune activity (multiple food intolerances or an autoimmune disease, for instance), I know that bacterial infections in the gut are likely wreaking havoc on thyroid function.

POOR ESTROGEN ELIMINATION

Another way poor digestive function contributes to hypothyroidism is by contributing to the excess estrogen accumulation. Dysbiosis and poor digestion prevents the body from successfully eliminating unnecessary estrogen, and toxic levels of this powerful hormone build.[267] This increases the risk for a number of undesirable outcomes, including hypothyroidism that won't show up on a blood test and an increase in breast and uterine cancer risk. Excess estrogen binds the thyroid-transport proteins so that thyroid hormones cannot get to the cells to do their jobs, causing hypothyroidism symptoms.

REPAIRING THE GUT BEGINS AT THE PLATE

A healthy GI tract is a tightly woven mesh of tissue that does not allow the absorption of bacteria, harmful foods, or undigested food particles into the bloodstream. However chronic inflammation brought on by poor diet, poor blood sugar control, and chronic stress loosens these junctures so that harmful substances and undigested food leak into the bloodstream. This is called *intestinal permeability*, but is more commonly known as *leaky gut*. Once in the bloodstream these particles are recognized as foreign invaders, or *antigens*, which the immune system attacks. Unfortunately for many people, especially those with insulin resistance who are most prone to having leaky gut, this response happens almost every time they eat, resulting in chronic inflammation and an immune system that never gets a break. This sets the stage for the development of an autoimmune disease such as Hashimoto's, when the beleaguered immune system confuses the thyroid gland with gluten, which was allowed in through the leaky gut.

The first step to repairing the GI tract is to remove the foods that are creating chronic immune responses with the elimination/provocation diet. This diet helps ferret out which foods are stoking your immune system, so that you know what to avoid until your gut integrity is restored. (Ideally, your holistic doctor or nutritionist will help you identify the culprits.) Unfortunately, these foods are typically people's favorites, such as ice cream, pasta, cheese, and bread. Also, because of the resemblance of the gluten molecules to thyroid tissue, I always have my patients with Hashimoto's immediately remove gluten from their diets.[268] [269]

To get started on the path toward restoring your gut health and managing your autoimmune or functional thyroid condition, you will start with the following diet.

THE ELIMINATION/PROVOCATION DIET

For a minimum of two weeks, but ideally three weeks or more, you must eliminate the following foods from your diet:

- Gluten
- Dairy (including butter and cream)
- Eggs
- Corn
- Soy
- Yeast

These are the most common problem foods for people with leaky gut. If there is another food that you eat frequently, you may need to include it on this list. For instance, nuts and seeds may also cause problems. Be strict, do not cheat, and enlist your family, friends, and coworkers to support or even join you. Eliminating potentially troubling foods will give your immune system and your gut a chance to rest and repair.

After a minimum of two weeks, you will reintroduce each food into your diet, one at a time. Wait at least 72 hours before reintroducing the next food. Do not introduce more than one food at a time. Keep a journal during this period to track symptoms.

Because it has had a chance to rest, your immune system will have sufficient strength to alert you to problem foods. Whereas you had no symptoms previously, reintroducing dairy after a break, for instance, could produce unpleasant reactions. Reactions vary from person to person, so keep a journal and pay close attention to what is happening physically, psychologically, and emotionally.

Some typical reactions to foods that are firing up your immune system include but are not limited to:

- Skin eruptions, eczema, acne
- Fatigue
- Joint pain
- Digestive complaints, such as indigestion, bloating, gas, heartburn, constipation, and diarrhea
- Lung or nasal congestion

- Anxiety
- Moodiness or irritability
- Headaches
- Cold sores

In order to address your autoimmune thyroid condition or functional hypothyroidism, you will need to eliminate the problem foods from your diet. It is possible after some concerted gut repair (discussed later in this chapter), that you may be able to reintroduce many of these foods into your diet. The exception, however, is gluten for people with Hashimoto's. Luckily this is a good time to go gluten-free. As you may have noticed at your local health food store, gluten-free foods are the fastest growing segment of the natural foods industry.

REPAIRING YOUR GUT – THE "4 R" PROGRAM FOR COLON HEALTH

Rare is the individual who walks into my office and doesn't need some degree of gut repair. Remember, 20 percent of thyroid activity depends upon healthy gut bacteria. Digestive dysfunctions drag down thyroid function in other ways too,[270] by skewing the conversion of T4 to T3, contributing to cellular resistance to thyroid hormones, or setting the stage for the development of autoimmune diseases such as Hashimoto's.

Ideally a nutritionist, or nutritionally oriented chiropractor or naturopath will help you restore your gut health. He or she can order specific tests to simplify the process, save you money on supplements, and save you time.

The 4-R Program for Colon Health

In my office I follow a gut restoration, colon health sequence called the "4 R" Program for Remove, Re-Inoculate, Replace, and Repair.

Remove

While my patients are following the elimination/provocation diet, I prescribe a gentle detoxification program that consists of multiple servings of a specially formulated, hypoallergenic protein powder mixed into water or a low-glycemic, hypoallergenic liquid. In addition to being high in rice protein (protein is essential for the body's ability to detoxify), this powder contains herbs and nutrients that promote fat digestion, gallbladder clearance, and liver detoxification. Vitamins and minerals, enzymes, probiotics, amino acids, and strong antioxidants are also essential for a good detoxification powder.

Several weeks of the elimination/provocation diet in conjunction with a high-quality detoxification powder clears up common digestive complaints such as gas, bloating, diarrhea, and constipation for many people. If a digestive problem still persists, I run a GI stool and salivary panel to see if parasites or other pathogens are causing problems. It's not uncommon to find infections by an amoeba, Giardia, roundworms, candida yeast, excess bacteria, or other pathogens affecting the person's gut health. How to eradicate these parasites and pathogens is beyond the scope of this book, and methods vary. There are situations in which I will recommend drugs instead of herbal remedies, because medications are ultimately more effective and easier on my patient. Herbal remedies, on the other hand, work well for many other conditions, including candida overgrowth[271] and h.pylori bacteria.[272]

Nutrients for the "Remove" phase include:

- Nutritional hypoallergenic protein powder and program (See Chapter Five.)

- Nutritional compounds to restore balance to an intestinal terrain propagated by yeast overgrowth, parasites, and harmful bacterial growth. Key ingredients include black walnut hull, caprylic acid, garlic, oregano oil, slippery elm, goldenseal, grapefruit seed, Pau D'Arco, Cat's Claw, guggul, long pepper fruit, Oregon grape root, berberis aristata extract, coptis chinensis extract, and yerba mansa. Please work with a qualified healthcare practitioner to safely and correctly use these nutrients in the right amounts.

Reinoculate

At this stage, I also recommend ample probiotics to inoculate the gut and replace an overabundance of bad bacteria with beneficial bacteria. I see many GI lab panels come back showing bacterial infection in the digestive tract. A good probiotic program is an important part of restoring balance, clearing out bad bacteria, and establishing healthy levels of the healthy bacteria necessary to convert T4 to T3.

Nutritional compounds for the "Reinoculate" phase include:

- A good source of beneficial bacteria, such as lactobacillus and bifidobacterium.

How Dysbiosis Contributes to Hypothyroidism

The GI tract plays an important role in activating thyroid hormones. About 20 percent of T4 is converted to T3 in the GI tract, in the forms of *T3 sulfate* (T3S) and *triidothyroacetic acid* (T3AC). T3S and T3AC remain inactive until they circulate through the GI tract where intestinal sulfatase turns them into active forms of T3.

Where does intestinal sulfatase come from? From healthy gut bacteria. Dysbiosis, an imbalance between pathogenic bacteria and beneficial bacteria, has a profoundly negative impact on the conversion of T3S and T3AC to active forms of T3.[273] [274] [275] This explains why many people suffering from GI dysfunction have low thyroid symptoms but normal lab results.

Gastric inflammation from dysbiosis or infection reduces active T3 in another way. The inflammation creates an alarm reaction, causing the adrenal glands to produce more cortisol. This hormone may further decrease active T3[276] [277] [278] levels while increasing levels of inactive T3.[279]

Replace

Once the gut has been cleaned up, we want it to stay that way, so I recommend digestive aids to compensate for mechanisms that have broken down over years of a poor diet and stressed-out lifestyle. These include supplemental hydrochloric acid to augment the stomach's own acid production to thoroughly digest proteins and ease the burden on the GI system. Supplementing with hydrochloric acid is especially important to those with hypothyroidism, since low thyroid activity hampers the stomach's production of its own acid.[280]

In addition to hydrochloric acid, I recommend enzymes. When gut health is poor, the pancreas loses the ability to secrete sufficient digestive enzymes. Ideally you will take your enzymes 15 to 20 minutes before your meal, or at least in the beginning. Take your hydrochloric acid toward the middle and end of the meal, as the acid can neutralize the effects of some digestive enzymes.

Thirdly, I like to support the gallbladder. Proper gallbladder function is essential for emulsifying and digesting fats, not to mention liver function.[281] Gallbladder removal because of gallstones and congestion is the most common surgery in the United States. By supporting your gallbladder, you no longer send irritating, undigested fats into the intestines, where they become rancid, cause inflammation, and contribute to bacterial infection.

If you have had your gallbladder removed, you should take a gallbladder nutritional compound for the rest of your life that includes the ingredients dandelion root, milk thistle seed extract, ginger root, phosphatidylcholine, and taurine.

By supporting the stomach with hydrochloric acid, the pancreas with digestive enzymes, and the gallbladder with a gallbladder decongestant, food goes into the intestines properly digested. This enhances the body's ability to extract nutrients from food, and prevents inflammation and infection from taking hold.

See Resources for more information on the following products mentioned.

Nutritional compounds for "Replace" phase include:

- Nutritional compounds to supply HCl and support the production of stomach acid. Key ingredients include betaine HCl, niacinamide, B6, pepsin, ox bile, and papain.

- Nutritional compounds to support healthy bile formation, secretion and flow. Key ingredients include dandelion root, milk thistle seed, ginger, taurine, beet concentrate, vitamin C, and phosphatidylcholine.

- Nutritional compounds to support digestion. Key ingredients include high levels of proteolytic and carbolytic plant enzymes.

Please work with a qualified health care practitioner to safely and correctly use these nutrients in the right amounts.

Repair

When a person has multiple food intolerances or allergies (or even environmental allergies), you can count on leaky gut being a problem. The preceding steps are integral to supporting leaky gut, however sometimes a more concerted effort is needed. In order to gauge progress, I like to use a lactoluse/mannitol test to establish the degree of permeability in the intestines. (Note: If fasting glucose is over 105, this test will be inaccurate.). This test, which is relatively inexpensive, involves swallowing a solution of two sugars and then collecting urine exactly six hours later.

Repairing leaky gut is a long road that requires patience and persistence. Abstaining from foods to which you are intolerant is vital, as is taking the nutritional compounds listed in the "Replace" section. Also, I find a "caveman diet" — that is, one free of grains and sugar and rich in fresh, green vegetables, homemade chicken broth, and high-quality proteins and fats — works best to support gut repair.

I recommend nutritional compounds that repair and rejuvenate the intestinal wall, until a lactulose/mannitol test shows the leaky gut is repaired. These compounds should contain herbs, nutrients, and amino acids that support gut repair and regeneration.

Nutritional compounds for the "Repair" phase include:
- Nutritional compounds to support gastric inflammation, increase mucous formation, and maintain healthy gastric lining. Key ingredients include deglycyrrhizinated licorice root, glutamine, flavanoids (catechin), bismuth citrate, gamma-oryzanol, rhubarb officiniale, and mastic gum.

- L-Glutamine powder: 1,500 mg three times a day

Please work with a qualified healthcare practitioner to safely and correctly use these nutrients in the right amounts.

ADRENALS AND LEAKY GUT

One important consideration when it comes to repairing leaky gut is adrenal health. Chronic stress and overworked adrenal glands profoundly weaken the integrity of gastrointestinal tissue.[282] Chapter Seven explores the causes and remedies of chronic adrenal stress, but it's important to mention here: **If chronic adrenal stress is not supported, it will cause a dramatic delay in supporting dysbiosis, leaky gut, and other gastrointestinal conditions.** This scenario will, in turn, make supporting functional hypothyroidism or managing an autoimmune thyroid condition difficult to impossible.

Flashforward:
Leaky gut, adrenal health and hypothyroidism

When faced with stress, whether it is from freeway traffic, blood sugar swings brought on by a sugary snack, or chronic gut inflammation, our adrenal glands release cortisol. As you can imagine, we Americans are constantly releasing cortisol in response to the endless barrage of stressors that make up our lives. Elevated cortisol levels weaken the immune barrier of the intestines, delay regeneration of intestinal tissue, and promote intestinal inflammation.[283] [284] [285] These conditions set the stage for dysbiosis, leaky gut and infections from pathogens, parasites, and yeast. In order to reverse your functional hypothyroidism or modulate your autoimmune thyroid condition, you must include adrenal support in your gut repair program.

When your lactuolose/mannitol tests comes back showing your gut is no longer leaky, it's time to see if you can reintroduce some eliminated foods back into your diet. Add one food at a time for three days. If you have no reactions, you can continue eating that food. If you have a reaction (review the list of possible reactions in the Elimination/

Provocation Diet section), that food needs to stay out of your diet. Continue adding one of the eliminated foods every three days.

The only exception is gluten, which must be permanently eliminated if you have Hashimoto's, especially if your HLA DQ gene test is positive for gluten intolerance or celiac disease (See Chapter Two.).

This is also the time to have another thyroid test. You may find yourself pleasantly surprised at the results. Restoring gut health alone can turn around a functional hypothyroid problem,[286] as well as successfully bring down TPO and TBG antibodies in people with Hashimoto's. Also thyroid medication works more effectively after you complete this program so you may need less of it. You will have more energy, a clearer, more focused mind and a happier, more even mood.

Lifestyle Changes Bring Rewards

Wayne was in his late 50s when he noticed he had gained quite a bit of weight and was exhausted all the time. He also took thyroid hormones and blood pressure medication. Through Dr. Steadman he learned he was insulin resistant and had high triglycerides, low vitamin D, and a sensitivity to gluten. Wayne adjusted his diet to be gluten-free, sugar-free, and low in carbohydrates. Dr. Steadman also gave him nutritional compounds to support his health. The diet was hard at first but Wayne has lost 38 pounds, no longer has gas and indigestion, and enjoys his newfound energy. He has lowered his medication dosages and hopes to get off them entirely. He even enjoys exercising now and says he feels agile and flexible.

Shane Steadman, DC, DACNB
Denver, CO

CHAPTER HIGHLIGHTS

- Hippocrates said, "All disease begins in the gut." I find this still true today, including in people with hypothyroidism and Hashimoto's. To support functional hypothyroidism or modulate an autoimmune thyroid condition, you must tend to your digestive health.

- Balancing blood sugar (Chapter Five) and ferreting out foods to which you are intolerant or allergic are the first steps to repairing your gut. Find what these foods are using the elimination/provocation diet.

- Begin restoring your gut health using the "4R" Program for Colon Health: Remove, re-inoculate, replace, and repair.

- A "caveman diet" that is high in fresh green vegetables, high quality proteins and fats, and homemade chicken broth is the recommended diet during the repair[26] phase. Grains, sweets, and processed foods are not advised during this period.

- A variety of nutritional compounds greatly speed along gut repair, and specific digestive aids are recommended before meals. Certain tests ordered by a qualified healthcare practitioner guarantee you the right support, which saves you time and money and speeds progress.

- After you have diligently worked at restoring gut integrity, you may be able to eat the foods you formerly eliminated. The exception is gluten in those with Hashimoto's.

- Surprise yourself with a thyroid test after your gut-health program. You may find your functional hypothyroidism is no longer an issue, and your autoimmune thyroid condition successfully modulated.

CHAPTER SEVEN

THE BELEAGUERED ADRENALS
AND THE BEATEN DOWN THYROID

Darlene had her thyroid checked annually as part of a regular exam, and it was always in good shape. After her third child, however, her TSH plummeted; it was quite low by functional medicine standards, but not low enough to warrant attention from her HMO physician. She also complained of trouble staying asleep, becoming shaky and lightheaded before meals, and getting very sleepy in the late afternoon. These were the classic symptoms of reactive hypoglycemia, and as a homeschooling mother of three children who also ran a small farm, the stress of caring for a new baby as well as a herd of dairy goats was formidable. The recent pregnancy, the hypoglycemia, and the increased workload created more stressors than her pituitary gland could handle. It began to poop out and communicate poorly with her thyroid gland, causing her TSH to drop. Had she not been so proactive in addressing the situation, she may very well have begun to experience a cascade of hypothyroid symptoms as well.

We've talked about how unstable blood sugar and poor gut health can lead to functional hypothyroidism or Hashimoto's. The adrenals, the two walnut-sized glands that sit atop the kidneys complete this circle. Because healthy thyroid function is so dependent upon healthy adrenal function, tending to them is integral to supporting the thyroid. Some factors affecting adrenal health are obvious, and obviously American — such as leading a stressed out life. Other factors are not so obvious but are just as taxing: Blood sugar swings, gut infections, food intolerances, chronic viruses, environmental toxins, and autoimmune conditions.[287] The body interprets all of these as alarm bells and directs the adrenal glands to pump out adrenal hormones. These hormones, cortisol in particular, trigger the body to release extra glucose into the bloodstream. The additional glucose is used to increase energy production to adapt to the demands of the stress. For many of us, this is a daily, ongoing reaction.

If you want to address your Hashimoto's disease or functional hypothyroidism, you're going to have to nurture these worn-out workhorses back to health.[288] Symptoms of adrenal stress run the gamut, from being too wired to too tired, but some common symptoms include:

- Fatigue
- Headaches with physical or mental stress
- Weak immune system
- Allergies
- Slow to start in the morning
- Gastric ulcers
- Afternoon headache
- Feeling full or bloated
- Craving sweets, caffeine, cigarettes
- Blurred vision
- Unstable behavior
- Becoming shaky or lightheaded if meals are missed or delayed
- Irritability before meals

- Eating to relieve fatigue

- Cannot stay asleep

- Cannot fall asleep

- Dizziness when moving from sitting or lying to standing

- Transient spells of dizziness

- Asthma

- Hemorrhoids

- Varicose veins

Adrenal imbalances are probably the most common health problems we see in functional medicine.[289] (Again, functional medicine is supporting a person from the standpoint of what constitutes health, not disease). We live in a society in which the prevailing diet is high in carbohydrates, synthetic sweeteners, artificial flavors, and synthetic additives and in which foods are loaded with compounds that alter human physiology, such as partially hydrogenated fats. This kind of a diet places tremendous stress on the body. Add to this the stress of endless to-do lists, deadlines, multitasking, early wake-up calls, and too few hours to accomplish everything. This has created an epidemic of adrenal related disorders, and since the adrenal glands so greatly affect the thyroid gland, it's no wonder thyroid problems affect an estimated 27 million people.[290]

ADRENAL STRESS AND HYPOTHYROIDISM

Low thyroid function is almost always secondary to some other condition, often adrenal stress.[291] Chronic adrenal stress does the following:

- Affects communication between the brain and the hormone glands. The hypothalamus and pituitary gland direct hormone production, including that of the thyroid. When the hypothalamus and pituitary weaken due to chronic adrenal stress, they are not able to communicate well with the thyroid gland.[292] [293] [294]

- Increases thyroid binding protein activity, so that thyroid hormones cannot get into cells to do their job.

- Hampers the conversion of T4 to active forms of T3 that the body can use.[295] [296] [297]

- Stymies the detoxification pathways through which unnecessary thyroid hormones exit the body, leading to thyroid hormone resistance.

- Causes cells to lose sensitivity to thyroid hormones.

- Weakens the immune barriers of the digestive tract, lungs, and brain; weakens the immune system; and promotes poor immune regulation.[298] [299] [300] These factors increase the risk for triggering Hashimoto's or exacerbating it.

These are some of the ways adrenal stress directly impacts thyroid function. What is more important, however, are the ways in which chronic adrenal stress affect other systems of the body, which in turn drag down thyroid function.[301] In the previous chapters I explained how poor blood sugar control and an unhealthy gut lead to hypothyroidism and Hashimoto's. The underlying factor in both these scenarios is chronic adrenal stress.

Adrenals and Blood Sugar
The adrenal hormone cortisol plays a big role in thyroid health. Cortisol raises blood sugar when it drops too low, which, when it happens repeatedly, exhausts the adrenal and thyroid glands, as well as the brain's control center, the hypothalamus and the pituitary gland. Over time, this exhaustion leads to functional hypothyroidism. Additionally, constant cortisol production weakens the GI tract, making it more susceptible to dysbiosis, inflammation, and infection,[302] creating a vicious cycle that weakens the thyroid.

Adrenals and Gut Inflammation
Gut inflammation and infections, as discussed in Chapter Six, create an alarm reaction in the body that causes the pituitary gland to increase cortisol production in order to help the body adapt to increased stress. The extra cortisol has the potential to shift higher

percentages of T4 into useless forms of inactive T3.[303] This is a situation in which a person's blood test results look normal, but she suffers from hypothyroidism symptoms.

Adrenals and Food Intolerances

A major cause of adrenal stress is the repeated ingestion of a food to which a person has an immune response. A person with dairy and gluten sensitivity, for instance, may eat those foods regularly without any obvious symptoms, and be totally oblivious to the fact that these foods are firing up the immune system until she does the elimination/provocation diet. This chronic immune response creates a chronic stress response that can increase the inactive form of reverse T3 and weaken the GI tract.

Adrenals and Progesterone

When the adrenal glands are in a constant state of alarm, continually releasing cortisol into the bloodstream, the pituitary gland becomes sluggish from overwork. As a result the reproductive system also suffers,[304] which leads to low progesterone in women [305] and low testosterone in men. Healthy thyroid activity depends upon appropriate levels of progesterone.

Adrenals and Estrogen

Too much estrogen creates excess thyroid binding proteins, the transport proteins that carry thyroid hormones through the bloodstream. As a result, not enough thyroid hormones can get into the body's cells. Prolonged, elevated cortisol runs down the liver's ability to detoxify discarded estrogens. As a result, estrogen circulates back into the bloodstream in a more toxic form, and becomes overly abundant, raising the thyroid binding protein level so that thyroid hormones cannot get into the cells.

Adrenals and Chronic Viruses

Just as with food intolerances or chronic inflammation, a chronic virus creates ongoing stimulation of the immune system. The pituitary gland perceives this as an alarm reaction, which calls on the adrenal glands to pump more cortisol into the bloodstream so the body can adapt to the demands of stress from the virus.[306] In time, pituitary and adrenal exhaustion lead to poor thyroid function.

Adrenals and Autoimmune Conditions

Again, chronic immune stimulation, as is the case with autoimmune diseases such as Hashimoto's, sets the stage for a prolonged cortisol elevation. Likewise, chronic cortisol elevation makes the immune system more prone to autoimmune disorders.[307] Managing an autoimmune condition supports healthy adrenal function, which can further dampen the autoimmune response.

Adrenals and Environmental Toxins

When a person begins having immune responses to environmental toxins, whether they are heavy metals[308] or synthetic chemicals, he or she is creating a chronic stressor for both the immune system and the adrenal glands, ultimately affecting thyroid health.

Hopefully by now you are thoroughly convinced how important adrenal health is to thyroid health. If you or a friend has ever consulted with a naturopath, nutritionist, or chiropractor, chances are he or she prescribed adrenal supplements. While such supplements are integral to an adrenal support program, you can see from the above how many other factors need to be addressed. **Adrenal health, like thyroid health, is always secondary to something else.** Medicine, even alternative medicine, likes to break the human body into separate components to be treated. The human body just doesn't operate that way. Every system affects every other system. Hormones, the immune system, digestive function and brain health are a tightly woven, interdependent matrix. Many of the above scenarios can create hypothyroid symptoms long before it shows up on blood tests and long after thyroid hormones have been prescribed.

Hypothyroidism and Fatigue

Allison struggled for ten years with fatigue so severe she could barely push a grocery cart, could no longer drive, and had to quit working or helping around the house. Her doctors ran tests but came up empty handed and instead offered her prescriptions for antidpressants, sleeping pills, and multiple hormones. One doctor told her that severe fatigue and memory loss were normal for her age. Another diagnosed Hashimoto's but didn't tell her about it for a year. Allison finally discovered Dr. Arthur, who interpreted her blood panels from a functional perspective. Dr Arthur put her on a diet eliminating gluten and other common immune triggers. He also managed her Hashimoto's appropriately and supported her low vitamin D status. Within only one month of following Dr. Arthur's protocol her depression vanished and she was back to her normal energy levels and able to work, visit with friends, and help around the house.
David Arthur, DC, DACNB
Denver, Colorado

THE DEAL BUSTERS TO SUPPORTING YOUR ADRENALS AND YOUR THYROID

For the rest of the chapter I will detail how to support your adrenal glands and address the physiologic effects of stress. Keep in mind the broad concepts discussed below. I call them the "deal busters." If you don't take care each of these conditions, you will not be able to support your adrenal glands. As a result, you will not be able to support your functional hypothyroidism or autoimmune thyroid condition.

• **Anemia** In the case of anemia, enough oxygen can't get to the cells for any metabolic progress to happen, including adrenal or thyroid support.

- **Unstable blood sugar** As you learned in Chapter Five, unstable blood sugar, whether it's too low or too high, is a significant stressor on adrenal health.

- **Gut infections** Poor gut function, inflammation, and infections are chronic stressors that overwork the adrenal glands and tax immune function.

- **Unidentified food intolerances and food allergies** Every time you eat a food that causes an immune reaction, even if you do not have noticeable symptoms, you are stressing the adrenal glands.

- **Essential fatty acid deficiency** The right fats in the right amounts are essential for hormone production, including adrenal and thyroid hormone.

- **Toxicity issues** Sometimes people develop immune reactions to environmental compounds, including heavy metals,[309] molds,[310] or chemicals.[311] If this situation goes unchecked, adrenal support is not possible.[312]

USING BLOOD TESTS TO ASSESS ADRENAL HEALTH

When a patient presents with symptoms or blood test results of hypothyroidism, I always order an Adrenal Salivary Index (ASI) test through DiagnosTechs Lab. To support the thyroid, it's important for me to get a clear picture of my patient's adrenal status using this test. Symptoms alone do not provide an accurate diagnosis, as symptoms can be the same for both over active and under active adrenal function. I also do not use urinary adrenal tests, for with hypothyroidism, the excretion of several adrenal hormones is decreased so that results can be inaccurate. The salivary panel provides the most useful, accurate, and comprehensive information.

The most important thing to know about the ASI test is that one ASI test is worthless. I repeat, one ASI test is worthless. It is the second and third test that tells me whether we're on the right track with a protocol. Adrenal health should improve on the protocol I give my patient. If it doesn't, I know something deeper is sabotaging the adrenals. Is it a parasite, like Giardia or roundworm? Is it a reaction to heavy metal toxicity (although we all have some degree of heavy metal toxicity, not all of us have an immune reaction to it)? Is it a chronic virus? Is it a food intolerance? Once I figure out and address what is taxing the adrenals, true thyroid support begins.

The ASI tells me how a person's adrenals are working throughout the day, by measuring adrenal hormone levels. The person takes the test kit home and collects samples of her saliva in the morning, at noon, in the afternoon, and at bedtime. Cortisol is secreted in a specific pattern according to your circadian rhythm over 24-hours, which should have you feeling awake and energetic in the morning and tired and ready for bed in the evening. Being in a chronic alarm or prolonged stress reaction will eventually disrupt your circadian rhythm. As you have probably already guessed, many people have abnormal circadian rhythms and experience insomnia, are "night owls," have problems staying asleep, don't sleep deeply, or wake up fatigued. These are all symptoms of adrenal stress. The ASI shows abnormalities in the circadian rhythm, charts key hormone levels, and pinpoints where problems arise along the spectrum of adrenal health.

The adrenal glands adapt to stress, whether it is chemical, emotional, or physical, in one of three stages. It was once thought these stages followed a sequence, starting with "alarm reaction" and ending in "exhaustion," but new research shows that is not always the case. For instance, a major trauma, such as a car accident, divorce, serious illness,[313] or death of a loved one, can send someone immediately into the adrenal exhaustion stage.

The three stages of adrenal dysfunction are:

Alarm reaction The adrenal glands become hyperactive to increase cortisol levels to adapt to the demands of stress.

Resistance stage The occurs in response to prolonged stress as the body steals pregnenolone from cholesterol to make more cortisol — a phenomenon known as *pregnenolone steal.* Normally pregnenolone helps make sex hormones such as progesterone and testosterone. As a result of pregnenolone steal, hormonal imbalances arise. It commonly causes PMS, infertility, male menopause, and polycystic ovary syndrome.

Exhaustion stage At this point the adrenals are exhausted and can no longer adapt to stress. The cofactors needed to make cortisol become depleted so cortisol levels drop too low. Because the adrenals no longer produce sufficient cortisol, the pregnenolone steal cycle stops.

The ASI measures where you are on the spectrum of adrenal health. The test requires four saliva samples retrieved throughout the same day. It's important not to expose yourself to adrenal stimulants or agents such as caffeine, ma huang, nicotine, licorice root, or adrenal glandulars on the day of the test and avoid herbs that impact adrenal function for at least four days before the test.

Also, the test should be performed during an average day that does not include abnormal stress, such as a day in divorce court, running a marathon, or riding roller coasters.

(Note: If you have been on corticosteroid drugs for up to three months prior, accurate levels may not be determined.)

The ASI measures the levels of cortisol, DHEA (a precursor hormone to cortisol, testosterone, and estrogen) and 17 hydroxyprogesterone, another cortisol a precursor. When looking at the ASI results, the most useful markers are the circadian rhythm and the ratio of cortisol to DHEA, both of which are compared to normal values.

A healthy circadian rhythm will show cortisol that is high in the morning and low at night. Someone who wakes up groggy but has insomnia will show the opposite. Some people's cortisol peaks and dips throughout the day, which means they've lost coordination between the adrenal glands and the brain.

The graph also charts the ratio between cortisol and DHEA, which shows, in specific detail, in which of stage of adrenal maladaption the person is.

Alarm Reaction   Cortisol and DHEA are high. This stage indicates an initial and acute response to stress. I usually see this pattern in healthy patients who are overworking themselves or in athletes who are overtraining.[314] This stage will usually resolve itself if the stressor is removed. Insulin resistance is common in this stage.

Nutritional Support   The objective is to support a healthy response to insulin resistance. Key ingredients include chromium, vanadium, alpha lipoic acid, mixed tocopherols, magnesium, biotin, zinc, inositol, and gymnema sylvestre.

- Nutritional compounds to also help the body adapt to the physiological stress responses. Key ingredients include panax ginseng, Siberian ginseng, ashwagandha, holybasil leaf extract, rhodiola rosea, punarva, and pantethine.

- Liposomal cream that delivers nutritional compounds to modulate the stress response. Key ingredient includes 2,000 mg a day of phosphatidylserine.

- Essential fatty acids support a healthy response to insulin resistance. Key ingredients include EPA and DHA from micro-emulsified fish oil, taurine, green tea extract, odorless garlic extract, and evening primrose oil.

Please work with a qualified healthcare practitioner to safely and correctly use these nutrients in the right amounts.

Progression of Alarm Reaction Cortisol is high while DHEA is normal. This early stage of alarm indicates further progression into the resistance stage even though the body is no longer in acute stress. The DHEA levels are no longer elevated because they are shifting into cortisol. Insulin resistance is common in this stage.

Nutritional Support

- Supporting a healthy response to insulin resistance is the goal. Key ingredients include chromium, vanadium, alpha lipoic acid, mixed tocopherols, magnesium, biotin, zinc, inositol, and gymnema sylvestre.

- Nutritional compounds to help the person adapt to the physiological stress responses. Key ingredients include panax ginseng, Siberian ginseng, ashwagandha, holybasil leaf extract, rhodiola rosea, punarva, and pantethine.

- Liposomal cream that delivers nutritional compounds to modulate the stress response. Key ingredient includes 2,000 mg a day of phosphatidylserine.

- Essential fatty acids to support a healthy response to insulin resistance. Key ingredients include EPA and DHA from micro emulsified fish oil, taurine, green tea extract, odorless garlic extract, and evening primrose oil.

Please work with a qualified healthcare practitioner to safely and correctly use these nutrients in the right amounts.

Resistance Cortisol is high and DHEA is low. This stage indicates the onset of the resistance stage and pregnenolone steal by cortisol, when DHEA is diverted to meeting the increasing demands of cortisol instead of toward making sex hormones. This sets the stage for major imbalances of the reproductive hormones. Insulin resistance is common in this stage.

Nutritional Support

- Supporting a healthy response to insulin resistance is the goal. Key ingredients include chromium, vanadium, alpha lipoic acid, mixed tocopherols, magnesium, biotin, zinc, inositol, and gymnema sylvestre.

- Nutritional compounds to help the person adapt to the physiological stress responses. Key ingredients include panax ginseng, Siberian ginseng, ashwagandha, holybasil leaf extract, rhodiola rosea, punarva, and pantethine.

- Liposomal cream that delivers nutritional compounds to modulate the stress response. Key ingredient includes 2,000 mg a day of phosphatidylserine.

- Essential fatty acids to support a healthy response to insulin resistance. Key ingredients include EPA and DHA from microemulsified fish oil, taurine, green tea extract, odorless garlic extract, and evening primrose oil.

Please work with a qualified healthcare practitioner to safely and correctly use these nutrients in the right amounts.

Progression of Resistance toward Exhaustion Cortisol is low and DHEA is low. This stage indicates the progression of resistance to adrenal exhaustion. In this stage the adrenals are at risk of losing the ability to produce cortisol and manage stress. Insulin resistance is common.

Nutritional Support
- Supporting a healthy response to insulin resistance is the goal. Key ingredients include chromium, vanadium, alpha lipoic acid, mixed tocopherols, magnesium, biotin, zinc, inositol, and gymnema sylvestre.

- Nutritional compounds to help the person adapt to the physiological stress responses. Key ingredients include panax ginseng, Siberian ginseng, ashwagandha, holybasil leaf extract, rhodiola rosea, punarva, and pantethine.

- Liposomal cream that delivers nutritional compounds to modulate the stress response. Key ingredient includes 2,000 mg a day of phosphatidylserine.

- Essential fatty to acids support a healthy response to insulin resistance. Key ingredients include EPA and DHA from microemulsified fish oil, taurine, green tea extract, odorless garlic extract, and evening primrose oil.

- Liposomal cream that delivers nutritional compounds to support low adrenal function. Key ingredients include licorice, B vitamins, and other nutrients to support adrenal health.

Please work with a qualified healthcare practitioner to safely and correctly use these nutrients in the right amounts.

Adrenal Exhaustion, Non-Adapted Cortisol is low, and DHEA is normal. This pattern demonstrates the onset of adrenal exhaustion, when the adrenal gland begins to fail and cannot produce either adequate cortisol or DHEA. Hypoglycemia is common.

Nutritional Support
- The objective is supporting healthy blood sugar balance. Key ingredients include chromium, bovine adrenal gland, choline bitartrate, bovine liver gland, bovine pancreas gland, inositol, L-carnitine, co-enzyme Q10, rubidium chelate, and vanadium aspartate.

- Nutritional compounds to help the person adapt to the physiological stress responses. Key ingredients include panax ginseng,

Siberian ginseng, ashwagandha, holybasil leaf extract, rhodiola rosea, punarva, and pantethine.

- Liposomal cream that delivers nutritional compounds to support low adrenal function. Key ingredients include licorice, B vitamins, and other nutrients to support adrenal health.

- Essential fatty acids to support a healthy response to hypoglycemia. Key ingredients include flaxseed oil, evening primrose oil, taurine, green tea extract, and odorless garlic extract.

Please work with a qualified healthcare practitioner to safely and correctly use these nutrients in the right amounts.

Inappropriate DHEA Cortisol is normal and DHEA is high. This pattern is not part of the progression to adrenal exhaustion. Patients in this stage should be evaluated for ovarian production of DHEA, the use of DHEA supplements or creams, or disturbances to the hormonal system caused by DHEA supplements or creams. This pattern could also indicate polycystic ovary syndrome (PCOS) or insulin resistance.

Adrenal Fatigue Cortisol is low and DHEA is low. This is the final stage of adrenal exhaustion in which the adrenals completely lose the ability to to produce cortisol or DHEA. This pattern is common in chronically ill patients. Hypoglycemia is common.
Nutritional Support
- The objective is to support healthy blood sugar balance. Key ingredients include chromium, bovine adrenal gland, choline bitartrate, bovine liver gland, bovine pancreas gland, inositol, L-carnitine, co-enzyme Q10, rubidium chelate, and vanadium aspartate.

- Nutritional compounds to help the person adapt to the physiological stress responses. Key ingredients include panax ginseng, Siberian ginseng, ashwagandha, holybasil leaf extract, rhodiola rosea, punarva, and pantethine.

- Liposomal cream that delivers nutritional compounds to support low adrenal function. Key ingredients include licorice, B vitamins, and other nutrients to support adrenal health.

- Essential fatty acids to support a healthy response to hypoglycemia. Key ingredients include flaxseed oil, evening primrose oil, taurine, green tea extract, and odorless garlic extract.

- Liposomal cream that delivers nutritional compounds to modulate the stress response. Key ingredient includes 2,000 mg a day of phosphatidylserine.

- In cases of extreme exhaustion, secondary support with sublingual pregnenolone* and sublingual DHEA* (see Resources) for 30 days may be necessary.

Please work with a qualified healthcare practitioner to safely and correctly use these nutrients in the right amounts.

*I rarely recommend hormones that are not sublingual. Hormone creams and pills can build up to excess levels in the fat tissue. Sublingual hormones need to be taken more frequently but do not create the risk for overload.

Fatigue and dysglycemia are common symptoms with all stages of adrenal fatigue; in fact, this condition is a driving factor of hypoglycemia. With stages one through four, insulin resistance is common. I see hypoglycemia more often in stages five through seven. However these are generalities and are not hard and fast rules. The ASI test reveals a few other things, such as the level of 17 hydroxyprogesterone, a precursor to cortisol. A high 17 hydroxyprogesterone and low cortisol levels mean that the adrenals have lost the ability to make cortisol.

Also included on the test are the Total SIgA (secretory antibodies) levels, and gliadin (gluten) SIgA levels. The Total SIgA indicates the impact of stress on the immune system, since these secretory antibodies make up the lining of the immune barrier in the digestive tract.[315] When the number is low, a person is more susceptible to food intolerances, parasites, and fungal and viral infections.[316]

The gliadin SIgA test screens for gluten intolerance, a powerful stressor that some researchers estimate affects as many as one in three people in the U.S. and creates ongoing adrenal stress. However, I do not place much weight on either of these tests, as a negative result can be due to a depressed immune system. The best test for food intolerances remains the elimination/provocation diet (See Chapter Six).

I also disregard the insulin result as it is too dependent on what the person ate on the day of the test.

Again, the most concerted adrenal support protocol will be worthless without determining why the adrenal stress occurs. For instance, is it a food intolerance? A chronic virus or parasite infection? If a person does not show significant improvement after one month on one of the above protocols, then I know I need to dig deeper for what is stressing the adrenals. This point also illustrates how useless one ASI test is and the value of a second or even a third test. As a bonus, I find my patients are much more compliant with their program if they know to expect a follow-up test.

SUPPORTING THE THYROID BY SUPPORTING THE ADRENALS

Adrenal stress is always secondary to something else, which is also the case for thyroid problems. So whether you are in adrenal exhaustion or your adrenals are over active, some fundamental practices will help restore adrenal health, which is integral to supporting thyroid health.

Avoid Adrenal Stimulators

If you are serious about supporting your thyroid and avoiding a lifetime dependence on medications, you may need to remove some favorite adrenal stressors, such as coffee, from your daily life. Failing to do so will provide little in the way of results. The following is a list of foods and chemicals that need to be completely avoided when making an attempt to restore adrenal health.

- Concentrated sugars
- Caffeine (Decaffeinated coffee is not acceptable because it is still 60 percent caffeinated; green tea is OK for less advanced stages)
- Nicotine (This is a tough one if you're addicted, but even just cutting down can make a big difference
- Alcohol

- Allergenic foods (Histamine, which is released when you eat a food to which you are allergic, is an adrenal stimulant)
- Partially hydrogenated fats, which inhibit adrenal hormone synthesis
- Artificial sweeteners, which block the synthesis of some adrenal hormones
- Overtraining (Athletes undercut their performance by training too hard.)
- Inadequate sleep

Stabilize blood sugar levels

When it comes to supporting the adrenals, diet is everything. If blood sugar levels are not stabilized (See Chapter Five), you will have little success in achieving adrenal health.[317] This is especially true for people who have hypoglycemia, those who are irritable before meals, get shaky and lightheaded when meals are missed, and who find eating relieves fatigue. Here is a recap to dietary guidelines as outlined in Chapter Five:

- Do not skip breakfast. Eat within one hour of waking.
- Eat a high quality, protein-based breakfast.
- Eat every two to three hours. Do not wait until you are hungry. Set your phone's alarm clock if need be.
- Snack with low-glycemic foods, such as nuts, seeds, or hard-boiled eggs. Avoid all fruit juices and carrot juice.
- Never consume high-glycemic foods or fruits without a source of protein or fat.
- Avoid all adrenal stimulants (listed above).
- Eat a well balanced diet consisting mostly of vegetables, quality meats, and healthy fats.

Exercise in your aerobic heart range

It is crucial to include walking, slow jogging, slow cycling, or other forms of exercise that involve endurance to support the adrenals. Aerobic exercise puts the emphasis on burning fat for energy production. Anaerobic exercise, such as weight lifting, burns sugar for energy. This exacerbates dysglycemia and stresses the adrenals as they struggle to normalize blood sugar. Aerobic exercise, on the other hand, not only decreases overly high cortisol levels,[318] but also relies on fat burning, which relieves the adrenals so they can rest and repair.

Practice relaxation techniques
Although everyone has different levels of and reactions to stress, daily life in the U.S. is universally recognized as stressful and hard on the adrenals. Eliminate the stressors that you can, then make practicing a relaxation technique in a quiet and restful atmosphere a daily habit. Here are two techniques with a good track record for reducing stress:

Positive Mental Imaging Think about the stressful events of the day. Put yourself back in the moment, using as many senses as possible (how did things sounds, smell, look, and feel?). Once you have the stressful event fixed in your mind, recreate the scenario, adding humorous and cartoon-like features to the people in the scene. For example, If your boss at work chastised you, picture your boss with a big clown nose and goofy ears, until the event becomes funny. Go through all the stressful events of the day, making them humorous. This discharges the negative emotion that builds stress.

Muscle Contraction/Relaxation Lie on your back with your eyes closed. Contract a group of muscles for two seconds. Start with your facial muscles and go up and down the body with different muscle groups, such as the quadriceps, hamstrings, calf muscles, toes, abdominals, pectorals, biceps, triceps, forearms, fingers, etc. Do this exercise until you have gone through each muscle group two to three times. Finish with deep, long breaths as long as you like.

Take time off
People underestimate how powerfully restorative regular time off is. It is important to schedule down time into your weeks and guard them fiercely. For example, since I teach many weekend seminars, I take Mondays off. If someone wants to meet with me on that day, I tell them I am booked all day. Ideally you will take an entire day off each week to do whatever you want. Do not use this day to catch up

on chores and errands. I know an entire day off can be impossible for mothers, so find childcare and take a half-day off. Knowing you can count on having that time to yourself each week is just as important as the time itself. People in adrenal stress always feel like they have something to do, and disengaging from that thought pattern is an important part of supporting the adrenals.

Adrenal Function During Pregnancy

Did you know that a pregnant mother can pass on adrenal dysfunction to her unborn child?[319] Studies show that in her third trimester of pregnancy a woman with adrenal exhaustion will draw adrenal hormones from the baby through the umbilical cord. As a result, the child is at risk for being born with compromised adrenal function.[320] Since adrenal dysfunction so greatly impacts immune and gut health, and since it is nearly universal these days, this helps explain the increasing rates of allergies, food intolerances, eczema, and autism among children,[321] not to mention maternal postpartum depression.

NUTRIENT AND HERBAL SUPPORT FOR ADRENAL HEALTH

To truly restore adrenal health and thus thyroid health, I look for what is causing adrenal stress, recommend the lifestyle changes explained above, and offer specific adrenal support based on a person's ASI test. Although someone in adrenal fatigue will need somewhat different support than someone with adrenal resistance, certain nutrients and herbs are recommended for *all* stages of adrenal dysfunction.

Essential Fatty Acids These include EPA and DHA from fish oils, and GLA from evening primrose, black currant, or borage oils. Essential fatty acids are necessary for cellular communication and the synthesis of hormones, including the adrenal and thyroid hormones. I do not recommend flax seed oil for those with insulin resistance as their bodies cannot convert it to EPA and DHA.

Phosphatidylserine (PS): Phosphatidylserine (PS) is a compound that makes up cell membranes and is a major nutrient for the brain. It is necessary for cell-to-cell communication, activating receptors on cell surfaces, and allowing nutrients to come into cells, and waste products to exit. Making PS in the body is a difficult and demanding process, requiring nutrients in which people are commonly deficient. Supplementing with PS has been shown to enhance cellular metabolism and communication; protect cells from oxidative damage; decrease anxiety; improve mood, motivation, and depression; and enhance memory and cognition.

The most clinically significant use for PS is its ability to lower elevated cortisol; however, I also recommend it for those with low cortisol. PS doesn't address the adrenal glands directly, but it helps the area of the brain that coordinates circadian rhythm and adrenal functions.

The problem is that PS is very expensive, and in order to be effective, eight or more capsules a day are required (we used to know that a patient was getting a therapeutic dose of PS when joint pain occurred). PS is now available in a cream, which allows for hundreds of milligrams to be delivered into the bloodstream, bypassing the digestive tract. This eliminates the need to take large quantities of expensive pills.

Adrenal Adaptogens These plant compounds normalize the hypothalamus-adrenal-pituitary (HPA) axis, improving communication between the brain and the adrenal glands and affecting how well the brain communicates with the thyroid. Adaptogens help adrenals that are both over active and under active. The most important adaptogens for the adrenals include panax ginseng, Siberian ginseng, ashwagandha, rhodiola, boerhaavia diffusa, and holybasil leaf extract.

Pantethine (B5) and B vitamins Pantethine, and B vitamins in general, are vital cofactors in the manufacturing of adrenal hormones. Pantethine has been shown to tone down excess release of cortisol in times of stress, and enhance the function of cortisol. People in adrenal stress tend to have a greater loss of B vitamins.

Nutrients that support insulin resistance In stages one through four of adrenal maladaption, in which cortisol is elevated, I also recommend nutrients that nutritionally support insulin resistance, since high cortisol leads to insulin resistance. These nutrients help the cells to regain their insulin sensitivity so that glucose can enter cells to produce energy. Although many people have insulin resistance in these stages, some don't so dysglycemia should be assessed and supported appropriately.

Nutrients that support hypoglycemia In stages five and seven, when the adrenals are exhausted, I recommend nutrients to support hypoglycemia. Low cortisol in stages of adrenal exhaustion often leads to hypoglycemia. Although many people have hypoglycemia in these stages, some don't so dysglycemia should be assessed and supported appropriately.

Glycyrrhizin I also recommend this for stages five and seven of adrenal exhaustion. This component of the licorice root increases the half-life of circulating cortisol — in other words, it makes what little cortisol you have last longer so the adrenal glands are less burdened. Glycyrrhizin has many other beneficial properties that are useful to the adrenal exhausted individual.

Please work with a qualified healthcare practitioner to safely and correctly use these nutrients in the right amounts.

When it comes to addressing functional hypothyroidism and managing Hashimoto's, nutritionally supporting blood sugar, digestion, and adrenal health is integral to supporting the thyroid. We are brainwashed to expect one pill or one doorway into treatment. In truth, the body's systems work in concert, with every organ and system affecting the rest. A breakdown in this matrix is what leads to hypothyroidism, and addressing the body as a whole leads to well being.

CHAPTER HIGHLIGHTS

- Thyroid health is very dependent upon adrenal health. To support the thyroid you must support the adrenals.

- Adrenal dysfunction is always secondary to something else. To support the adrenals you must address what is causing chronic adrenal stress.

- Some degree of adrenal dysfunction is extremely common in the U. S.

- Elevated cortisol associated with chronic adrenal stress leads to hypothyroidism in a number of ways, both directly and indirectly.

- The adrenal salivary index (ASI) test gives a clear picture of adrenal status, and using it rather than symptoms alone or urinary adrenal tests to make a diagnosis is best.

- One ASI test is useless. Follow-up tests determine progress.

- There are seven stages to adrenal dysfunction. Newer research shows they do not necessarily happen sequentially.

- A diet that stabilizes blood sugar and restores gut health is essential to adrenal health.

CHAPTER EIGHT

HOW THOSE HORMONE PILLS AND POTIONS ROB YOU OF THYROID HEALTH

If Suzanne Somers is on your radar, then you are probably familiar with hormone creams and supplements, those miracle cures that reverse aging, banish menopause symptoms, and put a twinkle in your eye. Where I live and work in San Diego, it seems there is an anti-aging clinic on every corner, all of which base their practices on hormone creams and pills. If you've gone to a doctor or naturopath with complaints of hypothyroid symptoms, you most likely were prescribed thyroid hormone medication without a second thought. And don't forget the birth control pill, a hormone medication so popular hardly anyone stops to ponder the consequences. Now they're even prescribing hormones to stop the inconvenience of menstruation. Why have hormone therapies become so popular? They work, right?

Well, sort of. They work up until they become excessive and create a slow, or sometimes rapid, cascade of health mishaps. Think of your body's hormones — not just estrogen and progesterone, but also insulin and thyroid and adrenal hormones as a row of dominos neatly lined up on their ends. Exogenous (meaning outside of the body) hormones, whether they are oral contraceptives, menopause creams, or inappropriately prescribed thyroid medications, are examples of the domino at the front of the line. With a gentle push, it falls forward, sending all the others crashing down, including thyroid function.

It has often seemed as if much of my practice was made up of rehabilitating refugees from the local anti-aging clinics. I have also helped reverse burn out from oral contraceptives, progesterone and estrogen creams, and synthetic and natural thyroid hormones. When nothing else worked, and my patients still suffered from hormone overload, it occurred to me to send their skin creams in for testing. Sure enough, some of the most popular skin creams on the market today are loaded with estrogen, which companies are not required to list on the label. Unfortunately, I am not able to reveal which creams they are — the economic repercussions for labs that test these creams would be swift and severe.

HOW EXOGENOUS HORMONES — HORMONE CREAMS, ORAL CONTRACEPTIVES AND ANTI-AGING HORMONES — CAN BECOME TOXIC

When it comes to the practice of functional medicine and returning the body to a state of wellness, hormone replacement therapy, including the inappropriate use of thyroid medications, can throw so many systems into disarray that an expert must do some probing to know where to begin undoing the damage.

When a person uses exogenous hormones, she is flooding her body with an unnatural amount of hormones. This causes dysfunction in a number of ways. For one, the receptor sites for that hormone on the cells become less active in an attempt at self-protection. Thyroid hormones can't get into the cells, even though they are abundant in the bloodstream,. As a result, a person can be on thyroid medication and yet have symptoms of hypothyroidism.

Hormone production also depends upon the finely tuned communication between the brain (the hypothalamus and pituitary glands) and the hormone glands, based on feedback the brain gets on hormone activity in the body. If the brain senses there is not enough of a particular hormone in the bloodstream, it tells the glands to make more. If it senses there is too much, a message goes out to slow production. When a person floods her system with hormone creams or pills, the brain gets the message no hormones are needed and the "feedback loop" between the brain and the gland slows down or becomes dormant. After a while, it shuts down completely and is forever lost. The gland atrophies and becomes useless, and those hormone creams or pills become a medical necessity. I have frequently seen this happen with the unnecessary and prolonged use of thyroid hormones.

Excess hormones become a health risk, especially in the case of estrogen for non-menopausal women. Hormone creams cause excess amounts of the hormone to accumulate in body fat, especially in obese persons. With the build up of any hormone, the liver is put under tremendous stress to break down those hormones so they can exit the body. Chronically overburdening the liver causes it to slow down, become congested, and falter in its many functions.

Poor liver function leads to all sorts of problems, including high cholesterol, inflammation, and poor immunity. But because the liver cannot properly break down the hormones for elimination, these hormones can go back into the bloodstream in an even more toxic form than when they entered the liver. This is especially true with estrogen, which can lead to breast cancer, endometriosis, premenstrual syndrome, fibrocystic breasts, ovarian cysts, cervical dysplasia, endometrial cancer, prostate carcinoma and hyperplasia, menopause and andropause ("male menopause"). Elevated estrogen also directly affects thyroid function by hampering the conversion of T4 to active forms of the thyroid hormone T3 in the liver, and by creating too many thyroid-binding proteins so that thyroid hormones can't get into the cells.

To make matters worse, if a doctor orders hormone tests for a person taking exogenous hormones, the results may show a hormone deficiency. Why? These tests only measure the natural hormones the body is making, and do not measure synthetic or non-natural forms of hormones. Additionally, the use of hormone creams and pills inhibits the production of natural hormones so that they *are* low. When the excessive or prolonged use of hormone creams and pills creates symptoms of hormone deficiency, and then inappropriate lab testing confirms the deficiency, what does your average doctor do? That's right, he prescribes even higher doses of hormones. This is just as much the case with thyroid hormones as it is with any other hormone.

Some hormone medications, like Premarin, are an exception. They will be partially metabolized into some of the natural hormones and thus may raise blood test results.

I have found ways to get around this situation. I check levels of follicle stimulating hormone (FSH) and luteinizing hormone (LH). Because these are the hormones that communicate with the brain's pituitary gland, I know synthetic hormones are still in the person's body when these levels are depressed.

Despite the risks and consequences, there are still cases when exogenous hormones are necessary. For instance, someone's thyroid function may be so far gone that thyroid medication is necessary. Or pre- and post-menopausal women who have completely lost the ability to make estrogen can preserve brain function with the use of exogenous estrogen.

DHEA

DHEA is a popular hormone supplement because it is a precursor to other hormones and supports immune function, brain function, and fat burning. However a need for DHEA dosing is a red flag: Low DHEA usually stems from adrenal disorders and pregnenolone steal (see Chapter Seven). Overdosing or long-term use of DHEA will convert into testosterone in females and estrogen in males. If a person needs extra DHEA, supplementation should not exceed 20 mg a day for longer than one month. As a matter of fact, 10 mg is a safe standard for most people, although even 5 mg can be appropriate. The safest form of DHEA delivery is sublingual.

DETOXING HORMONES

If your feedback loop between your brain and hormone glands is still working, it is possible to restore their healthy function by detoxifying your body of excess and synthetic hormones. This step is essential to restoring healthy thyroid function. If you are currently taking thyroid hormones, and your doctor believes it may be possible to wean you off them, it is absolutely essential that you follow the protocols outlined in this book, have your thyroid levels tested regularly, and work closely with your doctor.

For my patients I recommend detoxifying excess and synthetic hormones with combination herb and nutrient formulas, and supporting the pituitary at the same time with pituitary glandulars and cofactors. It's very important that you support the pituitary during the hormone detox.

Unfortunately, this can be a very unpleasant detox. Any woman who has dealt with the severe hormone fluctuations that accompany PMS, pregnancy, or perimenopause has an idea of what she's in for. All I can say is grit your teeth and get through it, because you will feel better, and you will be rewarded with the possibility of a life free of prescription hormones.

This detox lasts 30 to 90 days, depending on how long it takes to clear the hormones. The detoxifying herbs and nutrients work primarily by restoring function to the liver's detoxification pathways that are specific to breaking down hormones for elimination. They also decongest the liver and gallbladder and thin the bile to aid in hormone clearance.

(continued)

Hashimoto's and Hormonal Imbalances

A 45-year-old woman came to our office, complaining of fatigue, extreme moods swings, poor coordination, forgetfulness, sweating, weight gain, major hair loss, joint pain, herpes-like sores on her body, loss of her monthly cycle, constipation, and water retention for three years. Her doctor performed a thyroidectomy a year earlier, and she began thyroid replacement with Synthroid, Levoxl, and Cytomel — none of which gave her relief.

Her physician then diagnosed her with Wilson's temperature syndrome and treated her using the Wilson's syndrome protocol, monitoring her body temperature combined with time-released Cytomel. Again there was no change in the way she felt. An alternative MD then treated her with bio-identical hormones. Her hair loss increased, she gained weight, and she began having heavy, debilitating periods that kept her restricted to her home. We began using the protocols developed by Dr. Kharrazian. Comprehensive blood and immune tests showed she was suffering from an autoimmune thyroid condition [after thyroid removal there can still be enough tissue remaining to stimulate an autoimmune reaction] with a viral overload. She was placed on the autoimmune protocol.

The changes in her symptoms were immediate. Within a week her fatigue and mood swings were much better. Her husband was really pleased with the results. After about five weeks she noticed new hair growth on her scalp. As the autoimmune condition was being modulated, it was necessary to eliminate the elevated hormone levels in her body caused by the bio-identical hormones and poor liver detoxification. The Cytomel was also adjusted. Her MD was reluctant to do this because he was not familiar with the need to readjust dosages. But persistence paid off, adjustments were made, and she has been able to eliminate or reduce her symptoms.

David Peterson, DC
Wellness Alternatives
Town & Country, MO

HORMONE DETOX

For 30 to 90 days the following herbs, nutrients, and glandulars taken three times a day are key to clearing excess and synthetic hormones and restoring pituitary function.

Nutritional hypoallergenic protein powder I discussed using a high quality protein powder to support gut health in Chapter Six. I also recommend this product for the hormone detox. See the accompanying dietary protocol in Chapter Six.

Phase I and Phase II liver detoxifier: A healthy liver has the ability to turn fat soluble hormones into water soluble ones so they can exit the body. With hormone toxicity, liver function becomes impaired and needs support.

- Nutritional compounds to improve Phase I and II liver detoxification. Key ingredients include molybdenum chelate, milk thistle extract seed, dandelion root, gotu kola nut, panax ginseng, L-glutathione, glycine, N-acetyl-L-cysteine, and DL-methionine. Please work with a qualified healthcare practitioner to safely and correctly use these nutrients in the right amounts.

Phase II methylation support: One of the liver's detoxification pathways is called the methylation pathway. Oral contraceptives in particular deplete the body of the essential nutrients needed for methylation, hampering detoxification.

- Nutritional compounds to support healthy methylation reactions. Key ingredients include choline, trimethylglycine, MSM, beet root, and betaine HCl. Please work with a qualified healthcare practitioner to safely and correctly use these nutrients in the right amounts.

Liver and bile decongestant: When supporting the detoxification abilities of the liver, it's absolutely essential the gallbladder is clear, otherwise toxins can get trapped in the gallbladder and back up into the liver, sabotaging the detox and making matters worse.

- Nutritional compounds to support healthy bile formation, secretion, and flow. Key ingredients include dandelion root, milk thistle seed, ginger, taurine, beet concentrate, vitamin C, and phosphatidylcholine. Please work with a qualified healthcare practitioner to safely and correctly use these nutrients in the right amounts.

Estrogen metabolism: Women who have been taking oral contraceptives or using supplemental estrogen, such as estrogen creams, may need additional support to detoxify estrogen and restore cellular sensitivity to natural estrogen.

- Nutritional compounds to optimize estrogen metabolism and receptor site response. Key ingredients include daidzein, genistein, indole-3-carbinol, B6, black cohosh, dong quai, magnesium, and methylation cofactors. Please work with a qualified healthcare practitioner to safely and correctly use these nutrients in the right amounts.

Pituitary support: Since the use of exogenous hormones causes the pituitary gland to become sluggish, it's important to support the pituitary while clearing excess hormones. This is a good time to support the thyroid gland as well.

- Nutritional compounds to support the pituitary-thyroid axis. Key ingredients include porcine thyroid gland, porcine pituitary gland, rubidium sulfate, sage leaf extract, L-arginine, gamma oryzanal, magnesium, zinc, and manganese.

- Nutritional compounds to support the hypophyseal-ovarian axis to boost follicle stimulating hormone in order to promote estrogen production. Key ingredients include tribulus terrestris, Peruvian maca, panax ginseng, and zinc.

- Nutritional compounds to help support the hypophyseal-ovarian axis to stimulate luteinizing hormone and promote progesterone production. Key ingredients include chasteberry and shepherd's purse.

Please work with a qualified healthcare practitioner to safely and correctly use these nutrients in the right amounts.

CHAPTER HIGHLIGHTS

- The use of exogenous hormones — hormone creams, hormone pills, and oral contraceptives — in the long run cause problems of hormone deficiency. Why? By overwhelming the body with excess hormones, they shut down communication between the hormone glands and the brain. The cells become resistant to hormones in attempt at self-preservation and the glands atrophy.

- Toxicity of synthetic hormones doesn't show up on blood tests of hormones. As a result, when a person complains of symptoms related to hormone deficiency, many doctors simply prescribe more hormones, which compounds the problem.

- Excess hormones accumulate in body fat, bog down liver function, and suppress pituitary function.

- If the damage is not too far gone, it is possible to clear out excess hormones and restore pituitary health with a hormone detox. If it is too late, judicious use of exogenous hormones may be warranted.

CHAPTER NINE

DON'T FORGET ABOUT THE BRAIN

The outer edges of Marie's eyebrows have virtually vanished, her eyes and face are puffy, and she complains of always being tired, sleeping poorly, and having trouble losing weight. A typical diet for Marie, a mother of four, includes toast for breakfast, a bowl of pasta or a sandwich for lunch, followed by lentils for dinner. She's a regular at her local drive-through coffee kiosk, where she orders an extra-sweet grande Milky Way latte once or twice a day. Her cupboards and her car always contain a stash of candy, and she smokes about a half of a pack of cigarettes each day. Meanwhile, she has no knowledge of such concepts as hypoglycemia, poor adrenal function, hypothyroidism or neurotransmitter deficiencies, all of which she suffers from. Her high-carb diet subjects her to extreme insulin surges multiple times a day, which stresses her adrenals causing thyroid fatigue. Her excessive caffeine and nicotine consumption not only stresses her adrenals, but also depletes her of dopamine, a brain chemical essential for thyroid function. Her birth control pills also deplete her of dopamine, as well as raise her homocysteine levels, a formidable brain stressor. Although we all have some degree of ongoing brain degeneration, Marie's way of life and her current health has sped up the degeneration of her brain considerably. It's a factor that must be taken into consideration when addressing her thyroid health.

A doctor shouldn't evaluate thyroid function without considering the brain, which is saturated with thyroid hormone receptor sites. Is it any wonder why low thyroid function causes a mental fogginess and forgetfulness? When the hypothyroidism slows down metabolism, it takes the brain down with it. Also, a key component to healthy brain function is an abundance of *neurotransmitters*, brain chemicals that allow brain cells to communicate with one another. It's common for people to become deficient in the major neurotransmitters, such as serotonin or dopamine, which in turn impacts how the thyroid functions.

THE EFFECTS OF BRAIN CHEMISTRY ON THYROID FUNCTION

Interest in supporting brain function has exploded recently in the alternative health world. People are discovering the therapeutic power of amino acids, herbs, and nutrients that support the brain's neurotransmitters. We're increasingly understanding how the factors that lead to poor thyroid health — bad diet, unstable blood sugar control, adrenal stress, and gut infections — also lead to poor brain health, including brain tissue inflammation and degeneration, and a deficiency of neurotransmitters. When neurotransmitters become altered, brain function weakens and produces a host of symptoms that are surprisingly common in today's world, such as depression and poor memory.

By supplementing with amino acids and specific nutrients (while improving our diets and exercising more), we can boost the amount and activity of our brain's neurotransmitters, and hence many facets of health, including thyroid health. And by supporting our thyroid health we can help protect the health of our brain. Healthy thyroid function exerts a powerful protective effect on the brain.[322] [323] In fact, an unsupported thyroid condition guarantees some degree of brain degeneration in time.[324] [325] [326]

The master neurotransmitters are serotonin and dopamine, and research shows that deficiencies or breakdowns in the pathways of either one impact thyroid health in specific ways, such as hampering conversion of T4 to T3 and slowing down the brain's communication with the thyroid.[327] [328] [329] [330] [331] [332] [333] People with a deficiency will often have symptoms of depressed thyroid function with TSH below 1.8 and T4 below 6.

In addition to classic thyroid symptoms, these patients suffer from symptoms of either a serotonin or dopamine deficiency (or both).

Serotonin deficiency symptoms include:
- Loss of pleasure in hobbies and interests
- Feeling overwhelmed with ideas to manage
- Inner rage
- Paranoia
- Depression
- Not enjoying life
- Lack of artistic appreciation
- Depression with lack of sunlight
- Loss of enthusiasm for favorite activities
- Not enjoying favorite foods
- Not enjoying relationships
- Unable to fall into a deep, restful sleep
- Feelings of dependency on others
- More susceptible to pain
- Unprovoked anger

Dopamine deficiency symptoms include:
- Feelings of worthlessness
- Feelings of hopelessness
- Self-destructive thoughts
- Inability to handle stress
- Anger and aggression under stress

- Desire to isolate from others
- Unexplained lack of concern for family and friends
- Distracted easily
- Inability to finish tasks
- Need for caffeine to feel mentally alert
- Low libido
- Loss of temper for minor reasons

Clinically, the most common cause of both serotonin and dopamine deficiencies is poor blood sugar control (hypoglycemia, insulin resistance, or diabetes), a condition that affects the average American to some degree. To encourage brain health, I recommend nutrients to support a healthy response to insulin and balance blood sugar. (For more information on managing blood sugar, see Chapter Five.) Since poor adrenal health always accompanies dyglycemia, it is another major factor in brain degeneration and neurotransmitter deficiencies. In addition to blood sugar support, I also recommend adrenal adaptogens and phosphatidylserine. Although both nutrients support the adrenal glands, they have been shown to especially support brain health and neurotransmitter activity. (For more information on supporting the adrenals see Chapter Seven.) The use of a thyroid and pituitary support may also be useful to nutritionally support TSH production from the pituitary gland.

Dopamine is the feel-good neurotransmitter. That's why the substances that raise dopamine levels — chocolate, caffeine, nicotine, marijuana, and many recreational drugs — are so popular. Although these substances initially elevate dopamine levels, long-term use eventually causes dopamine deficiency.

Methyl donors, substances that nourish the brain in a process called methylation, are also crucial for dopamine synthesis. Methyl donor deficiency should be considered if you have low stomach acid, take anti-acid medication, or take an estrogen replacement, such as oral contraceptives, which deplete methyl donors. Sublingual methyl B-12 or nutrients that support healthy methylation are suggested for dopamine deficiency.

Although all the aspects covered in this book are fundamental to managing low thyroid function, it's always worth managing the neurotransmitter deficiency and its causes, too.[334] [335] I recommend supplementing with nutritional compounds that support the healthy response, activity, and synthesis of either dopamine or serotonin, depending on symptoms. The right nutrients can provide natural precursors to their respective neurotransmitters, improve the activity of serotonin and dopamine receptor sites, and provide cofactors necessary for neurotransmitter synthesis, in turn supporting thyroid health. Please work with a qualified healthcare practitioner to safely and correctly use these nutrients in the right amounts.

DOPAMINE'S INTIMATE CONNECTION WITH THE THYROID

Although all the brain's neurotransmitters are important for thyroid health, dopamine in particular has an intimate relationship with the thyroid. Dopamine stimulates the brain's hypothalamus to release TSH, impacts the production of T3 at the thyroid gland, and the conversion of T4 to T3 in the brain itself. It's that conversion to T3 that allows thyroid hormones to get into brain cells and keep them active so you are mentally alert and have a keen memory.[336] [337] [338] In return, thyroid hormones stimulate the production of dopamine in both the brain and the kidneys (the kidneys synthesize neurotransmitters to be used by the body). Low thyroid function decreases the release of dopamine from the midbrain, which makes it hard to maintain thyroid function.[339] As you can see, dopamine and thyroid hormones are so intertwined that a vicious cycle of deficiency develops easily. That's why I always consider dopamine deficiency when my patients have low thyroid function.

The amino acid precursor to dopamine is tyrosine. As you will recall, I warned those with low thyroid function against taking tyrosine if they are in an elevated stress response, as tyrosine stimulates the production of adrenal hormones that could suppress TPO production. Although it's true that tyrosine should not be given willy-nilly to everyone with low thyroid symptoms, when dopamine deficiency is evident, the judicious use of tyrosine clinically is warranted.

Lastly, if poor brain function is not enough to have you consider a dopamine deficiency, consider this: Hypothyroidism can put you at an increased risk for Parkinson's Disease, a disease that includes a profound dopamine deficiency. In fact, the clinician would be wise to distinguish early symptoms of Parkinson's disease from hypothyroidism and dopamine deficiency.[340]

Nutritional Support for low thyroid function due to neurotransmitter deficiency:

Serotonin support

- Nutritional compounds support serotonin response, activity and synthesis. Key ingredients include 5-HTP, St. John's Wort, SAMe, niacinamide, B6, methyl B12, and magnesium citrate.

Dopamine support

- Nutritional compounds to support healthy dopamine response, activity, and synthesis. Key ingredients include mucuna pruriens, beta-phenylethylamine (PEA), blueberry extract, D, L-phenylalanine (DLPA), N-acetyl-tyrosine, pyridoxal-5-phosphate (P-5-P), glutathione cofactors.

- Sublingual methyl B-12, or other nutrients to support healthy methylation. Key ingredients include choline, trimethylglycine, MSM, beetroot, and betaine HCl.

Hypoglycemia support

- Nutritional compounds to support healthy blood sugar balance. Key ingredients include chromium, bovine adrenal gland, choline bitartrate, bovine liver gland, bovine pancreas gland, inositol, L-carnitine, co-enzyme Q10, rubidium chelate, and vanadium aspartate.

Insulin resistance support

- Nutritional compounds to support a healthy response to insulin.. Key ingredients include chromium, vanadium, alpha-lipoic acid, mixed tocopherols, magnesium, biotin, zinc, inositol, and gymnema sylvestre.

Neurotransmitter balance from stress

- Nutritional compounds to help the body adapt to physiological stress responses. Key ingredients include panax ginseng, Siberian ginseng, ashwagandha, holy basil leaf extract, rhodiola rosea, punarva, and pantethine.

- Liposomal cream that delivers nutritional compounds to modulate the stress response. Key ingredient includes 2,000 mg a day of phosphatidylserine.

- Nutritional compounds to support the pituitary-thyroid axis. Key ingredients include porcine thyroid gland, porcine pituitary gland, rubidium sulfate, sage leaf extract, L-arginine, gamma oryzanal, magnesium, zinc, and manganese.

Please work with a qualified healthcare practitioner to safely and correctly use these nutrients in the right amounts.

CHAPTER HIGHLIGHTS

- The brain is saturated with thyroid receptors. Healthy thyroid function is integral to healthy brain function.

- Brain health and sufficiency of the neurotransmitters serotonin and dopamine are important for thyroid function.

- Clinically, poor blood sugar control is the most common cause of neurotransmitter deficiencies.

- There is an intimate relationship between dopamine and thyroid function.

CHAPTER TEN

THE 22 PATTERNS OF LOW THYROID FUNCTION

Although I introduced six patterns of low thyroid function that can be identified with blood tests in Chapter Four, I have actually identified 22 different factors that can cause low thyroid function. The medical literature refers to all of them and this book discusses most of them. Such a long list illustrates how sensitive the thyroid is to subtle and not-so-subtle metabolic shifts. Although the standard of health care has frequently been to correct some of these problems with thyroid medication, I believe it is wiser to correct the problem that caused the thyroid to falter in the first place. Poor blood sugar control, gut infections, adrenal problems, hormonal imbalances, irregular immune function, and poor brain function are factors that can depress the thyroid or drive an autoimmune thyroid condition. While prescription thyroid hormones might normalize blood test results, they won't address what caused the thyroid to malfunction in the first place, and dietary and lifestyle changes are almost always at the core of restoring thyroid health. Remember, the thyroid is like the engine light in your car. If it turns on, what would you rather do — remove the light or figure out what's wrong with the engine?

TWENTY-TWO PATTERNS OF LOW THYROID FUNCTION

1. Hypothalamus paraventricular defect relates to central nervous system deficiency of serotonin, leading to low TSH[341 342 343 344 345] The hypothalamus is the part of the brain that directs hormone function, including that of the thyroid, via the pituitary gland. Dysglycemia (hypoglycemia, insulin resistance, and diabetes) is the most common cause of a serotonin deficiency, which hampers communication between the brain and thyroid gland. People with this type of low thyroid function will have symptoms of serotonin deficiency, a TSH below the functional range of 1.8, and a T4 below 6.

Nutritional Support

Serotonin support

- Nutritional compounds to support serotonin response, activity, and synthesis. Key ingredients include 5-HTP, St. John's Wort, SAMe, niacinamide, B6, methyl B12, and magnesium citrate.

Blood sugar support

Low blood sugar

- Nutritional compounds to support healthy blood sugar balance. Key ingredients include chromium, bovine adrenal gland, choline bitartrate, bovine liver gland, bovine pancreas gland, inositol, L-carnitine, co-enzyme Q10, rubidium chelate, and vanadium aspartate.

Insulin resistance

- Nutritional compounds to support a healthy response to insulin resistance. Key ingredients include chromium, vanadium, alpha lipoic acid, mixed tocopherols, magnesium, biotin, zinc, inositol, and gymnema sylvestre.

- Botanical compounds to support a healthy response to insulin resistance. Key ingredients include banaba leaf extract, maitake mushroom, bitter melon, gymnema sylvestre leaf extract, and nopal cactus.

Adrenal/hypothalamus support

- Nutritional compounds to help the body adapt to physiological stress responses. Key ingredients include panax ginseng, Siberian ginseng, ashwagandha, holy basil leaf extract, rhodiola rosea, punarva, and pantethine.

- Liposomal cream that delivers nutritional compounds to modulate the stress response. Key ingredient includes 2,000 mg a day of phosphatidylserine.

Pituitary support of TSH

- Nutritional compounds to support the pituitary-thyroid axis. Key ingredients include porcine thyroid gland, porcine pituitary gland, rubidium sulfate, sage leaf extract, L-arginine, gamma oryzanal, magnesium, zinc, and manganese.

Please work with a qualified healthcare practitioner to safely and correctly use these nutrients in the right amounts.

2. Hypothalamus paraventricular defect relates to central nervous system deficiency of dopamine, leading to low TSH[346 347 348 349] The hypothalamus is the part of the brain that directs hormone function, including that of the thyroid, via the pituitary gland. Dysglycemia (hypoglycemia, insulin resistance, and diabetes) is the most common cause of a dopamine deficiency, which hampers communication between the brain and thyroid gland. Also, the importance of methylation cannot be overlooked with a dopamine deficiency and should be addressed as well. People with this type of low thyroid function have symptoms of dopamine deficiency, a TSH below the functional range of 1.8, and T4 below 6.

Nutritional Support

Dopamine support

- Nutritional compounds support healthy dopamine response, activity, and synthesis. Key ingredients include mucuna pruriens, beta-phenylethylamine (PEA), blueberry extract, D, L-phenylalanine (DLPA), N-acetyl-tyrosine, pyridoxal-5-phosphate (P-5-P), and glutathione cofactors.

Blood sugar support

Low blood sugar

- Nutritional compounds to support healthy blood sugar balance. Key ingredients include chromium, bovine adrenal gland, choline bitartrate, bovine liver gland, bovine pancreas gland, inositol, L-carnitine, co-enzyme Q10, rubidium chelate, and vanadium aspartate.

Insulin resistance

- Nutritional compounds to support a healthy response to insulin resistance. Key ingredients include chromium, vanadium, alpha-lipoic acid, mixed tocopherols, magnesium, biotin, zinc, inositol, and gymnema sylvestre.

- Botanical compounds to support a healthy response to insulin resistance. Key ingredients include banaba leaf extract, maitake mushroom, bitter melon, gymnema sylvestre, and nopal cactus.

Adrenal/hypothalamus support

- Nutritional compounds to help the body adapt to physiological stress responses. Key ingredients include panax ginseng, Siberian ginseng, ashwagandha, holy basil leaf extract, rhodiola rosea, punarva, and pantethine.

- Liposomal cream that delivers nutritional compounds to modulate the stress response. Key ingredient includes 2,000 mg a day of phosphatidylserine.

Pituitary support of TSH

- Nutritional compounds to support the pituitary-thyroid axis. Key ingredients include porcine thyroid gland, porcine pituitary gland, rubidium sulfate, sage leaf extract, L-arginine, gamma oryzanal, magnesium, zinc, and manganese.

Methylation support

- Sublingual methyl B12 and nutritional compounds to support healthy methylation reactions. Key ingredients include choline, trimethylglycine, MSM, beetroot, and betaine HCl.

Please work with a qualified healthcare practitioner to safely and correctly use these nutrients in the right amounts.

3. Hypothalamus paraventricular defect promoted by cytokines, leading to low TSH[350 351 352 353 354 355] Inflammation from gut infections, chronic viral infection, Lyme disease, food intolerances, molds, or environmental compounds can damage the hypothalamus and affect its ability to communicate with the thyroid gland. These patients typically will have low white blood cell counts, a TSH below the functional range of 1.8, and a T4 below 6.

Nutritional Support

Regulatory T-cell support
- Emulsified vitamin D and liposomal glutathione and superoxide dismutase cream.

TH-1 response or TH-2 response support
- Nutritional compounds to support the TH-1 response. Key ingredients include astragalus root extract, echinacea purpurea root, licorice root extract, porcine thymus gland, lemon balm, maitake mushroom, and pomegranate.

- Nutritional compounds to support the TH-2 response. Key ingredients include pine bark extract, grape seed extract, green tea extract, resveratrol, and pycnogenol.

For GI antigen support
- Nutritional compounds to support the immune system during minor bacterial, fungal, and parasitic infections and create a healthy digestive terrain. Key ingredients include golden seal extract, oregano oil extract, barberry extract, Oregon grape root, berberis aristata extract, coptis chinensis extract, and yerba mansa.

Please work with a qualified healthcare practitioner to safely and correctly use these nutrients in the right amounts.

4. Hypothalamus paraventricular defect promoted by elevated prolactin[356] [357] [358] [359] The hormone prolactin is very sensitive to shifts of dopamine, thyroid hormones, progesterone, and serotonin. These shifts can elevate prolactin, suppressing both TSH, and the luteinizing hormone (LH), leading to depression of the sex hormones in women and men. Prolactinoma, a benign pituitary tumor, may also elevate prolactin, again suppressing TSH.

Nutritional Support

Dopamine support

- Nutritional compounds support healthy dopamine response, activity, and synthesis. Key ingredients include mucuna pruriens, beta-phenylethylamine (PEA), blueberry extract, D, L-phenylalanine (DLPA), N-acetyl-tyrosine, pyridoxal-5-phosphate (P-5-P), and glutathione cofactors.

LH support in females

- Nutritional compounds help support the hypophyseal-ovarian axis to stimulate luteinizing hormone in order to increase progesterone production. Key ingredients include chaste berry and shepherd's purse.

LH support in males

- Nutritional compounds support the hypophyseal-gonadal axis to stimulate luteinizing hormone in men in order to boost testosterone production. Key ingredients include tribulus terrestris, Peruvian maca, panax ginseng, and zinc.

Please work with a qualified healthcare practitioner to safely and correctly use these nutrients in the right amounts.

5. Pituitary suppression from cortisol leading to low TSH[360] [361] [362] [363] [364] [365] This pattern (See Chapter Four) occurs when elevated cortisol from adrenal stress suppresses pituitary function and thus TSH levels. These patients will have a TSH below the functional range of 1.8, and T4 below 6. The main causes for this pattern are active infection, dysglycemia, unrelenting stress, and, most commonly, hypoglycemia or insulin resistance.

Blood sugar support

Low blood sugar

- Nutritional compounds to support healthy blood sugar balance. Key ingredients include chromium, bovine adrenal gland, choline bitartrate, bovine liver gland, bovine pancreas gland, inositol, L-carnitine, co-enzyme Q10, rubidium chelate, and vanadium aspartate.

Insulin resistance

- Nutritional compounds to support a healthy response to insulin resistance. Key ingredients include chromium, vanadium, alpha lipoic acid, mixed tocopherols, magnesium, biotin, zinc, inositol, and gymnema sylvestre.

- Botanical compounds to support a healthy response to insulin resistance. Key ingredients include banaba leaf extract, maitake mushroom, bitter melon, gymnema sylvestre, and nopal cactus.

Adrenal/hypothalamus support

- Nutritional compounds to help the body adapt to physiological stress responses. Key ingredients include panax ginseng, Siberian ginseng, ashwagandha, holy basil leaf extract, rhodiola rosea, punarva, and pantethine.

- Liposomal cream that delivers nutritional compounds to modulate the stress response. Key ingredient includes 2,000 mg a day of phosphatidylserine.

Pituitary support of TSH

- Nutritional compounds to support the pituitary-thyroid axis. Key ingredients include porcine thyroid gland, porcine pituitary gland, rubidium sulfate, sage leaf extract, L-arginine, gamma oryzanal, magnesium, zinc, and manganese.

Please work with a qualified healthcare practitioner to safely and correctly use these nutrients in the right amounts.

6. Thyroid tissue disorder related to thyroid peroxidase (TPO) autoimmune response:[366] TPO is the enzyme in the thyroid responsible for the production of thyroid hormones and is a common site for autoimmune attacks. A positive TPO antibody test suggests Hashimoto's disease.

Nutritional support

Regulatory T-cell Support

- Emulsified vitamin D and liposomal glutathione and superoxide dismutase cream.

TH-1 response or TH-2 response

- Nutritional compounds to support the TH-1 response. Key ingredients include astragalus root extract, echinacea purpurea root, licorice root extract, porcine thymus gland, lemon balm, maitake mushroom, and pomegranate.

- Nutritional compounds to support the TH-2 response. Key ingredients include pine bark extract, grape seed extract, green tea extract, resveratrol, and pycnogenol.

Please work with a qualified healthcare practitioner to safely and correctly use these nutrients in the right amounts.

7. Thyroid tissue disorder related to thyroglobulin (TGB) autoimmune response[367][368]

TGB is produced in the thyroid gland and is used to produce thyroid hormones. It is also a common site for autoimmune attacks. A positive TGB antibody tests suggests Hashimoto's.

Nutritional support

Regulatory T-cell Support:

- Emulsified vitamin D and liposomal glutathione and superoxide dismutase cream.

Nutrients that support TH-1 response or TH-2 response

- Nutritional compounds to support the TH-1 response. Key ingredients include astragalus root extract, echinacea purpurea root, licorice root extract, porcine thymus gland, lemon balm, maitake mushroom, and pomegranate.

- Nutritional compounds to support the TH-2 response. Key ingredients include pine bark extract, grape seed extract, green tea extract, resveratrol, and pycnogenol.

Please work with a qualified healthcare practitioner to safely and correctly use these nutrients in the right amounts.

8. Down-regulated TPO activity related to progesterone deficiency

Progesterone increases TPO activity.[369] This is why a woman's body temperature is higher when she ovulates — progesterone surges at ovulation, stimulating TPO activity and overall metabolism. Low progesterone can lead to low thyroid hormones, although their levels of TSH, T4, and T3 will not fall outside of normal lab ranges. Dysglycemia is a common culprit for low progesterone.

Nutritional Support

Pituitary/LH support

- Nutritional compounds help support the hypophyseal-ovarian axis to stimulate luteinizing hormone in order to boost progesterone production. Key ingredients include chaste berry and shepherd's purse.

Blood sugar support

Low blood sugar

- Nutritional compounds to support healthy blood sugar balance. Key ingredients include chromium, bovine adrenal gland, choline bitartrate, bovine liver gland, bovine pancreas gland, inositol, L-carnitine, co-enzyme Q10, rubidium chelate, and vanadium aspartate.

Insulin resistance

- Nutritional compounds to support a healthy response to insulin resistance. Key ingredients include chromium, vanadium, alpha lipoic acid, mixed tocopherols, magnesium, biotin, zinc, inositol, and gymnema sylvestre.

- Botanical compounds to support a healthy response to insulin resistance. Key ingredients include banaba leaf extract, maitake mushroom, bitter melon, gymnema sylvestre, and nopal cactus.

Adrenal/hypothalamus support

- Nutritional compounds to help the body adapt to physiological stress responses. Key ingredients include panax ginseng,

Siberian ginseng, ashwagandha, holy basil leaf extract, rhodiola rosea, punarva, and pantethine.

- Liposomal cream that delivers nutritional compounds to modulate the stress response. Key ingredient includes 2,000 mg a day of phosphatidylserine.

Adrenal Exhaustion support
- Liposomal cream that delivers nutritional compounds to support low adrenal function. Key ingredients include licorice, B vitamins, DHEA, and pregnenolone.

Please work with a qualified healthcare practitioner to safely and correctly use these nutrients in the right amounts.

9. Down-regulated TPO from deficiency of cofactors[370][371][372][373][374] Various nutrients are important for the manufacture and function of adequate levels of TPO, which is responsible for thyroid hormone production. Poor diet and gut function can lead to a deficiency in these nutrients (See Chapter Four).

Nutritional Support
TPO support
- Nutritional compounds to support healthy thyroid function. Key ingredients include porcine thyroid gland, ashwagandha, vitamin A, vitamin D, selenium, and zinc.

- Nutritional compounds to help support T4 to T3 synthesis. Key ingredients include guggulu, selenium, zinc, and antiperoxidative compounds.

Please work with a qualified healthcare practitioner to safely and correctly use these nutrients in the right amounts.

10. Down-regulated 5'deiodinase activity from deficiency of cofactors[375][376][377][378][379][380][381][382][383][384] The 5'deiodinase enzyme is responsible for converting T4 to T3, the only form of thyroid hormone the body can use. Poor diet and gut function can lead to a deficiency in the nutrients responsible for adequate function of this enzyme.

Nutritional Support
5'deiodinase support
- Nutritional compounds to support healthy thyroid function. Key ingredients include porcine thyroid gland, ashwagandha, vitamin A, vitamin D, selenium, and zinc.
- Nutritional compounds to help support T4 to T3 synthesis. Key ingredients include guggulu, selenium, zinc, and antiperoxidative compounds.

Please work with a qualified healthcare practitioner to safely and correctly use these nutrients in the right amounts.

11. Down-regulated 5'deiodinase from gastrointestinal dysbiosis and lipopolysaccharides[385] [386] [387] About 20 percent of the body's T3 depends on healthy gut flora for conversion. Dysbiosis and bacterial infections down-regulate the 5'deiodinase enzyme, which hampers this conversion.

12. Down-regulated 5'deiodinase activity from elevated cytokines[388] [389] [390] [391] [392] Inflammation from gut infections, chronic viral infection, Lyme's disease, food intolerances, molds, or environmental compounds can disrupt the conversion of T4 to T3. Inflammation elevates the levels of cytokines, which down regulates the 5'deiodinase enzyme. Because T3 levels do not affect TSH levels, it should be standard to measure T3. Normal TSH, normal T4, and a depressed T3 strongly suggest down-regulation of the 5'deiodinase enzyme.

13. Down-regulated 5'deiodinase activity from elevated cortisol[393] [394] [395] Elevated cortisol from chronic stress down-regulates the 5'deiodinase enzyme, inhibiting the conversion of T4 to T3. In the past it was believed T4 was shunted into irreversible and inactive T3. New research shows that there is not an increase in reverse T3, but rather poor clearance of reverse T3 due to elevated cortisol.[396] [397] [398]

14. Down-regulated 5'deiodinase activity from peripheral deficiencies of serotonin[399] Serotonin influences the hypothalamus-pituitary-thyroid axis, as well as T3 conversion. Peripheral serotonin deficiency down-regulates these functions.

15. Down-regulated 5'deiodinase activity from peripheral deficiencies of dopamine[400] Dopamine influences the hypothalamus-pituitary-thyroid axis as well as T3 conversion. Peripheral dopamine deficiency down regulates these functions.

16. Up-regulated 5'deiodinase activity from elevated testosterone[401] Elevated levels of testosterone in women create this pattern of too much T4 being converted into T3. The excess production of T3 overwhelms the cells and they develop a resistance to the thyroid hormone. This pattern is most often found in women with insulin resistance and PCOS or in men who use testosterone creams.

17. Elevations of thyroid binding globulin (TGB) leading to decreased production of thyroid hormones TGB is the protein responsible for transporting thyroid hormones. When TGB levels increase, the percentage of free-faction thyroid hormones drop. This is evidenced by a depressed T3 uptake or low free thyroid hormones, despite a normal TSH. This pattern is typically due to a source of exogenous estrogens, particularly oral contraceptives or Premarin.[402] [403] [404] [405]

Nutritional support
Estrogen clearance support
- Nutritional compounds to improve Phase I and II liver detoxification. Key ingredients include molybdenum chelate, milk thistle extract seed, dandelion root, gotu kola nut, panax ginseng, L-glutathione, glycine, N-acetyl-L-cysteine, and DL-methionine.

- Nutritional compounds to support healthy bile formation, secretion, and flow. Key ingredients include dandelion root, milk thistle seed, ginger, taurine, beet concentrate, vitamin C, and phosphatidylcholine.

- Nutritional compounds to support healthy methylation reactions. Key ingredients include choline, trimethylglycine, MSM, beetroot, and betaine HCl.

Please work with a qualified healthcare practitioner to safely and correctly use these nutrients in the right amounts.

18. Depression of thyroid-binding globulin (TGB) leading to increased production of thyroid hormones and resistance When TGB drops, the amount of free thyroid hormones rises. In this pattern, the TSH is normal. The free thyroid hormone elevation is typically subtle and does not create hyperthyroid symptoms. Instead, the person develops symptoms of hypothyroidism due to thyroid receptor-site resistance. This pattern is typically caused by elevations of estrogens associated with insulin resistance and may also be promoted by high testosterone,[406] such as occurs in women with insulin resistance or in men who use testosterone creams and medications.[407][408][409]

Nutritional support

Insulin resistance support

- Nutritional compounds to support a healthy response to insulin resistance. Key ingredients include chromium, vanadium, alpha-lipoic acid, mixed tocopherols, magnesium, biotin, zinc, inositol, and gymnema sylvestre.

- Botanical compounds to support a healthy response to insulin resistance. Key ingredients include banaba leaf extract, maitake mushroom, bitter melon, gymnema sylvestre, and nopal cactus.

- Nutritional compounds to support healthy insulin receptor sensitivity. Key ingredients include EPA, DHA, taurine, green tea extract, and odorless garlic extract.

- Nutritional compounds to help the body adapt to physiological stress responses. Key ingredients include panax ginseng, Siberian ginseng, ashwagandha, holy basil leaf extract, rhodiola rosea, punarva, and pantethine.

- Liposomal cream that delivers nutritional compounds to modulate the stress response. Key ingredient includes 2,000 mg a day of phosphatidylserine.

Testosterone clearance

- Nutritional compounds to improve Phase I and II liver detoxification. Key ingredients include molybdenum chelate, milk thistle extract seed, dandelion root, gotu kola nut, panax ginseng, L-glutathione, glycine, N-acetyl-L-cysteine, and DL-methionine.

- Nutritional compounds to support healthy bile formation, secretion and flow. Key ingredients include dandelion root, milk thistle seed, ginger, taurine, beet concentrate, vitamin C, and phosphatidylcholine.

- Nutritional compounds to support healthy methylation reactions. Key ingredients include choline, trimethylglycine, MSM, beetroot, and betaine HCl.

Please work with a qualified healthcare practitioner to safely and correctly use these nutrients in the right amounts.

19. Thyroid resistance promoted by an elevation of cytokines

Pro-inflammatory TH-1 cytokines have been shown to decrease a cell's sensitivity to thyroid hormones, causing symptoms of hypothyroidism.[410 411 412 413] This is especially apparent with people on thyroid replacement hormone medication who are still suffering from symptoms of low thyroid activity. The effect of a chronic inflammatory immune response on thyroid receptor sites should be considered in this case.

20. Thyroid resistance promoted by elevations of cortisol[414 415 416]

Chronic elevations in the adrenals hormone cortisol have been shown to decrease the sensitivity of cellular receptor sites to thyroid hormones.

Nutritional support

To dampen cortisol

- Nutritional compounds to help the body adapt to physiological stress responses. Key ingredients include panax ginseng, Siberian ginseng, ashwagandha, holy basil leaf extract, rhodiola rosea, punarva, and pantethine.

- Liposomal cream that delivers nutritional compounds to modulate the stress response. Key ingredient includes 2,000 mg a day of phosphatidylserine.

Please work with a qualified healthcare practitioner to safely and correctly use these nutrients in the right amounts.

21. Thyroid resistance promoted by deficiencies of vitamin A[417]

Thyroid hormone receptor sites must be sufficient in vitamin A in order to activate thyroid hormone. A deficiency in vitamin A hampers receptor site function so that the cell is resistant to thyroid hormones, leading to hypothyroidism symptoms. Vitamin A deficiency should be suspected with anemia, liver disease, cirrhosis, and alcoholism. The key clinical symptom of vitamin A deficiency is difficulty with night vision not related to astigmatism.

Nutritional support

Vitamin A with thyroid cofactors Nutritional compounds to support healthy thyroid function. Key ingredients include porcine thyroid gland, ashwagandha, vitamin A, vitamin D, selenium, and zinc.

22. Thyroid resistance promoted by homocysteine[418]

Elevated homocysteine has been shown to dampen the expression of thyroid hormones at the receptor site. Elevated homocysteine should always be considered in individuals who take antacid medications, oral contraceptives, and estrogen, or who have hypochlorydria and *H.pylori* infections. This pattern is difficult to identify since the patient has hypothyroid symptoms but normal blood tests. Since elevated homocysteine produces no symptoms, a blood test should be run to identify this pattern.

Nutritional support

Methyl donor support

- Nutritional compounds to support healthy methylation reactions. Key ingredients include choline, trimethylglycine, MSM, beetroot, and betaine HCl.

Please work with a qualified healthcare practitioner to safely and correctly use these nutrients in the right amounts.

CHAPTER HIGHLIGHTS

- I have identified 22 patterns of metabolic thyroid disorders that often produce normal blood test results.

- You cannot assess the thyroid without considering the impact the immune system, hormones, nutrition, and brain function has on the thyroid. Supporting hypothyroid symptoms involves addressing these factors.

- Low thyroid symptoms are like your car's engine light. Would you rather turn off the light with thyroid hormones that give you a normal blood test result or check the engine and fix it?

RESOURCES — WEBSITE

www.thyroidbook.com

On the website www.thyroidbook.com the person with low thyroid symptoms will find a list of qualified health care professionals around the country who have been educated in the principles discussed in *Why Do I Still Have Thyroid Symptoms?* These practitioners will use the right diagnostic tests and nutritional support to guide you safely and efficiently toward finding lasting relief from your low thyroid symptoms.

I have trained a team of practicing doctors to help me teach my functional medicine principles so this information can be brought to more practitioners around the country every year. My website is your starting point for surpassing outdated models of care in both conventional and alternative medicine. By applying these principles, you can supercharge your practice by offering genuine relief to a neglected patient population.

Supporting thyroid health is just one facet of what I research, practice, and teach. I will apply the functional principles introduced in *Why Do I Still Have Thyroid Symptoms?* to future books on other metabolic disorders. Please visit the website for updates on these upcoming projects.

Although a book is a good way to collect a wealth of information into one basket, functional medicine is hardly a static topic. My information is always evolving and being refined as I continue my own education. My blog http://drknews.com allows you to stay updated on new information, new concepts, and various facets of functional medicine.

I encourage patients and doctors to visit the website and post testimonials of your experiences using the functional medicine principles discussed in this book. Statistics show millions of Americans suffer needlessly from low thyroid symptoms. Your published testimonials will help fulfill my mission to bring this information to as many people possible. Together we have the potential to save countless numbers of people from prescription drugs and their damaging side effects or from missing out on a vibrant life experience due to chronic, irresolvable low thyroid symptoms.

RESOURCES —
NUTRITIONAL COMPOUNDS

Note: The Food and Drug Administration has not evaluated the statements below. These compounds are not intended to diagnose, treat, cure, or prevent any disease.

As my practice evolved, I needed products that supported the mechanisms I was discovering, and they simply didn't exist. Therefore, working with a staff of scientists and doctors, I formulated my own. I use products containing the following compounds regularly in my practice to nutritionally support Hashimoto's and address functional hypothyroidism.

The products I have formulated are available through a licensed or certified health care provider who has been trained by me on how to use them properly. It is important to work with a practitioner so that these nutritional compounds can be used safely and correctly to your benefit. Please visit my website at www.thyroidbook.com to find health care providers who can help you nutritionally support your thyroid health and for articles and resources to help you expand upon and stay updated on the concepts in this book.

1. INSULIN RESISTANCE: Nutritional compounds to support a healthy response to insulin

These nutrients support normal insulin receptor site sensitivity and intercellular signaling alterations. Insulin disorders are estimated to impact 20 percent of the population and are associated with many diseases, such as obesity, essential fatty acid defects, and alterations in metabolism. These herbs, vitamins, and minerals support healthy insulin receptor sensitivity and blood sugar metabolism.

KEY INGREDIENTS
RESEARCH COMMENTARY
CHROMIUM is an essential nutrient for insulin resistance, especially when one considers the evidence that chromium deficiencies are common in the United States and that chromium levels are depleted by a diet of refined carbohydrates and sugars. There is evidence that chromium deficiency results in insulin resistance.[7] [8] [9] Chromium, also known as "glucose tolerance factor," appears to optimize the impact of insulin on receptor sites and therefore improve glucose uptake.[10] [11] Studies have demonstrated that chromium normalizes postprandial glucose and insulin levels, glycated hemoglobin, and hypercholesterolemia. [12] [13] [14] [15] [16]

VANADIUM is an important mineral when it comes to managing insulin resistance. It appears to have insulin-like impact on receptor sites, and improves the transport of glucose transporter to the cell membrane to allow cells to intake serum glucose.[17] [18] [19] This physiologic impact is of great importance because most defects in insulin resistance involve intercellular transduction reactions that vanadium appears to enhance. Numerous studies have demonstrated the positive role vanadium plays in managing insulin resistance.[20] [21] [22]

ALPHA-LIPOIC ACID is a sulfur-containing substance that seems to improve insulin resistance by increasing the activation of glucose transporters (GLUT1 and 4) which enhance glucose disposal by sensitizing tissues to insulin and by restoring proper intracellular redox states which then reset signaling and response to insulin.[23][24][25][26] Alpha-lipoic acid has also shown to improve glucose metabolism, reduce serum lactate and pyruvate and improve mitochondrial oxidative phosphorylation.[27] Alpha-lipoic acid is also a powerful antioxidant that can help quench insulin-induced oxidative stress patterns.[28][29] Numerous studies have shown the positive impact of alpha-lipoic acid for insulin-resistant disorders.[30][31][32]

MIXED TOCOPHEROLS. Vitamin E (Tocopherols) has been shown to improve insulin sensitivity, improve serum triglycerides, and LDL and aid not only in the oxidative complications of diabetes, but also in the prevention of the disease.[33][34][35][36][37][38]

MAGNESIUM has been shown to improve insulin resistance. It appears to optimize insulin secretion, activate glucose transport for insulin-mediated glucose uptake and to improve insulin intercellular transcriptional response.[39][40][41] Furthermore, insulin resistance has been reported in individuals with low magnesium status.[42][43][44]

BIOTIN supplementation has been shown to improve insulin response to glucose load, lower post-prandial glucose levels, and up-regulate the enzyme glucokinase which is responsible for the first step in glucose utilization by the liver.[45][46][47][48]

ZINC is an important mineral in the support of insulin resistance. Zinc has protective effects against beta-cell destruction, improves insulin sensitivity, and plays an important role in insulin metabolism.[49] There have been strong correlations with low zinc status and increased risk for insulin resistance as well as evidence that diabetics excrete large amounts of zinc and therefore require supplementation.[50][51][52]

INOSITOL has shown the ability to re-establish normal myoinositol levels in deficient neurons and therefore may be helpful in cases of diabetic neuropathy.[53]

GYMNEMA SYLVESTRE has demonstrated positive impacts in managing insulin resistance. It has demonstrated the ability to reduce insulin requirements, decrease fasting blood sugar, enhance the action of insulin and even the ability to regenerate pancreas beta-cells.[1][2][3][4] It does not encourage the endogenous production of insulin and if given to healthy volunteers does not produce any blood sugar-lowering or hypoglycemic effects.[5][6]

2. INSULIN RESISTANCE: Botanicals to support a healthy response to insulin

These botanicals provide a nutritionally aggressive support system for insulin resistance. Essential fatty acids and adrenal support should be used to support stable and healthy cortisol levels.

KEY INGREDIENTS
RESEARCH COMMENTARY

Banaba Leaf Extract contains triterpenoid, lagerstroemin, flosin B, reginin A and corosolic acid, which have been shown to help regulate glucose levels. Studies indicate that these compounds produce glucose-lowering effects by enhancing peripheral glucose utilization[1][2]

Maitake Mushroom, or Grifola frondosa, appears to have glucose-stabilizing effects by improving peripheral insulin receptor site sensitivity. This response has been shown to simultaneously decrease circulating insulin and glucose concentrations.[3][4]Maitake also appears to contain soluble fiber in the immune-enhancing form of beta glucan, which may slow glucose absorption from the gastrointestinal tract[5] No serious adverse side effects have been recognized.[6]

BITTER MELON, or mormordica charantia, is the most popular plant used worldwide to support patients with diabetes.[7] [8] [9] Several clinical studies have been published demonstrating the glucose-balancing effect of bitter melon,[10] [11] [12] as well as profound impacts on the management of diabetes in animal studies .[13] Bitter melon, is well-tolerated and does not appear to have any adverse side effects, but it may not be appropriate for pregnant women.[14]

GYMNEMA SYLVESTRE has demonstrated positive impacts in managing insulin resistance. It has shown the ability to reduce insulin requirements, decrease fasting blood sugar, and enhance the action of insulin. It has even demonstrated the ability to regenerate pancreatic beta-cells.[15] [16] [17] [18] It does not encourage the endogenous production of insulin, and if given to healthy volunteers, does not produce any blood sugar-lowering or hypoglycemic effects.[19] [20]

OPUNTIA STREPTACANTHA LEMAIRE has compounds that have demonstrated glucose-stabilizing effects. It is theorized that this compound, derived from cactus stems, decreases glucose reabsorption. In small studies, there was a 41- 46 percent reduction of blood glucose with non-insulin-dependent diabetics. No adverse side effects are evident with this plant compound.[21] [22]

L-CARNITINE has the potential to support insulin sensitivity by enhancing whole-body glucose uptake and increasing glucose storage.[23] [24] [25]L-carnitine has been shown to support both peripheral nerve and vascular function in patients with diabetes.[26] In addition, it has been shown to significantly reduce total serum lipids and increase HDL cholesterol levels in diabetics.[27]

L-ARGININE'S activities, including its possible anti-atherogenic actions, may be accounted for by its role as the precursor to nitric oxide, or NO. NO is produced by all tissues of the body and plays a very important role in the cardiovascular system, immune system, and nervous system. L-arginine was credited with significantly managing lipid peroxidation in patients with diabetes mellitus.[28]

3. HYPOGLYCEMIA: Nutritional compounds to support healthy blood sugar balance

These nutrients improve the nutritive and biological conditions and support healthy blood sugar balance. Powerful antioxidants help support the body during high oxidative stress, especially when caused by oxidized blood glucose.

CHROMIUM, ADRENAL GLANDULAR, CHOLINE, LIVER GLANDULAR, PANCREAS GLANDULAR, PITUITARY GLANDULAR, INOSITOL, L-CARNITINE, CoQ10, RUBIDIUM, VANADIUM

4. ADRENAL ADAPTOGEN: Nutritional compounds to aid in the adaptation of physiological stress responses

These broad spectrum herbal adaptogens support healthy adrenal feedback loop function. Adaptogens are plant compounds that seem to have a normalizing impact on the Hypothalamus-Adrenal-Pituitary (HPA) axis under times of stress. An "adaptogen" was defined in 1957 by the Russian pharmacologist I.I. Berkman as a substance that fulfills three criteria. First, it must be innocuous and cause minimal disorders in the physiological functions of the organism. Second, it must have a non-specific action to increase resistance to adverse influences by a wide range of physical, chemical, and biochemical factors. Third, it has a normalizing action irrespective of the direction of the pathologic state.[1] Adaptogens seem to be useful during both adrenal hyperstress as well as adrenal hypofatigue. By definition, an adaptogen implies the capability for bi-directional or normalizing effects. The most important adaptogens for the adrenals include Panax Ginseng, Siberian Ginseng, Ashwagandha, Rhodiolia, Boerhaavia Diffusa, and Holybasil Leaf Extract.

KEY INGREDIENTS
RESEARCH COMMENTARY

PANAX GINSENG is also known as Korean ginseng and is probably one of the most recognized stress adaptogens. It appears that ginseng enhances fatty acid oxidation during prolonged exercise by sparing muscle glycogen.[2] The utilization of fatty acid metabolism over glycogen metabolism is an important role panax ginseng plays in adrenal stress syndrome. If metabolism is shifted into a state that can conserve glycogen levels by mobilizing fatty acids, tremendous stress is taken off the adrenals and blood sugar metabolism. Panax ginseng apparently supports metabolism so that an adequate supply of oxygen is available for working muscles, which will make non-esterfied fatty acids the preferential form of energy over glycogen. Panax ginseng has the ability to improve stamina, energy, and physical performance. Apparently the compounds in Panax ginseng improve the hypothalamus-pituitary-adrenal (HPA) feedback loop as well as reduce the suppression caused by cortisone on the immune system.[3] [4] [5] [6]

SIBERIAN GINSENG, also known as *eleutherococcus senticosus*, is an adaptogen. Most of the studies on Siberian ginseng were conducted in the Soviet Union. These studies demonstrated enhanced athletic performance in animals as well as the ability to optimize HPA axis performance under stress.[7] [8] [9] Studies have also demonstrated that Siberian ginseng has the ability to enhance work output under stressful conditions and to improve mental and physical responses under stress.[10]

ASHWAGANDHA is also known as *withania somnifera* and Indian ginseng. It is a very popular herbal adaptogen in Ayurvedic medicine. Many animal studies have been published on this adaptogen. It apparently has adaptogen-like glucocorticoid activity which makes it so helpful in adrenal stress syndromes.[11] Studies have found that ashwagandha has similar adaptogenic activity to panax ginseng.[12] It also has the ability to counteract some of the adverse physical responses to stress such as changes in blood sugar management.

HOLYBASIL LEAF EXTRACT is an adaptogen that supports an increased sense of well-being. Studies have shown that holybasil prevents the increase of plasma level of cortisol induced exposure to both chronic and acute stress, antagonized histamine, supports normal blood sugar levels, modulates HPA activity, increases physical endurance, has immunomodulatory activities, and enhances gastric mucosal strength.[13] [14] [15] [16]

RHODIOLA is an adaptogenic plant that has demonstrated central nervous system enhancement, and anti-depressant, anti-carcinogenic, and cardioprotective properties. It has shown the ability to increase the swimming speed of animals by 135-159 percent. The compounds in Rhodiola have shown the ability to prevent the stress-induced catecholamine activity, reduce adrenaline-induced arrhythmias in animals and prevent stress induced increases in cAMP and decrease cGMP in heart tissues of animals.[17] [18] [19] [20] [21] Rhodiola has also been shown to enhance cognitive function and reduce mental fatigue, as well as support immune function.[22] [23]

BOERHAAVIA DIFFUSA (PUNARVA) has the ability to support both adrenal over and under activation. In stressful conditions it has demonstrated the ability to buffer the elevations of serum cortisol and prevent the suppression of the immune system that takes place with elevated cortisol. On the other hand, Boerhaavia Diffusa has also demonstrated the ability to improve cortisol levels with end stage adrenal exhaustion.[24]

PANTETHINE is a major cofactor for adrenal hormone steroidogenesis and is a useful nutrient in stress conditions. Pantethine has demonstrated the ability to down-regulate the exaggerated secretion of cortisol under times of stress as well as the ability to support adrenal cortical function when needed.[25] [26] [27] [28]

5. ADRENAL BALANCING: Nutritional compounds to modulate the stress response

KEY INGREDIENTS
RESEARCH COMMENTARY

PHOSPHATIDYLSERINE (PS) is an endogenously produced phospholipid that is embedded in cell membranes and is the major phospholipids in the brain. Its general functions include supporting cellular chemical signal transmissions, activating cell surface receptors, and cellular exchange of nutrients and waste products.

The endogenous production of phosphatidylserine is a very difficult and energy consuming process. It requires the combination of L-serine, glycerphosphate, and two fatty acids, and the aid of methyl donors such as B-12, folic acid, S-adensylmethionine with essential fatty acids. Its arduous chemical synthesis that depends upon commonly deficient nutrients may explain why its exogenous intake has shown such great promise.

Exogenous supplementation of phosphatidylserine has shown the ability to enhance cellular metabolism and communication,[1] [2] [3] protect cells from oxidative damage,[4] decrease anxiety, improve mood, motivation and depression,[5] [6] [7] [8] enhance memory and cognition,[9] [10] [11] and decrease cortisol.[12] [13] [14] [15]

Perhaps the most clinically significant impact of PS is its ability to lower cortisol. An over active hypothalamus-pituitary-adrenal axis that induces hypercortisolemia has many adverse impacts on healthy metabolism. Elevated cortisol has been shown to induce insulin insensitivity, decrease TSH and T3 production,[16] [17] increase inactive reverse T3,[18] decrease phase II glucoronidation and sulfation, suppress pituitary function,[19] increase the potential for gastric and duodenal ulcers, lower intestinal secretory IgA,[20] [21] delay intestinal mucosal cell generation,[22] suppress immunity,[23] decrease bone density, induce depression,[24] encourage obesity,[25] [26] [27] and increase the risk for cardiovascular and neurodegenerative disorders.[28]

Therefore, the use of PS shows great promise in the management of disorders induced by the elevations of cortisol from chronic stress syndromes. Up until now, the use of PS was limited in clinical practice because very high doses of oral PS (up to 800 mg a day) are required to blunt the physiological stress response. This therapeutic dose of PS is very expensive and requires 8 or more capsules of intake per day, which makes it difficult for patient compliance. Many of the best responses of PS in clinical studies also used intravenous forms of delivery. This appeared to be the best form of delivery because it bypassed the gastrointestinal tract and was able to be delivered directly into the blood stream.

The new innovative form of PS delivery in a cream has now allowed clinicians to use the required amounts of PS to modulate the stress response. The PS cream allows hundreds of milligrams of PS to enter directly into the blood stream by bypassing the gastrointestinal tract. Transdermal delivery utilizes lipid spheres, known as liposomes, to transport PS through the skin and into the blood. Once there, the liposome shell around the PS substance degrades and makes PS available for active response in the blood stream.

6. ADRENAL EXHAUSTION: Liposomal cream that delivers nutritional compounds to support low adrenal function

These nutrients support individuals that have developed adrenal exhaustion. Adrenal exhaustion normally develops from chronic stress. The stress may be chemical, physical, or emotional, but it is usually a mixture of all three at some level. When the adrenals become exhausted they lose their ability to produce cortisol. This leads to hypoglycemia since the body depends on cortisol to stabilize blood sugar levels during the day. Cortisol also has anti-inflammatory, anti-allergic activity, and immuno-enhancing properties. As the adrenals become exhausted, the body's ability to synthesize all other hormones becomes compromised and all the negative concomitants associated with it may manifest clinically.

Putting these nutrients into a cream for transdermal delivery allows them to enter directly into the bloodstream and bypass the gastrointestinal tract and the liver. Transdermal delivery is a mechanism of delivery in which lipid spheres called liposomes surround the active compounds and act as a transport mechanism through the skin until it reaches the blood supply. Once there, the liposome shell around the active substance degrades and makes the compounds available for active response in the blood stream.

KEY INGREDIENTS
RESEARCH COMMENTARY

LICORICE (GLYCYRRHIZA GLABARA) The active ingredients in licorice include isoflavonoids, glycyrrhizin, chalcones, coumarins, sterons, amino acids, and lignins. These compounds have been shown to have cortisol sparring properties, estrogen modulating properties, anti-inflammatory and anti-allergic properties, immune stimulating activity, and anti-viral and anti-bacterial properties.

Glycyrrhizin has properties that are very helpful in restoring health to those that have adrenal exhaustion. Glycyrrhizin has the ability to down-regulate the enzyme 11-Beta-Hydroxylase which is responsible for converting active cortisol into a less active glucocorticoid, cortisone. Therefore this compound has the ability to increase the half-life of circulating cortisol. The end result is greater levels of circulating cortisol while taking the requirements off the adrenal glands for its production.[1] [2] [3]

The glycyrrhizin and lignins also exhibits modulating impacts on estrogen metabolism. The compound has demonstrated selective estrogen modulating properties therefore when estrogen levels are high it has the ability to inhibit estrogen action and when estrogen levels are low it has shown the ability to enhance the estrogenic response.[4] [5] This activity is important in the adrenal exhausted male or female since they usually suffer from altered estrogen metabolism.

The active components of licorice also have several independent supportive impacts on the immune system. It has shown anti-viral properties due to its ability to produce interferon production and inhibit viral RNA replication.[6] [7] Several studies using licorice have shown positive results with viral disorders such as well.[8] [9] [10] The isoflavonoid components of licorice saponins have displayed anti-microbial and anti-fungal activity.[11]

Licorice also has anti-inflammatory and anti-allergic activity.[12]

[13] These properties are very helpful with the adrenal exhausted patient because they are usually prone to allergies and sensitivities.

The flavonoid components of licorice have also shown profound abilities to heal peptic ulcers. These compounds work by stimulating the gastrointestinal defense mechanism that prevent ulcer formation and stimulate healing of the damage mucous membranes.[14] [15]

B VITAMINS are important for adrenal hormone synthesis. Patients that have been placed in an adrenal stress patterns have greater loss of B vitamins.[16] Therefore the use of B-vitamins in this cream is warranted.

DEHYDROEPIANDROSTERONE (DHEA) is made by the adrenal glands and is the precursor for testosterone and estrogen. DHEA levels become suppressed with chronic stress. The adrenal's ability to produce DHEA is compromised during chronic stress because the glands will produce cortisol to stabilize energy and blood sugar levels at the expense of synthesizing DHEA. This can cause many negative impacts on physiology since DHEA has been shown to improve memory, lower cholesterol, strengthen the immune system, prevent bone loss, and optimize insulin receptor function.[17] [18] [19] [20] [21]

PREGNENOLONE is produced by the adrenal glands and is a precursor to cortisol. The adrenal glands store pregnenolone and convert it to other hormones such as progesterone or DHEA as required by the body. When a person develops adrenal exhaustion they are in need of precursor such as pregnenolone to help make adrenal and reproductive hormones. Pregnenolone has shown in several studies to improve memory, cognition, and mood as well as act as a powerful antioxidant.[22] [23] [24]

7. GLUTATHIONE/SOD CREAM: Nutritional compounds to reduce inflammation and oxidative stress

GLUTATHIONE (GSH) AND SUPEROXIDE DISMUTASE (SOD) are considered to be the most important antioxidants known to the human species. These antioxidants are vital for cellular health and protect the cell against oxygen radicals and mitochondrial oxidative stress. The status of glutathione is considered the single most accurate indicator of the health of the cell. Antioxidant levels become depleted in inflammatory and degenerative conditions and their depletions creates a vicious cycle of further oxidative stress and degeneration.

In addition to antioxidant depletion from oxidative stress, antioxidants like GSH and SOD become exhausted from exposure to everyday environmental chemicals and toxins, cigarette smoke, pharmaceutical drugs, exercise, inappropriate diet, blood sugar disorders, trauma, and alcohol intake.

Numerous health disorders and alterations in physiology have been associated with GSH and SOD depletion. GSH levels powerfully influence healthy immune functions and cellular signaling. Research has shown that T and B lymphocytes require adequate GSH for differentiation and cellular activation. Numerous studies have shown the importance of GSH levels in immunomodulatory function and its central role in a healthy functioning immune system. The importance of optimizing glutathione reserves in immune-related conditions cannot be overemphasized.

Neurodegenerative disorders have been associated with alteration in glutathione and antioxidant status. Since the tissues of the nervous system are highly oxygenated and are composed of unsaturated fatty acids, they are prone to lipid peroxidation in instances of GSH and SOD depletion. Research has shown dramatically low levels of glutathione in conditions such as Parkinson's and Alzheimer's. Since glutathione and superoxide dismutase quench the lipid peroxidation process associated with neurodegeneration, <u>its use in chronic neurological disorders must be considered.</u>

GSH and SOD are important substrates for hepatic detoxification. GSH is important for Phase II conjugation, and both SOD and GSH are important for Phase I oxidation/reduction reactions. When hepatic reserves of glutathione become depleted, detoxification potentials become hindered and the body becomes more susceptible to exogenous and endogenous toxins. Studies have shown that glutathione depletion <u>contributes and is linked to liver disease, cirrhosis, hepatitis, fatty liver, and alcohol-damaged liver.</u>

Antioxidants, particularly GSH and SOD, should be considered for heart health. Atherosclerosis has been associated with decreased GSH peroxidase levels, oxidative stress, and lipid peroxidation. Exogenous glutathione has demonstrated the ability to reduce lipid peroxidation, optimize eicosanoid balance, and ultimately help protect the endothelium against damage.

The use of GSH and SOD in a liposomal delivery cream is a breakthrough in antioxidant therapy and should be considered in cases that require antioxidant therapy, such as inflammatory disorders.

This cream is best delivered on the bottoms of the feet.

8. VITAMIN D: Emulsified vitamin D and cofactors

The conversion of vitamin D (cholecalciferol) into active vitamin 25(OH) D includes many cofactors such as magnesium, biotin, pantethine, calcium, and boron. Along with vitamin D, these cofactors support immune system separately or through strengthening the physiological effects of vitamin D. Calcium and magnesium are of importance in intracellular metabolic functions regulated mainly via hormonal signals.

Magnesium - a predominantly intracellular ion,[57] is involved in modulating cellular events during inflammation.[58] Magnesium deficiency may lead to peripheral resistance to vitamin D.[59] Vitamin A has important role in the immune system and its deficiency is associated with altered immune function and cytokine dysregulation,[60][61] such as impaired TH-1 response.[62] Vitamin B6 has synergistic beneficial effects on the immune system and sugar metabolism via different pathways. Studies show that a vitamin B6 deficiency can decrease antibody production and suppress the immune response. B6 participates in the maintenance of glutathione status (as a cofactor for glutathione reductase). It is shown that its deficiency can reduce cell numbers in lymphoid tissues and cause functional abnormalities in the cell mediated immune response. [63][64]

Vitamin B-6 is important in hemoglobin synthesis and increases the amount of oxygen carried by hemoglobin.[64] B6 participates in sugar metabolism and helps maintain blood sugar within a normal range.[65][66] Glyco-Modulating effects of vitamin D and B6 are consistent with lipid modulating effects of Biotin and pantethine in dysglycemic states.[67]

EPA and DHA show anti-inflammatory activities by regulation of pro-inflammatory substances such as PGE2, LTB4, TNF-alpha, IL-1, and lipooxigenase (LOX), so that they can be protective against inflammatory problems including cardiovascular, neurodegeneration and diabetes (DMT1).[68][69][70][71]

Genistein and carnosic acid help improve vitamin D utilization and metabolism. Genistein can optimize the 1,25 hydroxy D3 synthesis and therefore promote increased utilization of vitamin D into an active form.[1] Carnosic acid from rosemary leaf extract has demonstrated the ability to potentiate the effects of vitamin D.[2]

SUMMARY OF VITAMIN D RESEARCH

Vitamin D and Autoimmune Diseases

Autoimmune diseases are now classified as T-Helper 1 or T-Helper 2 subset dominant to indicate if either the cell-mediated or humoral immune system has become over active. The balance of TH-1/TH-2 cells appear to be strongly influence by regulatory T-cells. Vitamin D appears to have some influence on the activity of regulatory T-cells and the balance of TH-1/TH-2 cells.[24][25][26][27] Vitamin D appears to help against autoimmune mediated thyroid dysfunction.[28][29] Vitamin D appears to be helpful for autoimmune induced diabetes.[30] Numerous papers have been published linking autoimmune to vitamin D.[31][32][33][34]

Vitamin D and Chronic Muscle Pain

Vitamin D deficiencies may cause chronic diffuse nonspecific musculoskeletal pain that is associated with both muscle and bone pain.[35][36] In a study in which 150 patients presented to a hospital in Minneapolis with complaints of chronic nonspecific musculoskeletal pain, 140 had vitamin D deficiencies when evaluated with a serum 25(OH) D test.[37] Ethnicities with darker skin appear to be at more risk for vitamin D insufficiencies in general, but specifically as it relates to chronic nonspecific musculoskeletal pain. The study found that 16 percent of Asians, 24 percent of Anglo Americans, 40 percent of Hispanics and Native Americans, and 50 percent of African Americans with chronic nonspecific musculoskeletal pain demonstrate severe vitamin D deficiencies.[38]

Vitamin D and Diabetes

Individuals with hypovitaminosis D are at higher risk of insulin resistance and metabolic syndrome.[39] Research has demonstrated preventative roles for vitamin D for type I diabetes mellitus.[40] [41]

Vitamin D and Neurodegenerative Disorders

Vitamin D has demonstrated many influential roles in neurodegenerative disease such as multiple sclerosis.[42] [43] Vitamin D supplementation has exhibited diminished relapse rates.[44] [45] [46]

Vitamin D Bone Metabolism and Osteoporosis

The link between vitamin D and healthy bone metabolism is well known. Vitamin D is important for regulation of both calcium and phosphorus absorption and metabolism.[47] There is a direct relationship between serum 25 (OH) D levels and bone in health in both males and females for all age groups.[48]

Vitamin D in Pregnancy, Infancy, and Childhood

Associations with vitamin D insufficiency during pregnancy and low birth weight have been published.[49] Research has also shown that there are increased maternal bone density losses during pregnancy when vitamin D deficiency is present.[50] Adequate maternal vitamin D status is important for proper tooth and metabolism and also reduces the risk of the development of type I diabetes.[51] Inadequate vitamin D intake in infancy can lead to unhealthy bone metabolism and increased risk of fractures.[52]

VITAMIN D DOSAGES AND DEFICIENCIES

Vitamin D Dosages

Current vitamin D dosage guidelines are based solely on the

maintenance of bone health and do not account for the influence of vitamin D for other physiological functions.[3] Many experts on Vitamin D research have considered the current dosage requirements for vitamin D to be obsolete.[4] Levels as twenty times the RDA for vitamin D have been shown to be safe when used for several months.[5][6][7]

The primary source for vitamin D for most people is solar ultraviolet-B (UVB). In the absence of exposure to sunlight, a minimum of 1,000 IU of vitamin D3 is required to maintain a healthy concentration of 25-hydroxyvitamin D3 in the blood.[8] However, despite exposure to adequate sunlight, the prevalence of vitamin D deficiency is high.[9][10][11][12][13] Dietary sources of vitamin D include sources such as fatty fish, which, in conjunction with other societal factors, has led to gross deficiency in the United States.[14][15][16][17][18]

Factors that can cause Vitamin D deficiencies

Many factors are involved with the promotion of vitamin D deficiencies, which include a lack of sunlight exposure and inadequate consumption of vitamin D rich foods such as oily fish. Gastrointestinal inflammatory disorders reduce absorption of vitamin D. Cortisol elevations or use of cortisone can deplete vitamin D levels. Ethnicities with darker skin and individuals with obesity are more at risk for vitamin D insufficiencies.[19][20][21] Also, as individuals become older, they become less efficient in photo production to use sunlight to process vitamin D. [22][23]

EMULSIFICATION DESCRIPTION

Physiologically, emulsification occurs as a principal step toward fat digestion and absorption on a daily basis along with every meal involving the biliary system.

Bioavailability of vitamin D has been shown to increase when emulsified. Vitamin D is absorbed in the jejunum and in lesser amounts in the ileum. Emulsified vitamin D guarantees the homogenized, well-dispersed vitamin D-containing droplets in the jejunum, which is even more important in those with biliary malfunction.

9. TH-1 SUPPORT: Nutritional compounds to support the TH-1 response

These compounds have been shown to support the TH-1 response. They also support healthy immune system function, and can be used as nutritional support during an infection. Although there is no treatment specific to viral infections, some of the compounds in this formula have demonstrated the ability to support healthy cellular and humeral immunity. Support has been shown for healthy phagocytic activity of macrophages and monocytes, as well as the natural killer cells, neutrophils and lymphokines.

KEY INGREDIENTS
RESEARCH COMMENTARY

ASTRAGALUS membranaceus is a traditional Chinese medical herb with documented immune-supporting properties. *Its* physiological impact has been demonstrated as the ability to increase interferon production and inhibit viral ribonuclease systems, therefore enhancing anti-viral responses.[1][2][3][4] It enhances the phagocytic activity of macrophages and monocytes,[5] modulates T-cell activity and increases the production of natural killer cells.[6][7]

Clinical studies in China have shown it to be effective during viral infections, compromised immunity due to chemical and radiation exposure.[8][9][10] Research on astragulus has also demonstrated its ability to enhance antibody responses to T-dependent antigens,[11] as well as reduce the severity and duration of the common cold.[12]

ECHINACEA Hundreds of studies have been performed on echinacea, demonstrating its effectiveness in supporting the immune system. It has been shown to have numerous physiological impacts, such as immunostimulatory, anti-inflammatory, anti-viral, and anti-bacterial properties.[13][14]

The anti-viral properties of echinacea have been attributed to its role in supporting the cytotoxic killing of virus-infected cells and the release of interferon. It may also possess the ability to inhibit hyaluronidase and block virus receptors on the surface of cells. Echinacea has also been shown to increase the number of neutrophils, lymphokines, and promote non-specific T-cell activation.[15][16][17][18]

GLYCYRRHIZA GLABRA (LICORICE ROOT EXTRACT) The active components of glycyrrhiza glabra have several independent supportive impacts on the immune system. They have shown anti-viral properties due to their ability to increase interferon production and inhibit viral RNA replication.[19][20] Several studies using licorice have shown positive results with viral disorders.[21][22][23]
The isoflavonoid components of licorice saponins have displayed anti-microbial and anti-fungal activity.[24]

MELISSA OFFICINALIS (also known as lemon balm) is derived from the mint family of plants. It contains rich polyphenols, which have been shown to exhibit anti-viral and anti-bacterial activity. It appears to improve both humoral and cellular immune responses.[25][26] Melissa officinalis has demonstrated the ability to inhibit viral replication and be supportive in the management of viruses such as herpes simplex outbreaks.[27][28]

MAITAKE MUSHROOM has been shown to have numerous health promoting properties in regards to immune function. It has demonstrated the ability to activate natural killer cells and macrophages, as well as enhance humoral and cellular immunity.[29][30][31]

PUNICA GRANTUM (POMEGRANATE) has been shown to have many immune-enhancing and modulating properties. It has been used for centuries in Asian, Indian, and Middle Eastern plant-based therapies. The flavonoids, polyphenols, and tannins in this plant have been shown to decrease oxidative markers such as malondialdehyde, hydroxyperoxides, and conjugated dienes. It has shown the ability to increase the activities of the enzymes catalase, superoxide dismutase, and glutathione peroxidase.[32][33] Punica grantum has also demonstrated the potential to provide properties that may act as viral entry inhibitors and inhibit viral replication.[34][35]

10. TH-2 SUPPORT: Nutritional compounds to support the TH-2 response

These compounds support a healthy TH-2 response. They also provides nutritional support during inflammation and provide a rich source of antioxidants.

KEY INGREDIENTS
RESEARCH COMMENTARY

PINE BARK EXTRACT is a bioflavonoid rich source of proanthocyanidins with powerful antioxidant properties. These compounds demonstrate anti-inflammatory activity by increasing T-Helper 2 cytokines. It has demonstrated immunomodulatory effects on human and animal studies of autoimmune conditions such as lupus and asthma. Pine bark extract has also demonstrated protective properties for the thymus gland.

GRAPE SEED EXTRACT has a rich source of the proanthcyanidin flavonoids that exhibit antioxidant and anti-inflammatory properties. These compounds have demonstrated a modulating decreased production of immunostimulatory cytokines.

GREEN TEA EXTRACT contains polyphenolic compounds with antioxidant properties that have enhancing potential on the anti-inflammatory TH-2 system. These compounds also exhibit immunomodulatory suppression of the cell mediated TH-1 inflammatory response.

RESVERATROL The polyphenol resveratrol has demonstrated modulating properties of T-helper and T-suppressor cells and inhibits the release of inflammatory cytokines.

PYCNOGENOL° has demonstrated anti-inflammatory properties due to its ability to decrease the activation and production of T-Helper 1 cytokines, nuclear factor kappa B, and inflammatory leukotrienes. It has also been shown to inhibit mast cell activation and the release of histamine.

11. CLEANSING PROTEIN POWDER: Nutritional hypoallergenic protein powder product and cleansing program

Certain nutritional factors play extremely important roles in the proper functioning of the cellular cleansing processes. The body's natural detoxifying ability will deteriorate if these nutrients are deficient or lacking at the cellular level. In addition, certain botanicals and botanical extracts have been shown to strengthen the cells and maximize the processes that are involved in detoxification reactions. These nutrients provides the necessary nutritional compounds and the botanical extracts that have been recognized to be pivotal in the body's *natural abilities to neutralize and expel toxins.* They can be extremely beneficial to those patients who demonstrate gallstone type symptoms, imbalanced hormonal patterns, PMS, menopause, or any other condition in which optimizing the clearance of hormones is indicated. They can also help to normalize the digestive processes in people that have had their gallbladder removed.

MACRONUTRIENTS: Vegetable proteins are often considered to be incomplete to meet human needs for essential amino acids. *Among the plant proteins, soy and rice provide sound nutrition, but rice protein offers additional benefits.* Soy protein often is difficult for people to digest and may pose allergy risks, plus some simply do not like the taste. Rice protein actually is utilized more efficiently by the body than soy. Volunteer subjects eating diets in which the protein was derived virtually exclusively from rice, when compared with those eating both rice and chicken showed no significant difference in nitrogen balance, indicating that their protein intake was sufficient. Many individuals are allergic or sensitive to dietary protein from different sources, such as wheat, soy, etc. Rice protein is a hypoallergenic protein and suitable for use by those with food allergies and has even been used for tube feeding of infants, the elderly, and the severely ill.

MICRONUTRIENTS: Certain vitamins and minerals that are required as cofactors in ***enzymatic reactions*** involved in hepatic detoxification processes. Vitamin B6 (P-5-P), vitamin D3, mixed carotenoids, zinc and manganese gluconate, selenium amino acid chelate, magnesium citrate, chromium and molybdenum picolinate, calcium, and potassium citrate are examples. A number of amino acids such as N-Acetylcysteine, Methionine, Taurine, L-Glutamine, Glutamic Acid, necessary for a variety of biochemical reactions including, sulfation and methylation to support *phase I* and *II* detoxification reactions.

OTHER NUTRITIONAL COMPOUNDS, AND BOTANICALS: Strong antioxidants such as quercitin, grape seed extract, green tea extract, herbs, and herbal extracts such as milk thistle seed extract improve hepatic cell growth and recovery, and increase bile solubility. Glutathione and Glycine enhance conjugation reactions. Lysine further improves amino acid balance in rice protein. Digestive enzymes such as invertase, cellulase, maltase, and amylase improve digestion and absorption of the nutrients. Additional herbal and nutritional compounds such as Jerusalem artichoke, Marshmallow, Gamma Oryzanol, Rutin, Hesperidin, MSM (Methyl Sulphonyl Methane), Evening Primrose Oil, and Medium Chain Triglycerides round out the support.

KEY INGREDIENTS
RESEARCH COMMENTARY

MEDIUM CHAIN TRIGLYCERIDES (MCTs) are derived from coconut oil and range in length from 6 to 12 carbons. Their lengths allow for an easily absorbed energy source for people with malabsorption syndromes. Unlike other long-chain fatty acids, they do not require pancreatic enzymes or bile acid for absorption. MCTs are rapidly utilized by gastrointestinal mucosa cells for energy and may aid gastrointestinal regenerative processes and provide a useful source of energy for people that suffer from malabsorption.[1] [2]

GAMMA-ORYZANOL is an ester of ferulic acid that is isolated from rice bran oil. It has demonstrated powerful antioxidant ability in experimental studies.[3] [4] Gamma-oryzanol has demonstrated effectiveness in numerous gastrointestinal disorders including, ulcers, irritable bowel syndrome, gastritis, and even non-specific gastrointestinal conditions. In addition to having an anti-inflammatory impact, it also seems to have normalization properties over the gastrointestinal nervous system.[5] [6] [7]

BIOTIN is an important vitamin that is important for the utilization of fats and amino acids by the body, but may become depleted in individuals that suffer from unhealthy gastrointestinal flora. A major portion of human biotin supply is provided by healthy intestinal microflora. In cases of dysbiosis, biotin deficiency may become apparent. Biotin is important for strong nails, healthy hair, it aids in the synthesis of fatty acids, it enhances insulin sensitivity, and aids in the removal of the amine groups in the metabolism of amino acid important for cell growth and replication.[8]

GLUTAMINE is the preferred fuel source for the cells of the small intestines and has shown to be helpful in improving the regeneration and repair of the intestinal lining. It has shown to increase the number of cells in the small intestine, the number of villi on those cells, and the height of the villi. Glutamine reduces permeability of the lining which may accompany "leaky gut" patterns that may lead to inflammation and the development of delayed food intolerances.[9] [10] [11]

LACTOBACILLI ACIDOPHILUS has long been noted for the role it plays as a probiotic organism to maintain healthy gastrointestinal environment. These healthy organisms, part of the normal gastrointestinal microflora, have been shown to inhibit growth and attachment of adverse non-beneficial bacteria and pathogens. L acidophilus produces metabolic byproducts known as bacteriocins that inhibit and antagonize unhealthy bacteria.[12] [13] [14]

JEURUSALEM ARTICHOKE AND INULIN are prebiotics and provide a good source of short-chain fatty acids known as fructooligosaccharides (FOS). These prebiotics have shown the ability to improve healthy bacteria, especially Bifidobacteria, and also reduce the colonization of unhealthy bacteria. In addition to improving gastrointestinal bacterial microecology, they increase the levels of short-chain fatty acids such as butyrate, and improve liver function and the elimination of toxic compounds.[15] [16]

MARSHMALLOW ROOT is used to support repair and quench inflammation of the intestines. It enhances mucosal cell secretions, improves microflora ecology, and coats the intestinal tract to protect injured cells.[17]

QUERCITIN is a very powerful anti-inflammatory flavonoid because it directly inhibits the initial cellular mediators in the inflammatory cascade such as arachadonic acid, present with inflammatory disorders of the upper or lower bowel. It also directly inhibits the manufacture and release of histamines that are involved with allergic responses.[18] [19]

GRAPE SEED EXTRACT contains very powerful anti-inflammatory flavonoids called proanthocyanidins (PCO) that have shown to prevent the release of compounds that promote inflammation and allergy such as histamines, serine proteases, prostaglandins, and leukotrienes.[20]

RUTIN AND HESPERIDEN are natural antioxidants with powerful antioxidant and healing properties important in inflammatory conditions of the gastrointestinal tract. Their primary impact is on quenching the inflammatory prostaglandin cascade by inhibiting the pro-inflammatory enzymes responsible for producing inflammatory prostaglandins and leukotrienes.[21]

EVENING PRIMROSE increases the production of prostaglandin E2 series, which promotes healing and repair of the gastrointestinal tract. This may be important in cases of gastric ulcers or in cases which increased gastrointestinal permeability exists.

MILK THISTLE (SILYBUM MARIANUM) has the ability to increase the solubility of bile and its use has been shown to significantly reduce biliary cholesterol concentrations and bile saturation index.[22] It has potent antioxidant activity, which supports phase I detoxification and prevents the depletion of hepatic glutathione which is important for phase II detoxification.[23][24][25] Silybum marianum has anti-inflammatory chemical properties that are inhibitors of inflammatory prostaglandins and leukotriens as well as chemical properties that promote protein synthesis for the replacement of damaged liver cells. [26][27][28][29]

ENZYME BLEND The enzymes used in this formula are amylase, cellulose, glucanase, and protease. These are the enzymes of the intestinal brush border and provide digestive support with reduced potential for the enzymes to create further destruction of the intestinal lining. Enzyme blends that are not found in the small intestine brush border may have the potential to digest the healthy gastrointestinal lining in compromised individuals.

12. GUT HEALTH: Nutritional compounds to support gut health

These compounds have shown the ability to increase the number of villi and cells of the small intestine, manage gastric inflammation, increase mucous formation, and maintain healthy gastric lining.

KEY INGREDIENTS
RESEARCH COMMENTARY

DEGLYCYRRHIZINATED LICORICE ROOT (DGL)
DGL is a popular and substantially studied, natural compound that provides flavonoids shown to heal the gastric lining. Many different mechanisms have been demonstrated with regard to its restorative properties, including stimulation and differentiation of glandular cells, mucous formation and secretion, and the growth and regeneration of the stomach and intestinal cells.[1][2][3][4]

GLUTAMINE

Glutamine is the preferred fuel source for the cells of the small intestine, and has been shown to be helpful in the regeneration and repair of the intestinal lining. It has demonstrated the ability to increase the number of cells in the small intestine, the number of villi, as well as the height of the villi. Glutamine also reduces permeability of the lining linked with "leaky gut," inflammation and food intolerances.[5] [6] [7]

FLAVONOIDS (CATECHIN)

The flavonoid catechin has demonstrated properties that inhibit the enzyme histadine decarboxylase, thereby supporting anti-ulcer activity. Several studies have demonstrated the positive impacts of catechin on ulcerative states.[8] [9] Flavonoids such as catechin have also been shown to inhibit H. pylori in a clear-cut concentration-dependent manner.[10]

BISMUTH CITRATE

Bismuth is a naturally occurring mineral that exhibits activity against H. pylori and is used in the treatment of ulcers. Two double-blind placebo-controlled studies have demonstrated the safe and effective use of bismuth in managing gastric inflammation.[11] [12]

GAMMA-ORYZANOL

Gamma-Oryzanol is an ester of ferulic acid that is isolated from rice bran oil. It has been demonstrated as a powerful antioxidant in experimental studies.[13] [14] Gamma-Oryzanol has proven effective in numerous gastrointestinal disorders including ulcers, irritable bowel syndrome, gastritis, and even non-specific gastrointestinal conditions. In addition to having an anti-inflammatory impact, it also seems to have normalization properties over the gastrointestinal nervous system.[15] [16] [17]

RHUBARB OFFICINALE

Rhubarb is a plant-based compound that provides astringent anthraquinones and flavonoids. It may provide support in healing the gastrointestinal tract during ulcerative conditions. In one double-blind study of 312 cases, it demonstrated the ability to change pre and post-stool occult blood tests with a 90 percent efficacy rate within 56 hours.[18]

MASTIC GUM

Mastic is a resinous exudate obtained from the stem and the main leaves of Pistacia lentiscus. It is used as a food ingredient in the Mediterranean region. Clinically, mastic has been effective in the treatment of benign gastric ulcers and duodenal ulcers.[19] [20] [21]

13. GUT INFECTIONS: Nutritional compounds to support the immune system during minor bacterial, fungal, and parasitic infections and create a healthy digestive terrain

These herbal extracts have been shown to support the immune system during minor bacterial, fungal, and parasitic infections. They also work to create a healthy terrain.

KEY INGREDIENTS
RESEARCH COMMENTARY

BERBERINE-CONTAINING BOTANICALS
(BERBERIS VULGARIS, BERBERIS AQUIFOLIUM, BERBERIS ARISTATA, HYDRASTIS CANADENSIS, COPTIS CHINENSIS)

Plants with high berberis alkaloids have been used in both Chinese and Ayurevedic medicine for centuries. These plants appear to demonstrate significant antimicrobial activity against a variety of bacteria,[1] [2] [3] [4] fungi,[5] [6] protozoans,[7] [8] [9] helminthes,[10] chlamydia,[11] [12] and viruses.[13] Berberine has demonstrated the ability to inhibit the growth of Giardia lamblia, Trichomonas, and Entamoeba histolytica.[14] These plants have also demonstrated anti-inflammatory properties, such as the inhibition of arachidonic acid-induced thromboxane A3 release and the ability to activate macrophages.[15] [16]

YERBA MANSA is not related to the berberine-containing plants chemically or botanically, but it is used to treat similar conditions. The active compound in Yerba mansa is methyleugenol, an antispasmodic. It is similar in chemical structure to the compounds found in nutmeg, which are used to treat irritable stomach.[17] It also appears to have anti-inflammatory effects and is used to treat inflammation of the mucous membranes.[18] This plant has also been shown to have anti-fungal properties.

14. LIVER DETOXIFICATION: Nutritional compounds to improve Phase I and II liver detoxification

Healthy detoxification is of utmost importance, especially during any metabolic disorders. The management of thyroid, adrenal, or menopausal patterns will prove to be ineffective and ambiguous if detoxification imbalances are overlooked. If detoxification pathways are compromised or are down-regulated, the potential for metabolic disorders exist. For example, numerous studies have demonstrated the adverse impact of compromised detoxification on neurological disorders,[1] [2] [3] chemical sensitivities, [4] adverse drug reactions,[5] [6] [7] and fatigue.[8] [9]

The ultimate goal of hepatic detoxification is to transform compounds that are fat-soluble or lipophilic chemicals from an endogenous source such as hormones, intercellular mediators, neurotransmitters, bacteria, intestinal bacteria endotoxins, and antigen-antibody complexes; as well as exogenous compounds such as drugs, pesticides, environmental toxins, and drugs into water-soluble compounds. Water-soluble compounds can then be eliminated as urine by the kidneys, as sweat by our sweat glands, and into fecal matter from bile. The steps involved to carry out this process have been named Phase I and Phase II. Phase I detoxification involves the cytochrome 450 enzymes. Phase I enzymes directly neutralize some chemicals, but most are converted to intermediate forms that are then processed by phase II conjugation enzymes.

Phase II detoxification typically involves conjugation of Phase I intermediates, however some toxins are directly acted upon by Phase II enzymes. This conjugation reaction either neutralizes the toxin or makes the toxin more easily excreted through the urine, sweat, or bile. There are six main Phase II pathways which include: glutathione conjugation, glycine (amino acid) conjugation, methylation, sulfation, acetlyation and glucuronidation. This formula contains herbs, nutrients, and amino acids to support healthy Phase I and II detoxification.

KEY INGREDIENTS
RESEARCH COMMENTARY

DANDELION (TARAXACUM OFFICINALE) Dandelion root has physiologic impacts on both the liver and gallbladder. It impacts the liver by promoting the production of bile and its delivery to the gallbladder. It impacts the gallbladder by causing contraction and release of stored bile.[11] [12] [13]

MILK THISTLE (SILYBUM MARIANUM) has the ability to increase the solubility of bile and its use has been shown to significantly reduce biliary cholesterol concentrations and bile saturation index.[14] It has potent antioxidant activity which supports phase I detoxification and prevents the depletion of hepatic glutathione which is important for phase II detoxification.[15] [16] [17] Silybum marianum has anti-inflammatory chemical properties that are inhibitors of inflammatory prostaglandins and leukotrienes as well as chemical properties that promote protein synthesis to replace damaged liver cells. [18] [19] [20] [21]

CENTELLA ASITICA has active constituents known as triterpenoid compounds that have impacts on cells and tissues that are important in detoxification. It has even shown the ability to improve histological findings of liver cirrhosis.[22] [23] It also supports hepatic detoxification due to its physiological impact on enhancing venous circulation. Centella Asitica has shown the ability to improve venous disorders such as chronic venous insufficiency and venous hypertension.[24] [25] Improved venous circulation has influential roles in optimizing detoxification that are generally overlooked.

PANAX GINSENG has shown in several studies to have numerous positive impacts on hepatic function. It has shown to reverse fatty liver in animals, and demonstrate profound anti-hepatotoxic properties.[26] [27] It has shown the ability to promote Kupffer cells and shown to increase nuclear, ribosomal, and messenger RNA biosynthesis. Its use in a formula to support hepatic detoxification appears mandatory.[28] [29] [30]

GLUTATHIONE CONJUGATION SUPPORT Glutathione is a tripeptide amino acid that consists of glycine, cysteine, and glutamic acid and is hence also known as gamma-glutamylcysteinylglycine. In addition to playing an important part in phase II conjugation, it is responsible as the main reducing agent and primary cellular agent of the cells. Glutathione helps maintain the structure of red blood cell membranes and other cellular proteins, it also helps maintain the cytoplasm in a reduced state. Glutathione is also responsible for the synthesis of leukotrienes and functions as a carrier in the transport of sulfur containing amino acids into the cell.

As a phase II detoxifier it conjugates with phase I substrates to produce water-soluble mercaptates that are excreted in the urine. Glutathione is a tripeptide amino acid that depends upon adequate levels of essential nutrients such as B6, riboflavin, choline, methionine, cysteine or n-acetlycysteine, vitamin C, beatine, glycine, glutamic acid, potassium, copper, zinc and selenium. Numerous studies have shown that taking these essential nutrients will enhance glutathione levels. [31] [32]

METHYLATION CONJUGATION SUPPORT Methylation involves conjugating phase I end products with single-carbon compounds. Methylation requires methionine, beatine, ascorbic acid, alpha tocopherol, choline, pyradoxyl-5-phosphate, trimethlyglycine, magnesium, methylcobalamin and folic acid.

ACETYLATION CONJUGATION SUPPORT Acetylation pathways conjugate toxins with acetyl-CoA and two carbon compounds. Acetylation pathways are dependent on pantothenic acid, thiamin, and vitamin C.[33]

GLUCURONIDIATION CONJUGATION SUPPORT
Glucuronidation involves combining toxins and end products with glucuronic acid. This pathway is supported by B-vitamins, magnesium,

and glycine, which help support the uronic acid pathway that synthesizes glucuronic acid.

SULFATION CONJUGATION SUPPORT   Sulfation involves combining toxins and end products with sulfur-containing amino acids. An important step in sulfation is the conversion of sulfites to sulfates by the molybdenum dependent enzyme sulfite oxidase. Therefore, the mineral molybdenum and the sulfur-contaning amino acids such as N-acetyl-cysteine, glycine, and methionine are important for sulfation conjugation support.

15. METHYLATION: Nutritional compounds to support healthy methylation reactions

These nutrients support healthy methylation reactions. Methylation is the biochemical reaction responsible for the transfer of one-carbon molecules. This chemical reaction is a crucial step in many important biochemical pathways and is dependent on essential nutrients to act as cofactors. Altered methylation reactions have been associated with elevated homocysteine, dementia, depression, compromised Phase II detoxification, birth defects, etc. These nutrients should be considered by all women that use oral contraceptives as they are depleted while on the birth-control pill.[1][2][3][4][5][6][7][8]

CHOLINE, TRIMETHYLGLYCINE, MSM, BEET ROOT, METHYL B12, AND BETAINE HCL

16. GALLBLADDER/BILE: Nutritional compounds to support healthy bile formation, secretion and flow

These nutrients are useful anytime a detoxification program is indicated. Once the liver has detoxified chemicals, they are delivered to the gallbladder for bile secretion into the feces for elimination. If bile synthesis or secretion is compromised, hepatic detoxification of toxins, adverse chemicals, or hormones will not be eliminated. This may have adverse impacts on many functional metabolic pathways.

Unhealthy bile synthesis and elimination can cause intolerance to fried foods, flatulence several hours after meals, excessive burping after meals, etc. These nutrients may also be used by people that have had their gallbladder removed. If the gallbladder is removed the cystic duct acts as a reservoir for bile, therefore optimal synthesis and elimination of bile is essential.

Healthy bile synthesis and elimination can also be of be of great value in balancing hormonal patterns due to bile's ability to enhance clearance of hormones. These nutrients should be considered in PMS, menopause, or any other condition in which optimizing the clearance of hormones is indicated.

KEY INGREDIENTS
RESEARCH COMMENTARY

DANDELION (TARAXACUM OFFICINALE) Dandelion root has physiologic impacts on both the liver and gallbladder. It impacts the liver by promoting the production of bile and its delivery to the gallbladder. It impacts the gallbladder by causing contraction and release of stored bile.[1] [2] [3]

MILK THISTLE (SILYBUM MARIANUM) has the ability to increase the solubility of bile and its use has been shown to significantly reduce biliary cholesterol concentrations and bile saturation indexes.[4] It has potent antioxidant activity which supports phase I detoxification and prevents the depletion of hepatic glutathione which is important for phase II detoxification.[5] [6] [7] Silybum marianum has anti-inflammatory chemical properties that are inhibitors of inflammatory prostaglandins and leukotriens as well as chemical properties that promote protein synthesis to replace damaged liver cells. [8] [9] [10] [11]

GINGER (ZINGIBER OFFICINALE) contains chemical compounds that have been shown to increase bile secretion and to reduce hepatic cholesterol levels by up-regulating the enzyme cholesterol-7-alpha-hydorxylase which is the rate limiting enzyme in bile acid synthesis.[12] [13] [14]

NUTRITIONAL COMPOUNDS THAT SUPPORT BILIARY STATSIS The nutrients taurine, beatine (beet concentrate), vitamin C, and lecithin (phosphatidylcholine) have been shown to be lipotropic agents. These nutrients support pathways of bile synthesis.[15] [16] [17]

17. THYROID HORMONE SYNTHESIS: Nutritional compounds to help support T4 to T3 synthesis

These nutrients support healthy peripheral thyroid metabolism and glutathione synthesis.

KEY INGREDIENTS
RESEARCH COMMENTARY

COMMIPHORA MUKU (GUGGULU) The guggulsterones compounds in this herb have been shown to stimulate the healthy synthesis of T3 hormones.[1] They also appear to have the ability to balance LDL cholesterol and decrease lipid peroxidation.[2] Commiphora's ability to support T3 production, its ability to balance cholesterol, and its antiperoxidative effects make it a very useful herb to consider to balance T3 patterns.

SELENIUM is the major cofactor for the enzyme 5'deiodinase, which is responsible for converting T4 into T3 as well as degrading rT3. Studies have confirmed lower production T3 in individuals with lower selenium status.[3] [4] [5] Numerous studies have demonstrated increased T3 synthesis as well as decreased reverse T3 production with selenium.[6] [7] [8] [9] [10]

ZINC It has been shown that low zinc status compromises T3 production.[11] Studies have also demonstrated that zinc supplementation improves thyroid hormone production.[12] [13] [14] [15] These effects may be due to the cofactor role zinc plays with type I 5'deiodinase. In addition, zinc may play a role in reducing thyroidal antibodies.[16]

ANTIPEROXIDATIVE COMPOUNDS Lipid peroxidation and antioxidant enzyme systems have been shown to play a profound role on its impact on peripheral thyroid hormone conversion. Numerous studies have demonstrated that peroxidation and oxidative stress significantly alters thyroid metabolism.[17] [18] [19] [20] [21] [22] This formula contains compounds that help support peroxidation directly and indirectly via glutathione synthesis.[23] [24]

18. THYROID FUNCTION: Nutritional compounds to support healthy thyroid function

These nutrients support T3 and T4 production, healthy thyroid hormone receptor binding, and energy-producing metabolism, which is useful during low thyroid function.

KEY INGREDIENTS
RESEARCH COMMENTARY

PORCINE THYROID GLANDULAR is derived from Argentina in which the animals are range fed and are free of hormones and chemicals and exceed USDA guidelines. The glandulars are kept clean and healthy. This provides high quality glandular tissue that contains the needed amino acids, fatty acids, co-enzymes, and other supporting material for the thyroid. Porcine glandular tissue, as opposed to other types of tissue such as bovine, is the best source to support the thyroid.

WITHANIA SOMNIFERA (ASHWAGANDHA) contains compounds that have been shown to have a stimulatory impact on both T3 and T4 hormone synthesis. It also has been shown to reduce hepatic lipid peroxidation and increase the activity of superoxide dismutase and other antioxidant systems.[1] [2] This is important because numerous studies have demonstrated that peroxidation and oxidative stress significantly alters thyroid metabolism.[3] [4] [5] [6] [7] [8] Withania somnifera also exerts adaptogen-like glucocorticoid activity which makes it helpful in thyroid imbalances that are negatively influenced by the stress hormone cortisol.[9] [10] Cortisol has the potential to lower TSH, suppress peripheral T3 conversion, increase inactive rT3 production, and antagonize the effects of thyroid signaling at the genome.[11] Since Withania somnifera has demonstrated abilities to increase T3 and T4 hormone levels, decrease peroxidation and act as an adaptogen to modulate the release of cortisol it should always be considered as a powerful agent to use when supporting the thyroid.

VITAMIN A Once thyroid hormones bind to receptor sites, a series of biochemical reactions called intercellular transduction are initiated. This intercellular transduction response carries the message of binding to the nuclear receptors. Once the nuclear receptor has been activated, it will respond by producing proteins that express enhanced metabolic rate and energy production. Vitamin A appears to influence thyroid hormone nuclear receptors. Thyroid hormone nuclear transcription activation involves vitamin A dependent, retinoic acid-specific receptors.[12]

VITAMIN D Elevated autoimmune thyroid antibodies are a very common pattern associated with the etiology of thyroid disorders. Vitamin D has shown to be an effective immune modulator and even shown to suppress autoimmune activity.[13]

SELENIUM is the major cofactor for the enzyme 5'deiodinase which is responsible for converting T4 into T3 as well as degrading rT3. Studies have confirmed lower production T3 in individuals with lower selenium status.[14] [15] [16] Numerous studies have demonstrated increased T3 synthesis as well as decreased rT3 production with selenium. [17] [18] [19] [20] [21]

ZINC It has been shown that low zinc status compromises T3 production.[22] Studies have also demonstrated that zinc supplementation improves thyroid hormone production.[23] [24] [25] [26] These effects may be due to the cofactor role zinc plays with type I 5'deiodinase. In addition, zinc may play a role in reducing thyroidal antibodies.[27]

19. THYROID-PITUITARY AXIS: Nutritional compounds to support the pituitary-thyroid axis

The pituitary releases TSH in order to stimulate the thyroid to produce thyroid hormones. If the pituitary is suppressed, usually as a result of excess thyroid hormones, contraceptives, or elevated cortisol from stress, it may not secrete proper amounts of TSH. These nutrients are used in the functional model to support this feedback system.

MAGNESIUM, ZINC, MANGANESE, THYROID GLANDU-LAR (PORCINE), PITUITARY GLANDULAR (PORCINE), RUBIDIUM, SAGE LEAF EXTRACT (SALVIA OFFICINALIS), L-ARGININE HCL, GAMMA ORYZANAL

20. HYPOPHYSEAL-GONADAL AXIS: Nutritional compounds to support the hypophyseal-ovarian axis to stimulate follicle stimulating hormone in order to stimulate estrogen production

These nutrients can be used in both males and females to optimize hypophyseal-gonadal function. These compounds work synergistically to optimize fertility, virility, and vitality. They have been shown to support Leuteinizing Hormone (LH) and testosterone production, as well as spermatogenesis. In females they may support Follicle Stimulating Hormone (FSH) and estradiol levels.

KEY INGREDIENTS
RESEARCH COMMENTARY

TRIBULUS TERRESTRIS is a popular herb used to support sexual weakness in both males and females. It seems to have opposite impacts on physiology on males versus females. In males, Tribulus has shown to support spermatogenesis, increase the number of Sertoli cells in the testis, and increase LH and testosterone with no change in FSH levels. In females Tribulus appears to support healthy concentration of FSH and estradiol. Therefore, the primary role of Tribulus appears to be the support of the hypophyseal-gonadal axis in both males and females.[1] [2] [3] [4] [5] [6]

LEPIDIUM MAYENIL (PERUVIAN MACA) is an herb that has been used historically to enhance fertility in males, females, and livestock. It appears to have positive impacts on spermatogenesis, fertility, and hormone levels. Aphrodisiac and anti-stress properties of this herb have also been reported.[7] [8] [9] [10]

PANAX GINSENG has a long history of its use in supporting fertility and virility in both sexes. It has shown the ability to improve libido, support healthy testosterone concentrations, promote the growth of the testis, and improve spermatogenesis.[11] [12] [13] [14]

ZINC has always played an important role in healthy hormone metabolism. Most of the research on the impact of zinc is the role it has shown to play with male infertility and testosterone concentrations. Zinc supplementation has shown to improve both fertility and serum testosterone concentrations when levels of zinc are deficient.[15] [16] [17]

21. PROGESTERONE METABOLISM: Nutritional compounds to help support the hypophyseal-ovarian axis to stimulate leutinizing hormone in order to simulate progesterone production

These nutrients have been shown to support a healthy release of leuteinizing hormone and the output of progesterone. They also support a healthy estrogen/progesterone ratio, the body's ability to produce progesterone, and the ability to manage premenstrual syndrome.

KEY INGREDIENTS
RESEARCH COMMENTARY

CHASTEBERRY (VITEX ANGUS-CASTUS) contains numerous glycosides and flavonoids that appear to have an optimizing impact in luteal phase function. In some studies it has demonstrated the ability to increase progesterone levels while lowering estrogen levels, because of its ability to increase leuteinizing hormone (LH) while supporting a decrease in follicle-stimulating hormone (FSH).[1] [2] [3] [4]

CHASTEBERRY is also shown to posess modulating effects on prolactin.[5] This is important because hyperprolactenemia is associated with corpus luteum insufficiency and abnormal levels of progesterone in the second half of the menstrual cycle.[6] Studies on Chasteberry have also demonstrated its role in normalizing abnormal cycles,[7] improving premenstrual syndrome,[8] [9] supporting fertility,[10] and optimizing luteal phase function.

SHEPHERD'S PURSE (CASELLA BUSA-PASTORIS) contains compounds that increase uterine tone as well as hemostatic properties. It appears to be helpful in dysfunctional uterine bleeding associated with progesterone deficiency. Shepherd's Purse has also been used to treat hemorrhoids and diarrhea.[11] [12] [13] [14]

22. ESTROGEN METABOLISM: Nutritional compounds to optimize estrogen metabolism and receptor site response

These nutrients are recommended for healthy estrogen balance in both men and women. Estrogen dominance is a very common hormonal imbalance that exists in all industrialized countries. Estrogen dominance can be determined by elevated levels of estrogen, or by the progesterone/estrogen ratio in women, or the testosterone/estrogen ratio in men. These nutrients are useful in cases that require maintaining healthy estrogen metabolism such as premenstrual syndrome, menopause, etc. They can also be used to support estrogen balance during follicular phase or luteal phase variations.

KEY INGREDIENTS
RESEARCH COMMENTARY

ISOFLAVONES (DAIDZEIN AND GENISTEIN) Soy contains compounds called isoflavones. The biological active isoflavones include the compounds daidzein and genistein. Isoflavones have been classified as phytoestrogens because of their estrogenic properties, however this classification may not be appropriate. The term "Selective Estrogen Receptor Modulator" is the term that has gained recent acceptance due to the adaptive nature of these compounds on estrogen receptor sites. Isoflavones are not just compounds that have the ability to bind to estrogen receptors and induce an estrogen-like response. Their pharmacology is much more advanced. It appears that isoflavones have the ability to exert both agonistic and anti-agonistic effects on estrogen receptor sites depending on the circumstance. For example, isoflavones have demonstrated an estrogenic effect on receptor sites in tissues absent of proper estrogen levels, and an anti-estrogenic effect on receptor sites in the presence of excess estrogen.[1]

This explains their acknowledged clinical effectiveness in both low and high estrogen cases. These compounds have also been shown to have modulating impacts on estrogen metabolism that are not direct receptor mediated due to their impact on sex hormone-binding globulin (SHBG). Isoflavones have the ability to support the production of SHBG, which has the ability to bind to the cell surface receptors resulting in the regulation and the bioavailability and activity of hormones.[2] Isoflavones have also demonstrated in studies to have many positive impacts on both male and female metabolism,[3] [4] [5] antiviral properties,[6] anti-inflammatory properties,[7] antioxidant properties,[8] [9] and cardioprotective properties.[10]

INDOLE-3-CARBINOL Estrogen hormones are metabolized initially in the liver by hydroxylation at phase I of the detoxification process. This hydroxylation takes place primarily on one of three carbons. The 2-carbon, which yields 2-hydroxyestrone (2-OH), the 4-carbon which yields 4-hydroxyestrone (4-0H) or on the 16-alpha-carbon which yields 16-alpha-hydroxyestrone (16-alpha-OH).

The 2-OH metabolite has a very weak estrogenic response and is therefore the preferential estrogen metabolite. On the other hand,

16-alpha-OH and the 4-OH exert a powerful and persistent mitogenic estrogen receptor response. Therefore, modifying metabolism to yield more 2-0H metabolites and less 16-alpha-OH and the 4-OH metabolites would be optimal, especially for those that are estrogen dominant. A natural compound derived from cruciferous vegetables called Indole-3-Carbinol (I3C) has the ability to shift the ratio of 2-OH to 16-alpha-OH in favor of 2-OH. I3C promotes 2-OH formation by inducing phase I cytochrome P450-1A1 and P450-1A2, which facilitates 2-hydroxylation of estrogen. In addition, I3C also has shown some ability to decrease 4-OH production. Improving the ratios of phase I hydroxylation metabolites may have positive impacts on the influence of healthy estrogen metabolism. [11] [12] [13] [14] [15] [16] [17]

PYRIDOXAL-5-PHOSPHATE (B6) Vitamin B-6 has been shown to reduce tissue hypersensitivity to estrogen. Evidence shows that vitamin B6 interacts with the steroid hormone receptor complex and the binding of this complex to DNA. This binding will then turn off the transmission of the hormonal signal to the nucleus of the cell. A B-6 deficiency may explain why there may be exaggerated symptoms of estrogen dominance with normal or slightly increased estrogen levels. It may not be the level of estrogens causing estrogen excess symptoms, but rather the exaggerated transcriptional response that induces the expression of estrogen excess symptoms and patterns. An active form of B-6 such as pyridoxal-5-phosphate should be considered anytime a nutritional approach is used to optimize estrogen or other hormonal patterns.[18]

BLACK COHOSH (CIMICIFUGA RACEMOSA) contains triterpene glycosides which have estrogen modulating impacts on metabolism. The active components of black cohosh appear to improve estrogen deficient type symptoms without the adverse risks of estrogen replacement therapy. It has shown to decrease hot flashes, increase blood flow to the pelvic area, relieve spasms, and improve hormone related mood depression, but it does not stimulate the uterine tissues the way estrogen does or alter the release of prolactin or follicle-stimulating hormone. Therefore, it lacks the complete properties of estrogen, which makes it a safe and natural compound to use in support of estrogen balance.[20] [21] [22] [23] [24]

DONG QUAI (ANGELICA SINENSIS) is another herb that has "Selective Estrogen Receptor Modulator" properties. It contains compounds that exhibit estrogenic expression. However, their activity is as low as a 1:400 ratio compared to human estrogens and have no true estrogen impact on cells. It is its chemical influence on receptor sites that have made this herb useful in both estrogen deficient and estrogen excess cases. In estrogen deficient patterns, angelica compounds have the ability to exert some influence on estrogen receptor site expression and improve symptoms of low estrogen. In estrogen excess type patterns, angelica compounds have the ability to compete with estrogens on receptor sites and reduce the influence of estrogen receptor binding. Therefore, it may be useful in both excess and deficient type patterns.[25] Angelica has many other favorable qualities including qualities as a hemotonic for treating anemia, analgesic properties, anti-inflammatory and anti-allergenic actions, cardioprotective influence, mild laxative property, as well as its ability to increase vagina lubrication.[26] [27] [28] [29] [30] [31]

MAGNESIUM is an essential nutrient for the phase II detoxification of estrogens. Once estrogens are hydroxylated by phase I detoxification they become catechol estrogens with the potential to become oxidized to quinone estrogens. Quinone estrogens can induce genotoxic damage and promote carcinogenesis.[32] Magnesium is an essential cofactor for the enzyme catechol-O-methyltransferase (COMT) which converts catechol estrogens into water soluble metabolites before they become potential carcinogenic quinone estrogens.[33] Magnesium also helps phase II glucuronidation by up-regulating the enzyme glucuronyl transferase which helps detoxify estrogens.

METHYLATION COFACTORS Vitamin B12 and folic acid help support the essential methylation detoxification pathway which helps convert the estrogens to methyl ester metabolites which can then be excreted via bile elimination or urination.

23. TESTOSTERONE BALANCE: Nutritional compounds to help prevent the conversion of testosterone into estrogen

An enzyme called aromatase functions by converting testosterone into estrogen. This occurs normally in peripheral tissue, especially in body fat. Aromatase over activity is very common, especially in men. As a matter of fact, it is the most common cause of andropause. Andropause refers to a physiological state in which the production of androgen dominant hormones such as testosterone decline. Functional andropause takes place when the ratios between testosterone and other hormones shift. The most common cause of functional andropause occurs when there is a difference in the ratio between serum levels of testosterone and estrogen. For example, a normal serum testosterone to estrogen ratio may be 50:1. Some men with andropause appear to have an 8:1 ratio. These men may have normal lab ranges of testosterone, but their state of estrogen dominance is expressing a low testosterone state. This is usually due to over active aromatase function which creates a metabolic shift that metabolizes testosterone into estrogens. [1] [2] [3]

When an individual has over activity of aromatase they will have an abnormal testosterone to estrogen ratio and express signs and symptoms of low androgens such as loss of libido, inability to maintain erections, loss of muscle mass, increase in body fat, sweating attacks, depression, high blood sugar and insulin, high blood pressure, and high cholesterol. [4] [5] Many times these patients' abnormal metabolism is missed because only a bioassay of testosterone is completed. [6]

KEY INGREDIENTS
RESEARCH COMMENTARY

CHRYSIN CREAM Chrysin (5,7-dihydroxyflavone) is a compound that belongs to the flavonoid family. The flavonoid chrysin has shown a unique ability to prevent the conversion of testosterone into estrogens by inhibiting the enzyme aromatase. [7] [8] [9] [10] [11] [12] This is crucial in normalizing hormone shifts in which testosterone is converted into estrogens.

Recent advances in flavonoid delivery have allowed a cream to be developed to increase tissue exposure to chrysin. A cream delivery is far superior to oral intake of chrysin for several reasons. First, the absorption of chrysin via the gastrointestinal tract is difficult and the use of a cream allows delivery of the flavonoid directly into the blood stream by bypassing the gastrointestinal tract.[13] Second, the cream can be applied directly to adipose tissue, which is the location of most the aromatase enzyme. The chrysin cream form of delivery incorporates advanced delivery mechanisms that use lipid spheres called liposomes to deliver the flavonoid directly to the tissue where it is needed.

In addition to chrysin's role as an aromatase inhibitor, flavonoids such as chrysin are widely distributed in plants and have a characteristic molecular structure. These compounds have also shown to have antioxidant, [14] [15] anti-inflammatory, [16] [17] anti-histamine, [18] anti-viral, [19] and anti-carcinogenic properties.[20] [21] [22] The use of chrysin in a cream far exceeds only aromatase down-regulation activity.

24. SEROTONIN: Nutritional compounds to support serotonin response, activity and synthesis

These compounds provide amino acids and cofactors required for serotonin production, and that have been shown to inhibit serotonin catabolism.

KEY INGREDIENTS
RESEARCH COMMENTARY

5-HYDROXYTRYPTOPHAN (5-HTP) is an amino acid precursor to serotonin. Supplementation with 5-HTP has been shown clinically to increase serotonin levels. It has also been shown as an effective compound for mood swings, persistent nightmares, and more.[1] [2] [3] [4] [5] [6] [7] [8]

ST. JOHN'S WORT is also known as Hypericum perforatum and the active constituents include hyperforin, hypericin, and tannins. The botanical compounds have shown to increase serotoninergic activity be acting as a selective serotonin reuptake inhibitor. St. John's Wort has been shown to be an effective compound for certain mental states.[9] [10] [11] [12] [13] [14] [15] [16] [17]

S-ADENOSYLMETHIONINE (SAME) is a methyl donor in the brain and can transfer the methyl group of S-adenosylmethionine to the hydroxy group of N-acetyl-serotonin. A minimum of 10 placebo-controlled studies have demonstrated that SAMe has few reported side effects.[18] [19] Administration of SAMe has shown the ability to increase 5-hydroxyindoleacetic acid and serotonin.[20] [21] [22] SAMe has shown to be an effective mood enhancer.[23] [24] [25]

SEROTONIN COFACTORS Niacinamide, P-5-P, methylcobalamin, folic acid, and magnesium are essential nutritional cofactors for serotonin synthesis.

25. DOPAMINE: Nutritional compounds to support serotonin response, activity and synthesis

These compounds provide amino acids and cofactors required for serotonin production, and that have been shown to protect dopaminergic neurons.

KEY INGREDIENTS
RESEARCH COMMENTARY

MUCUNA PRURIENS is commonly known as cowhage and its active components include L-Dopa, tyrptamine alkaloids, lecithin, and tannins. It is postulated that the L-Dopa amino acid compounds in the botanicals are converted into dopamine in the brain. It has been used as a botanical for neurological disorders since ancient days and recent research has demonstrated that the botanical has Anti-Parkinson influences due to its precursor compounds. Additionally, the active components in Mucuna pruriens have protective impacts on the substantia nigra and nigrastriatal pathways.[1] [2] [3] [4] [5] [6]

BETA-PHENYLETHYLAMINE (PEA*)* is an endogenous monamine alkaloid and crosses the blood-brain barrier easily. It acts as a neuromodulator in the nigrostriatal dopaminergic pathway and stimulates the release of dopamine. PEA also has influences on beta endorphins that have been attributed to feeling of pleasure. Chocolate contains a rich source of PEA and it is this mechanism that is theorized to cause the feelings of love, pleasure, and satisfaction via dopamine activation. PEA supplementation has shown to improve attention and enhance mood.[7][8][9][10][11]

BLUEBERRY EXTRACT contains a rich and potent source of antioxidants, particularly the Anthocyanin compounds. These compounds have proven effective in free radical quenching areas of the dopamine rich neurons of the central nervous system.[12][13][14][15]

D, L–PHENYLALANINE (DLPA) is an essential amino acid precursor for the production of dopamine. It is required from the diet form sources such as meat, fish, eggs, and dairy products. The L-form of phenylalanine is converted into catecholamines such as dopamine. The D-form of phenyalanine is used to produce the dopamine modulator phenylethylamine. The combination of both forms of phenylalanine are referred to as DLPA and found to be an effective mood enhancer, and reduces pain perception. DLPA prevents the breakdown and degradation of endorphins.[16][17][18][19][20][21]

N-ACETYL-TYROSINE is an amino acid that serves as a precursor for dopamine production. Oral supplementation with tyrosine results in increased plasma and brain levels of the compound. Tyrosine supplementation has demonstrated the ability to change plasma neurotransmitter levels. Tyrosine is converted into dopamine by the enzyme tyrosine hydroxylase in the brain. Additionally, tyrosine depletion by dietary means produces symptoms of decreased dopamine in both human and animal studies.[22][23][24][25][26][27]

PYRIDOXAL-5-PHOSPHATE (P-5-P) the active form of vitamin B6 is pyridoxal-5-phosphate (P-5-P) and under nutrition of[28] this compound promotes loss of dopamine in the corpus straitum. It appears that dopaminergic neurons of the nigrostriatal tract may be vulnerable to long-term P-5-P deficiency. Additionally, P-5-P deficiency prolongs the time course of evoked dopamine release from the rat striatum.[29][30][31][32]

GLUTATHIONE COFACTORS The substania nigra is extremely sensitive to oxidative stress by hydroxy radicals. Glutathione has demonstrate promise in protecting these neuronal tissues responsible for producing dopamine. The essential nutritional substrates for the synthesis of glutathione are selenium, and N-acetyl-cysteine.[33][34][35]

GLOSSARY

Antigen presenting cell (APC): A cell created when a macrophage attaches to an intruder and acts like a burglar alarm, summoning the rest of the immune system to come help

B-cells: Immune cells that make antibodies against antigens in order to remember the antigen

Celiac disease: A form of gluten intolerance that involves an autoimmune response in the small intestine

Circadian rhythm: A cycle of cortisol excretion that should be higher in the mornings and low in the evenings so that one wakes up alert and is tired before bed

Cortisol: A hormone secreted by the adrenal glands

Cytotoxic T-cells: Immune cells sent to destroy an antigen

Dopamine: An excitatory brain neurotransmitter

Endocrine glands: Hormone-producing glands

Exogenous hormones: Hormones not made by the body, such as oral contraceptives or estrogen creams

Gliadin: The portion of gluten that causes an immune reaction in those with gluten intolerance or celiac disease

Gluten: The protein found in wheat and wheat-like grains, including spelt, kamut, rye, barley, triticale, and oats

Gluten ataxia: A disease in which gluten triggers neurological problems

Growth hormone (GH): A hormone that regenerates cells and tissues

Hashimoto's disease: An autoimmune disorder in which the immune system attacks and destroys the thyroid gland

Hypochlorhydria: A condition in which the stomach produces too little stomach acid, or hydrochloric acid (HCl)

Hypoglycemia: Blood sugar that is chronically low

Hypothalamus: A tiny, cone-shaped structure located in the lower center of the brain that communicates between the nervous and endocrine systems

Hypothyroidism: When the thyroid is under active

Hyperthyroidism: When the thyroid is over active

Insulin resistance (also knows as Metabolic Syndrome, or Syndrome X): When cells refuse entry to insulin and thus glucose, resulting in high blood sugar

Intestinal permeability (leaky gut): When the junctures of the intestinal wall loosen, allowing undigested food and other substances into the bloodstream

Leaky gut (intestinal permeability): When the junctures of the intestinal wall loosen, allowing undigested food and other substances into the bloodstream

Macrophages: Immune cells that engulf an antigen and stimulate an immune response

Natural killer cells: Immune cells sent to destroy an antigen

Pituitary gland: A gland in the brain that is like an air traffic controller, directing the endocrine system

Polycystic ovarian syndrome (PCOS): The most common female hormone disorder in the United States that presents as elevated insulin, elevated testosterone and multiple ovarian cysts

Pregnenolone steal: When the body steals pregnenolone, a precursor to the sex hormones, from cholesterol to make more cortisol in response to chronic stress

Reactive hypoglycemia: Low blood sugar that occurs two to five hours after eating

Serotonin: An inhibitory brain neurotransmitter

TH-1: T-helper cells involved in an innate, or immediate, immune response

TH-2: T-helper cells involved in a humoral, or delayed, immune response

TH-1 dominance: An immune imbalance in which the TH-1 pathway is over abundant or over active

TH-2 dominance: An immune imbalance in which the TH-2 pathway is over abundant or over active

T-helper cells: Immune cells that help direct immune activity

T-regulator cells: Immune cells that direct immune activity

T-suppressor cells: Immune cells that stop an immune reaction when necessary

Tetraidothyronine 5' deiodinase: An enzyme that removes one molecule of iodine from T4

Thyroid binding globulins: Proteins that transport thyroid hormones through the bloodstream

Thyroid follicles: Small spheres of hormone-producing cells within the gland

Thyroglobulin: A protein involved in thyroid hormone production

Thyroglobulin antibodies (TGB Ab): Immune cells that indicate the immune system is attacking TGB in the thyroid gland

Thyroid peroxidase (TPO): An enzyme in the thyroid responsible for thyroid hormone production

Thyroid peroxidase antibodies (TPO Ab): Immune cells that indicate the immune system is attacking TPO in the thyroid gland

Thyroid-stimulating hormone (TSH): A hormone secreted by the pituitary gland to stimulate thyroid activity

Thyrotropin releasing hormone (TRH): A hormone sent from the hypothalamus to the pituitary gland to stimulate thyroid activity

Thyroxine (T4): A thyroid hormone named for its four molecules of iodine

Triiodothyronine (T3): A thyroid hormone named for its three molecules of iodine, and the most predominate and active form of thyroid hormone the body can use

Reverse T3 (rT3): A form of thyroid hormone the body cannot use

T3 acetic acid: A thyroid hormone that has the potential to become useful if acted upon by healthy bacteria in the digestive tract

T3 sulfate: A thyroid hormone that has the potential to become useful if acted upon by healthy bacteria in the digestive tract

REFERENCES FOR
NUTRITIONAL COMPOUNDS

1. INSULIN RESISTANCE

[1] Shanmugasundaram ERB, et al. Use of Gynema sylvestre leaf extract in the control of blood glucose in insulin-dependent diabetes mellitus. *J Ethanopharmacol* 1990; 30: 281-294.

[2] Persaud SJ, Al-Majed H, Raman A, Jones PM. Gymnema sylvestre stimulates insulin release in vitro by increased membrane permeability. *J Endocrinol* 1999; 163(2):207-12.

[3] Shanmugasundaram ERB, et al. Possible regeneration of the islet of Langerhans in streptozoticin-diabetic rats given Gynema sylvestre leaf extracts. *J Ethnopharmacol* 1990 30; 265-279.

[4] Shanmugasundaram KR, et al. Enzyme changes and glucose utilization in diabetic rabbits: the effect of Gymnema sylvestre, R.Br. *J Ethnopharmacol* 1983; 7(2):205-34.

[5] Kaskaran K, et al. Antidiabetic effect of a leaf extract from Gymnema sylvestre in non-insulin dependent diabetes mellitus patients. *J Ethnopharmacol* 1990; 30: 295-305.

[6] Khare AK, Tondon RN, Tewari JP. Hypoglycemic activity of an indigenous drug (Gymnema sylvestre, 'Gurmar') in normal and diabetic persons. *Indian J Physiol Pharmacol* 1983;27(3):257-8.

[7] Striffler JS, Polansky MM, Anderson RA. Overproduction of insulin in the chromium-deficient rat. *Metabolism* 1999;48:1063-1068.

[8] Striffler JS, Polansky MM, et al. Chromium improves insulin response to glucose in rats. *Metabolism* 1995;44:1314-1320.

[9] Anderson RA, Polansky MM, Bryden NA, Canary JJ. Supplemental-chromium effects on glucose, insulin, glucagon, and urinary chromium losses in subjects consuming controlled low-chromium diets. *Am J Clin Nutr* 1991:54:909-916.

[10] Offenbacher EG, Pi-Sunyer FX. Beneficial effect of chromium-rich yeast on glucose tolerance and blood lipids in elderly subjects. *Diabetes* 1980;29:919-925.

[11] Riales R, Albrink MJ. Effect of chromium chloride supplementation on glucose tolerance and serum lipids including high-density lipoprotein of adult men. *Am J Clin Nutr* 1981;34:2670-2678.

[12] Evans GW, Browman TD. Chromium picolinate increases membrane and rate of insulin internalization. *J Inorg Bio* 1992;46:243-250.

[13] Roeback, Jr. JR, Hla KM, Chambless, et al. Effects of chromium supplementation on serum high density lipoprotein cholesterol levels in men taking beta-blockers. *Ann Intern Med.* 1991:115:917-924.

[14] Anderson R, Cheng N, Bryden, et al. Beneficial effects of chromium for people with type II diabetes. *Diabetes* 1996;45:124A.

[15] Anderson RA, Cheng N, Bryden NA, et al. Elevated intakes of supplemental chromium improve glucose and insulin variables in individuals with type 2 diabetes. *Diabetes* 1997;46:1786-1791.

[16] Levine R, Streeten D, Doisy R. Effect of oral chromium supplementation on the glucose tolerance of elderly human subjects. *Metabolism* 1968;17:114-125.

[17] French RJ, Jones PJ. Role of vanadium in nutrition: metabolism, essential and dietary considerations. *Life Sciences* 1992;52:339-346.

[18] Shechter, Li Meyerovitch, et al. Insulin-like actions of vanadate are mediated in an insulin receptor independent manner via non-receptor protein tyrosine kinases and protein phosphotyrisine phosphates. *Mol Cell Biochem* 1995;153(1-2):39-47.

[19] Halberstm M, Cohen N, Shlimovish P, et al. Oral vanadyl sulfate improves insulin sensitivity NIDDM but not in obese nondiabetic subjects. *Diabetes* 1996;45:659-665.

[20] Boden G, Chen X, Ruiz J, et al. Effects of vanadyl sulfate on carbohydrate and lipid metabolism in patients with non-insulin dependent diabetes mellitus. *Metabolism* 1996;45:1130-1135.

[21] Cohen N,Halberstam M, Shlimovih P, et al. Oral vanadyl sulfate improves hepatic and peripheral insulin insensitivity in patients with non-insulin dependent diabetes mellitus. *J Clin Invest 1995;95:2501-2509.*

[22] Goldfine AB, Simonson DC, Folli F, et al. Metabolic effects of sodium metavandate in humans with insulin-dependent and noninsulin-dependent diabetes mellitus in vivo and vitro studies. *J Clin Enco and Meta* 1995;80(11);3311-3319.

[23] Shang H, Osada K, Maebashi M, et al. A high biotin diet improves the impaired glucose tolerance of long-term spontaneously hyperglycemic rats with non-insulin dependent diabetes mellitus. *J Nutr Sci Vitamin* 1996;42:517-526.

[24] Jacob S, Henriksen EJ, Schiemann AL, et al. Enhancment of glucose disposal in patients with Type 2 diabetes by alpha-lipoic acid. *Arzneim-Rosch Drug Res* 1995;45(2):872-874.

[25] Jacob S, Streeper RS, Fogt DL, et al. The antioxidant alpha-lipoic acid enhances insulin-stimulated glucose metabolism in insulin resistant rate skeletal muscle. *Diabetes* 1996;45:1024-1029.

[26] Streeper RS, Henriksen EJ, Jacob S, et al. Differential effects of lipoic acid stereoisomers on glucose metabolism in insulin resistant skeletal muscle. *Am J Physiol* 1997;273:E185-E191.

[27] Konard T, Vicini P, Kuster K, et al. Alpha-lipoic acid treatment decreases serum lactate and pyruvate concentrations and improves glucose effectiveness in lean and obese patients with type 2 diabetes. *Diabetes Care* 1999;22(2):280-287.

[28] Rudich A, Tirosh A, Potashinik R, Khamaisi M, Bashan N. Lipoic acid protects against oxidative stress induced impairment in insulin stimulation of protein kinase B and glucose transport in 3T3-L1 adipocytes. *Diabeologia* 1999;42:949-957.

[29] Kawabata T and Packer L. Alpha-lipoate can protect against glycation of serum albumin, bu nto low density lipoprotein. *Biochem Biophys Res Comm* 1994;203:99-104.

[30] Jacob S, Ruus P, Hermann R, et al. Improvement of insulin-stimulated glucose-disposal in type 2 diabets after repeated patenteral administration of thioctic acid. *Exp Clin Endocrinol Diabetes* 1996;104:284-288.

[31] Jacob S, Ruus, Herman R, et al. Oral administration of RAC-alpha-lipoic acid modulates insulin sensitivity in patients with type-2 diabetes: a placebo-controlled pilot trial. *Free Radic Biol Med* 1999;27:309-314.

[32] Nagamstsu M, et al. Lipoic acid improves nerve blood flow, reduces oxidative stress, and improves distal nerve conduction in experimental diabetic neuropathy. *Diabetes Care* 1995;18:1160-1167.

[33] Paolisso G, D'Amore A, Galzenano D. Daily vitamin E supplementations improve metabolic control but not insulin secretion in elderly type II diabetic

patients. *Diabetes Care* 1993;16:1433-1437.

[34] Salonen JT, Jyyssonen K, Tuomainen TP. Increased risk of non-insulin diabetes mellitus at low plasma vitamin E concentrations. A four year follow-up study in men. *Br Med J* 1995;311:1124-1127.

[35] Barbagallo M, Dominquez LJ, Tagliamonte MR, et al. Effects of vitamin E and glutathione on glucose metabolism: role of magnesium. *Hypertension* 1999; 34:1002-1006.

[36] Paolisso G, D'Amore A, Guigliano D, et al. Pharmacologic doses of vitamin E improves insulin action in healthy subjectsand in non-insulin-dependent diabetic patients. *Am J Clin Nutr* 1993;57:650-656.

[37] Paolisso G, Gambardella A, Giugilano D, et al. Chronic intake of pharmacological doses of vitamin E might be useful in the therapy of elderly patients with coronary heart disease. *Am J Clin Nutr* 1995;81:848-852.

[38] Jain SK, McVie R, Jaramillo JJ, et al. Effect of modest vitamin E supplementation on blood glycated hemoglobin and triglyceride levels and red cell indices in type I diabetic patients. *J Amer Col Nutr* 1996;15(5);458-461.

[39] Paolisso G, Ravussin E. Intercellular magnesium and insulin resistance; results in Pima Indians and Caucasians. *J Endocrinol Metab* 1995;80:1382-1385.

[40] Paolisso G, Sgambato S, Pizza G, et al. Improved insulin response and action by chronic magnesium administration in aged NIDDM subjects. *Diabetes Care* 1989;12;265-269.

[41] Paolisso G, Sgambato S, Gambardell A, et al. Daily magnesium supplements improve glucose handling in elderly subjects. *Am J Clin Nutr* 1992;55:1161-1167.

[42] Nadler JL, Buchanan T, Natarajan R, et al. Magnesium deficiency produces insulin resistance and increased thromboxane synthesis. *Hypertension* 1993;21:1024-1029.

[43] Humphries S, Kushner H, Falkner B. Low dietary magnesium is associated with insulin resistance in a sampling of young, nondiabetic Black Americans. *Am J Hypertens* 1999;12:747-756.

[44] Dominguez LJ, Barbagallo M, Sowers JR, Resnick LM. Magnesium responsiveness to insulin and insulin-like growth factor I in erthrocytes from normotensive and hypertensive subjects. *J Clin Endocrinol Metab* 1998;83:4402-4407.

[45] Reddi A, DeAngelis B, Frank O, et al. Biotin Supplementation improves glucose and insulin tolerances in genetically diabetic KK mice. *Life Science* 1998;42:1323-1330.

[46] Kutosikos D, Fourtounas C, Kepetanaki A, et al. Oral glucose tolerance test after high-dose i.v. bioitin administration in normoglucemic hemodialysis paitents. *Ren Fail* 1996;18:131-137.

[47] Shang H, Osada K, Maebashi M, et al. A high biotin diet improves the impaired glucose tolerance of long-term spontaneously hyperglycemic rats with non-insulin-dependent diabetes mellitus. *J Nutr Sci Vitamin* 1996;42:517-526.

[48] Maebashi M, Makino Y, Furukawa Y, et al. Therapeutic evaluation of the effect of biotin on hyperglycemia in patients with non-insulin dependent diabetes mellitus. *J Clin Biochem Nutr* 1993;14:211-218.

[49] Hegazi SM. Effects of zinc supplementation on serum glucose, insulin, glucagons, glucose-6-phosphate, and mineral levels in diabetics. *J Clin Biochem Nutr* 1992;12:209-215.

[50] Mooradian AD, Morley JE. Micronutrient status in diabetes mellitus. *Am J Clin Nutr* 1987;45:877-895.

[51] Chen MD, Lin PY, Lin Wh. Investigation of relationship between zinc and obesity. *Kao Hsiung I Hsueh Tsa Chih* 1991;7:628-634.

[52] Singh RB, Niaz MA, Rastogi SS, et al. Current zinc intake and risk of diabetes

and coronary artery diseasse and factors associated with insulin resistance in rural and urban populations of North India. *J Am Col Nutr* 1998;17:564-570.

[53] Leslie RDG, Elliot RB. Early environmental events as a cause of IDDM. *Diabetes* 1994;43:843-850.

[54] Urberg M, Zemel MB. Evidence of synergism between chromium and nicotinic acid in the control of glucose tolerance in elderly humans. *Metabolism* 1987;36:574-576.

[55] Pocoit F, Reimers JI, Anderson HU. Nicotimaminde – biological action and therapeutic potential in diabetes prevention. *Diabetologia* 1993;36:574-576.

[56] Clearly JP. Vitamin B3 in the treatment of diabetes mellitus: case reports and review of the literature. *J Nutr Med* 1990;1:217-225.

[57] Pozzilli P, Andreani D. The potential role of nicotinimide in the secondary prevention of IDDM. *Diabetes Metabol Rev* 1993;9:219-230.

[58] Anderson HU, Jorgensen KH, Egeberg J. Nicotinamide prevents interleukin-1 effects on accumulated insulin release and nitric oxide production in rat islets of langerhans. *Diabetes* 1994;43:770-777.

[59] Heller W, Mushi HE, Gaebel G, et al. Effect of L-carnitine on post-stress metabolism in surgical patients. Infusiosther Klin Ernahr 1986;13:268-276.

[60] Gunal AI, Celiker H, Donder E, Gunal SY. The effect of L-carnitine on insulin resistance in hemodialysed patients with chronic renal failure. *J Nephrol* 1999;12:38-40.

[61] Mingrone G, Greco AV, Capristo E, et al. L-carnitine improves glucose disposal in type 2 diabetic patients. *J Am Coll Nutr* 1999;18:77-82.

[62] Greco AV, et al. Effect of propionyl-L-carnitine in the treatment of angiopathy: Controlled double blind trial versus placebo. *Drugs Exp Clin Res* 1992;18:69-80.

[63] Abdel-Aziz MT, Abdou MS, Soliman K, et al. Effects of L-carnitine on blood lipid patterns in diabetic patients. *Nutr Rep Int* 1984;29:1071-1079.

2. INSULIN RESISTANCE BOTANICALS

[1] Kakudat T, Sakane L, Takihara T, Ozaki Y, Takeuchi H, and Kuroyanagi M. Hypoglycemic effects of extracts from Lagerstroema speciosa L. leaves in genetically diabetic KK-AY mice. *Biosci Biotechno Biochem*, 1996; 60:204-208.

[2] Murakami C, Myoga K, Kasai R, Othani K, Kurowkasca T, Ishibashi S, Dayrit F, Padolina WG, and Yamaski K. Screening of plant constituents for effect on glucose transport activity in Erlich ascites tumor cells. *Chem Pharm Bull* (Tokyo), 1993;41:2129-2131.

[3] Kubo K, Aoki H, and Nanba H. Anti-diabetic activity present in the fruit body of Grifola frondosa (Maitake). *Biol Pharm Bull*,1994; 17:1106-1110.

[4] Manohar V, Talpur N, Echard BW, Leiberman S, and Preusss HG. Effects of water soluble extract of maitake mushroom on circulating glucose/insulin concentrations in KK mice. *Diabetes, Obesity and Metabolism*, 2001.

[5] Mizuno T and Zhuang C. Maitake, Grigola frondosa; pharmacologic effects. *Food Reviews Int*, 1995;11:135-149.

[6] Therapeutic Research Faculty. Maitake. In: *Natural Medicines*. Comprehensive Database. Stockton, CA, 2001; pp 699-700.

[7] Marles,RJ, Farnsworth,NR: Plants as sources of antidiabetic agents. *Economic and Medical Plant Research* 6:149-187, 1993

[8] Marles,RJ, Farnsworth,NR: Antidiabetic plants and their active constituents. *Phytomed* 2:137-189, 1995

[9] Grover,JK, Yadav,S, Vats,V: Medicinal plants of India with anti-diabetic potential. *J Ethnopharmacol.* 81:81-100, 2002

[10] Shapiro,K, Gong,WC: Natural products used for diabetes. *J Am Pharm Assoc* (Wash.) 42:217-226, 2002

[11] Yeh,GY, Eisenberg,DM, Kaptchuk,TJ, Phillips,RS: Systematic review of herbs and dietary supplements for glycemic control in diabetes. *Diabetes Care* 26:1277-1294, 2003

[12] Basch,E, Gabardi,S, Ulbricht,C: Bitter melon (Momordica charantia): a review of efficacy and safety. *Am J Health Syst Pharm* 60:356-359, 2003

[13] Nag,B, Medicherla,S, Sharma,SD: Orally active fraction of momordica charantia, active peptides thereof, and their use in the treatment of diabetes. US Patent 6,391,854:1-14, 2002

[14] Basch,E, Gabardi,S, Ulbricht,C: Bitter melon (Momordica charantia): a review of efficacy and safety. *Am J Health Syst Pharm* 60:356-359, 2003

[15] Shanmugasundaram ERB, et al. Use of Gynema sylvestre leaf extract in the control of blood glucose in insulin-dependent diabetes mellitus. J Ethanopharmacol 1990; 30: 281-294.

[16] Persaud SJ, Al-Majed H, Raman A, Jones PM. Gymnema sylvestre stimulates insulin release in vitro by increased membrane permeability. *J Endocrinol* 1999; 163(2):207-12.

[17] Shanmugasundaram ERB, et al. Possible regeneration of the islet of Langerhans in streptozoticin-diabetic rats given Gynema sylvestre leaf extracts. *J Ethnopharmacol* 1990 30; 265-279.

[18] Shanmugasundaram KR, et al. Enzyme changes and glucose utilization in diabetic rabbits: the effect of Gymnema sylvestre, R.Br. *J Ethnopharmacol* 1983;7(2):205-34.

[19] Kaskaran K, et al. Antidiabetic effect of a leaf extract from Gymnema sylvestre in non-insulin dependent diabetes mellitus patients. *J Ethnopharmacol* 1990; 30: 295-305.

[20] Khare AK, Tondon RN, Tewari JP. Hypoglycemic activity of an indigenous drug (Gymnema sylvestre, 'Gurmar') in normal and diabetic persons. *Indian J Physiol Pharmacol* 1983;27(3):257-8.

[21] Therapeutic Research Faculty. Prickly Pear Cactus. In : Natural Medicines. Comprehensive Database. Stockton, CA, 2001; pp 858-859.[22] Frait-Munari AC, Gordillo Be, Altamirano P, and Ariza CR. Hypoglycemic effect of Opuntia streptacantha Lemiare in NIDDM. *Diabetes Care* 1988; 11:63-66.

[23] Heller W, Mushi HE, Gaebel G, et al. Effect of L-carnitine on post-stress metabolism in surgical patients. *Infusiosther Klin Ernahr* 1986;13:268-276.

[24] Gunal AI, Celiker H, Donder E, Gunal SY. The effect of L-carnitine on insulin resistance in hemodialysed patients with chronic renal failure. *J Nephrol* 1999;12:38-40.

[25] Mingrone G, Greco AV, Capristo E, et al. L-carnitine improves glucose disposal in type 2 diabetic patients. *J Am Coll Nutr* 1999;18:77-82.

[26] Greco AV, et al. Effect of propionyl-L-carnitine in the treatment of angiopathy: Controlled double blind trial versus placebo. *Drugs Exp Clin Res* 1992;18:69-80.

[27] Abdel-Aziz MT, Abdou MS, Soliman K, et al. Effects of L-carnitine on blood lipid patterns in diabetic patients. *Nutr Rep Int* 1984;29:1071-1079.

[28] Lubec B, Hayn M, Kitzmü ller E, et al. L-arginine reduces lipid peroxidation in patients with diabetes mellitus. Free Rad Biol Med 1997;22:355-357.

3. N/A

4. ADRENAL ADAPTOGENS
[1] Shibita S, et al. Chemistry and pharmacology of Panax. *Economic and Medicinal Plant Research* 1985; 1:217-284.

[2] Avakia EV, Evonuk E. Effects of Pannax ginseng extract on tissue glycogen and adrenal cholesterol depletion during prolonged exercise. *Planta Medica* 1979; 36: 43-48.

[3] Shibata S, Tanaka O, Shoji, Saito H, Chemistry and pharmacology of Panax. In: *Economic and Medicinal Plant Research* vol. 1. London: Acadmic Pr;1985.

[4] Huong NT, Matusomoto K, Watanabe H. The antistress effect of majoniside-R2, a major saponin component of Vietnemase ginseng: neuronal mechanisms of action. *Methods Find Exp Clin Pharmacol* 1998;20(1):65-76.

[5] Gaffny BT, Hugel HM, Rich PA. Pannax ginseng in Eleutherococcus senticosus may exaggerate an already existing biphasic response to stress via inhibition of enzymes which limit the binding of stress hormones to their receptors. *Med Hypotheses* 2001;56(5):56-72.

[6] Fulder SJ. Ginseng and the hypothalamic-pituitary control of stress. *Am J Chinese Med* 1981;9(2):112-118.

[7] Nishibe S, et al. Phenolic compounds from stem bark of Acanthopanax senticosus and their pharmacological effect in chronic swimming stressed rats. *Chem Pharm Bull* 1990;38:1763-1765.

[8] Golotin VG, et al. Effect of ionol and eleutherococcus on changes of the hypophysea-adrenal system in rats under extreme conditions. *Vopr Med Khim* 1989;35:35-37.

[9] Filaretov AA, et al. Effects of adaptagens on the activity of the pituitary-adrenocortical system in rats. *Biull Eksp Biol Med* 1986;101:573-574.

[10] Fransworth NR, et al. Siberian ginseng (Eleutherococcus senticosus): Current status of an adaptogen. *Econ Med Plan Res* 1985;156-215.

[11] Eleskka M, et al. Withania somnifera, a plant with a great therapeutical future. *Rev Med Chir Soc Med Nat Iasi* 1989;93:349-350.

[12] Grandhi A, et al. A comparative pharmacological investigation of Ashwagandha and Ginseng. *J Ethnopharmacol* 1994;44:131-135.

[13] Kapoor LDL: Handbook of Ayuvedic Medicinal Plants, CRC Press: NY, 1990 (337-338)

[14] Sembulingam K, et al. *Indian J Physiol Phamacol.* 1997; 41(2);139-143.

[15] Wichtl MW. *Herbal Drugs and Phytopharmaceuticals.* Ed. N.M. Bisset. Stuttgart: Medpharm Scientific Publishers

[16] Wagner H, et al. Plant Adaptagens, *Phytomedicne* Vol 1 1994, pp. 63-76.

[17] Azizova AP, Seifulla RD. The effect of elton, leveton, fitoton and adapton on the work capacity of experimental animals. *Eksp Klin Farmakol* 1998;61:61-63.

[18] Maslova LV, Kondrat'ev Blu, Maslov LN, Lishmanov IuB. The cardioprotective and antiadrenergic activity of an extract of Rhodiola rosea in stress. *Eksp Klin Farmakol* 1994;57:61-63.

[19] Maimeskulova LA, Maslov LN. The anti-arrhyhmia action of an extract of Rhodiola rosea and of n-tyrosol in models of experimental arrhythmias. *Eksp Klin Farmakol* 1998;61:37-40.

[20] Afanas'ev SA., Alekseeva ED, Bardamova IB, et al. Cardiac contractile function following acute cooling of the body and the adaptagenic corrections of its disorders. *Biull Eksp Biol Med* 1993;116:480-483.

[21] Lishmanov IuB, Trifonova ZhV, Tsibin AN, et al. Plasma beta-endorphin and stress hormones in stress and adaptation. *Buil Eksp Biol Med* 1987;103:422-424.

[22] Spasov AA, Wikman GK, Mandrikov VB, et al. A double-blind placebo-controlled pilot study of the stimulating and adapatogenic effect of Rhodiola rosea SHR-5 extract on the fatigue of students caused by stress during an examination period with repeated low-dose regimen. *Phytomedicine* 2000;7(2):85-89.

[23] Darbinyan V, Kteyn A, Panossian A, et al. Rhodiola rosea in stress induced fatigue – a double blind cross-over study of a standardized extract SHR-5 with a repeated low-dose regimen on the mental performance of healthy physicians during night duty. *Phytomedicine* 2000;7(5):365-71.

[24] Mungantiwar AA, Nair AM, Shinde UA, Saraf MN. Effect of stress on plasma and adrenal cortisol levels and immune responsiveness in rats: modulation by alkaoidal fraction of Boerhaavia difuasa. *Fitoterapia* 1997;6:498-500.

[25] Kosaka C, Okdio M, Keneyuki, et al. Action of panathine on the adrenal cortex of hypophysectomized rats. *Horumon to Rinsho* 1973; 21:517-525.

[26] Onuki M, Hoshino H. Effects of pantehine on the adrenocortical fuction. Experimental results using rabbits. *Horumon To Rinsho* 197018: 601-605.

[27] Koska M, Kikui S, Fujiwara T. Kimoto T. Aciton of panathine on the adrenal cortex. *Horumn ToRhinsho* 1966;14:843-847.

[28] Onuki M, Suzawa A. Effect of panthine on the function of the adrenal cortex. Clinical experience using panatethine in cases under steroid hormone treatment. *Horumon To Rhinsho* 1970;18:937-940.

5. MODULATE ADRENAL STRESS RESPONSE

[1] Crook TH, Petrie W, Wells C, Massari DC, Effects of phosphatidylserine in Alzheimer's Disease. *Psychopharmacol Bull* 1992;28:61-66.

[2] Ameducci L, Crook TH, Lippi A, et al. Use of phosphatidylserine in Alzheimer's Disease. *Ann Ny Acad Sci* 1991;640:245-249.

[3] Cenacchi T, Bertoldin T, Farina C, et al. Cognitive decline in the elderly: A double-blind, placebo controlled multicenter study on efficacy of phosphatidylserine administration. *Aging Clin Ecp Res* 1993;5:123-133.

[4] Latorraca S, Piersanti P, Tesco G, et al. Effects of phosphatidylserine on free radical susceptibility in human diploid fibroblasts. *Neurol Transm Park Dis Dement Sect* 1993;6:73-77.

[5] Maggioni M, Picotti GB, Bondiolotti GP, et al. Effects of phosphatidylserine therapy in geriatric patients with depressive disorders. *Acta Psychiatr Scand* 1990;81:265-270.

[6] Brambilli F, Magioni M. Blood levels of cytokines in elderly patients with major depressive disorder. *Acta Psychiatr Scand* 1998;97:309-313.

[7] Brambilla F, Maggioni M, Panerai AE, et al. Beta-endorphin concentration in peripheral blood mononuclear cells of elderly depressed patients effects on phosphatidylserine therapy. *Neuropsychobiology* 1996;34:18-21.

[8] Palmieri G. Double-blind controlled trial of phosphatidylserine in patients with senile mental deterioration. *Clin Trials J* 1987;24:73-83.

[9] Kidd PM, Phosphatidylserine; membrane nutrient for memory. A clinical and mechanistic assessment. *Altern Med Rev* 1996;1:70-84.

[10] Cenacchi T, Betoldin R, Farina C, et al. Cognitive decline in the elderly. A double blind, placebo-controlled multicenter study on efficacy of phosphatidylserine administration. *Aging* 1993;5:123-133.

[11] Crook TH, Tinklenberg J, Yesavage J, et al. Effects of phosphatidylserine in age-associated memory impairment. *Neurology* 1991;41:644-649.

[12] Monteleone P, Mag M, Beinat, et al. Blunting of chronic phosphatidylserine administration of the stress-induced activation of the hypothalamic-pituitary-adrenal axis in healthy men. *Eur J Clin Pharmacol* 1992;41:385-388.

[13] Monteleone P, Beintat L, Tanzillo C, et al. Effects of phosphatidylserine on the neuroendocrine response to physical stress in humans. *Neuroendocrinology* 1990;52:243-248.

[14] Nerozzi D, Aceti F, Melia E, et al. Early cortisol escape phenomenon reversed by phosphatidylserine in elderly normal subjects. *Clinical Trial J* 1989;26:33-38.

[15] Fahey TD, Pearl MS. The hormonal and perceptive effects of phosphatidylserine administration during two weeks of resistive exercise-induced overtraining. *Biol Sport* 1998;15:135-144.

[16] LoPresti, JS and Nicoloff, JT. Thyroid response to critical illness. Endocrinology of Critical Disease. Human Press. Totowa. NJ. 1997. pp 157-173.

[17] Strakis, CA and Chrousos, GP. Neuroendocrinology and Pathophysiology of the Stress System, *Ann Ny Acad Sci*, Vol. 771, pp. 1-18,1995.

[18] Stockigt, JR. Update on the Sick Euthyroid Syndrome, in Baverman, LE ed., Diseases of the Thyroid, Humana Press, Totowa, NJ, 1997, pp. 49-68.

[19] Van Der Pomp G., et al. Elevated basal cortisol levels and attenuated ACTH and cortisol responses to a behavioral challenge in women with metastatic breast cancer. *Psychoneuroendocrinology,* 21(4). 361-374,1996.

[20] Guhad, FA, et al. Salivary IgA as a marker of social stress in rats. *Neurosci Lett,* 216(2). 137-140,1996.

[21] Cunningham-Rundies, C., et al. *Proc. Nat Acada. Sci USA.* 75:3387,1978.

[22] Scott, H., et al. *Scan. J. Gastroenterol.* 15:81, 1980.

[23] Daynes, R., et al. *Eur J Immunol.* 20:793,1990.

[24] Maggioni M, Picotti GM, Bondiolotti GP, et al. Effects of phosphatidylserine therapy in geriatric patients with depressive disorders. *Acta Psychiatr Scan* 1990;81:265-270.

[25] Havel PJ. Leptin production and action: relevance to energy balance in humans. *Am J Clin Nutr.* 1998;67(3):355-358.

[26] Freidman JM. Leptin, leptin receptors, and the control of body weight. *Nutr Rev.* 1998;56(2):S38-S46.

[27] Brindly DN. Role of glucocorticoids and fatty acids in the impairment of lipid metabolism observed in metabolic syndrome. *Int J Obes Relat Metab Disord* 1995;19(Suppl 1):S69-75.

[28] Bergh, F.T., et al. Dysregulation of the hypothalamo-pituitary-adrenal axis is related to the clinical course of MS. *Neurology* 53; 772-777,1999.

6. ADRENAL SUPPORT FOR ENERGY LEVELS

[1] Bensky D et al: Chinese Herbal Medicine Materia Medica revisited edition. *Eastland Press*: WA 1993.

[2] Huang, CH: The Pharmacology of Chinese Herbs, 2nd Edition, *CRC Press*: NY 1999

[3] Epstien M, Espiner E, Donald R, et al. Effect of eating licorice on the rennin-angiotensin aldosterone axis in normal subjects. *Br Med J* 1977; 1:488-490.

[4] Kumagai A, Nishino K, Shimomura A, et al. Effect of glycyrrhizin on estrogen action. *Endocrinol Japan* 1967;9:421-424.

[5] Kraus S. The anti-estrogenic action of beta-glycrrhetinic acid. *Exp Med Surg* 1969; 27:411-420.

[6] Abe N, Ebina T, Ishida N. Interferon induction by glycyrrhizic acid. *Experientia* 1980; 36:304-305.

[7] Pompei R, et al. Antiviral activity of glycyrrhizic acid. *Experientia* 1980; 36:304.

[8] Csonka G, Tyrrell D. Treatment of herpes genitals with carbonoxolone and cicloxolone creams. A double blinded placebo controlled trial. *Br J Ven Dis* 1984; 60:178-181.

[9] Hattori T, Ikematsu S, Kioto A, et al. Preliminary evidence for inhibitory effect of glycyrrhizin on HIV replication in patients with AIDS. *Antiviral Res* 1989; 11:255-261.

[10] Suzuki H, Ohta Y, Takino T, et al. Effects of glycyrrhizin on biochemical tests in patients with chronic hepatitis – double blind trial. *Asian Med J* 1984; 26:423-438.

[11] Mitscher L, Park Y, Clark D. Antimicrobial agents from higher plants. Antimicrobial isoflavonoids from Glycyrrhiza glabra. *J Natural Products* 1980; 43: 259-269.

[12] Kuroyanagi T, Sato M. Effect of prednisolone and glycyrrhizin on passive transfer of experimental allergic encephalomyelitis. *Allergy* 1966; 15:67-75.

[13] Kroes BH, et al. Inhibition of human complement by b-glycyrrhetinic acid. *Immunology* 1997; 90:115-20.

[14] Goso Y, Ogata Y, Ishihara K, Hotta K. Effects of traditional herbal medicine on gastric mucin against ethanol-induced gastric injury in rats. *Comp Biochem Phsyiol* 1996; 113C: 17-21.

[15] Glick L. Deglycrrhizinated liquorice in peptic ulcer. *Lancet* 1982; ii: 817.

[16] Bhatt HR. Antagonistic effectsof pentagastrin and cortisol on plasma level, urinary excretion and hepatic and renal uptake of vitamin B12 after intravenous injection in the cat. *J Physiol* 296, 1979.

[17] Regelson W, Lori R, Kalimi M, Dehydroepiandrosterone (DHEA) the "Mother Steroid" I: Immunologic Action. *Ann NY Acad Sci* 1994; 719: 553-563.

[18] Nestler JE, Clore JN, Blackard WG. Dehydroepiandrsterone: the "missing link" between hyperinsulinemia and atherosclerosis. *FASEB J* 1992; 6: 3073-3075.

[19] Leiter E, Beamer W, Coleman D, Longcope C. Androgenic and estrogenic metabolites in serum mice fed dehydroepiandrosterone: relationship to antihyperglycemic effects. *Metabolism* 1987; 36:863-869.

[20] Loria R Inge T, Cook S, et al. Androstenediol regulates systemic resistance against lethal infections in mice. *Arch of Virology* 1992; 127:103-115.

[21] Haffner SM, Valdez R, et al. Decreased testosterone and DHEA-S concentrations are associated with increased insulin and glucose concentrations in non-diabetic men. *Metabolism* 1994; 43:599-603.

[22] Robert E. Pregnenolone – From Selye to Alzheimer and a model of the prengnenolone sulfate binding site on the GABA receptor. *Biochem Pharmacol* 1995; 49: 1-16.

[23] Mathis C, Paul S, et al. The neurosteroid pregnenolone blocks NMDA-induced deficits in a passive avoidance task. *Psychopharm* 1994; 116;201-6.

[24] George J, Gudotti A, et al. CSF neuroactive steroids in affective disorders: pregenenolone, progesterone and DBI. *Biol Psychiatry* 1994; 35:775-80.

7. GLUTATHIONE/SOD CREAM

Witschi A, et al. The systemic availability of oral glutathione. *Euro J Clin Pharmacol* 1992; 43:667-669.

Cross CE, et al. Oxygen Radicals and human disease. *Ann Intern Med* 1987;107:526-545.

Biaglow JE, et al. Role of glutathione and other thiols in cellular response to radiation and drugs. *Drug Metab Rev* 1989;20:1-12.

Ji LL. Oxidative stress during exercise: implications of antioxidant nutrients. *Free Rad Biol Medi* 1995;18(6):1079-1086.

Fidelus RK. Glutathione and lymphocyte activation: a function of aging and auto-immune disease. *Immunology* 1987;61:503-508.

Droge W, et al. Functions of glutathione and glutathione disulfide in immunology and immunopathology. *FASEB J* 1994;8:1131-1138.

Kinscheref R, et al. Effect of glutathione depletion and oral N-acetyl-cysteine treatment on CD4+ and CD8+ cells. *FASEB J* 1994;8:448-451.

Wu D, et al. In vitro glutathione supplementation enhances interleukin-2 production and mitogenic response of peripheral blood mononuclear cells from young and old subjects. *J Nutr* 1994;124:655-663.

Fidelus, et al. Glutathione and lymphocyte activation: a function of aging and auto-immune disease. *Immunology* 1987; 61:503-508.

Buhl, et al. Systemic glutathione deficiency in symptom-free HIV-1 seropositive individuals. *Lancet* 1989(Dec 2);1294-1298.

Adams JD, et al. Alzheimer's and Parkinson's Disease. Brian levels of glutathione, glutathione disulfide, and vitamin E. *Mol Clin Neuropathol* 1991;14:213-226.

Jenner P. Oxidative damage in neurodegenerative disease. *Lancet* 1994 (Sept 17);796-798.

Kidd PM. Liver biotransformation of xenobiotics, food, and drugs to free radical oxidants. In:Levine SA, Kidd PM. Antioxidants Adaptation and Its Role in Free Radical Pathology. San Leandro, CA: *Biocurrents*; 1985:222-281.

Seifert CF, et al. Correlation of acetaminophen and ethanol use, plasma glutathione concentrations and diet with hepatotoxicity. *Pharmacotherapy* 1994;14:376-377.

Shigesawa, et al. Significance of plasma glutathione determination of patients with alcohol and non-alcoholic liver disease. *J Gastroenterol Hepatol* 1992;7:7-11.

Loguercio C, et al. Alteration of erythrocyte glutathione, cyteine, and glutathione synthetase in alcoholic and non-alcoholic cirrhosis. *Scan J Clin Lab Invest* 1992;52:207-213.

Altomore E, et al. Hepatic glutathione content in patients with alcoholic and non-alcoholic liver disease. *Life Sci* 1988;43:991-998.

Stamler JS, Slivka A. Biological chemistry of thiols in the vasculature and in vascular related disease. *Nutr Revs* 1996;54:1-30.

Buchanan MR, Brister SJ. Altering vessel wall fatty acid metabolism: a new strategy for antithrombotic treatment. *Sem Throm Hemostasis* 1993;19:149-57.

Kidd PM. Cell membranes, endothelia, and atherosclerosis and the importance of dietary fatty acid balance. *Alternative Med Rev* 1996;1(3):148-167.

8. VITAMIN D

Moschakis T et al: Microstructural evolution of viscoelastic emulsions stabilised by sodium caseinate and xanthan gum. Procter Department of Food Science, University of Leeds, Leeds LS2 9JT, UK
J Colloid Interface Sci. 2005 Apr 15;284(2):714-28

Liu HX et al; Promotion of intestinal drug absorption by milk fat globule membrane
Department of Hospital Pharmacy, Toyama Medical and Pharmaceutical University, Japan. *Yakugaku Zasshi.* 1991 Sep;111(9):510-4

[1] Cross D, et al. Phytoestrogens and vitamin D metabolism: A new concept for the prevention and therapy of colorectal, prostate, and mammary carcinomas. *J Nutrition.* 2004; 134: 127-1212.

[2] Danilenko M, et al. Carnosic acid and promotion of monocytic differentiation of HL60-G cells initiated by other agents. *J Natl Cancer Inst.* 2001, 93(16): 1224-1233.

[3] Standing Committee on the Scientific Evaluation of Dietary Reference Intakes, Food and Nutrition Board, Institute of Medicine. Dietary Reference Intakes for Calcium, Phosphorus, Magnesium, Vitamin D, and Fluoride. Wasington, DC: The National Academies Press; 1997.

[4] Grant W & Holick M. Benefits and Requirements of Vitamin D for Optimal Health: A Review. *Alt Med Rev*, 2005;10:94-108.

[5] Vieth R. Why the optimal requirements for vitamin D3 is probably much higher than what is officially recommended for Vitamin D. *J Nutr* 2005;135:317-322.

[6] Veith R, Chan PC, MacFaralane GD. Efficacy and safety of vitamin D3 intake exceeding the lowest observed adverse effect level. *Am J Clin Nutr* 2001;73:288-294.

[7] Veith R, Kimbeall S, Hu A, Walfish PG. Randomized comparison of the effects of the vitamin D3 adequate intake versus 100 mcg (4,000 IU) per day on biochemical responses and the wellbeing of patients. *Nutr J* 2004;3:8.

[8] Hoick M. Vitamin D: importance in the prevention of cancers, type I diabetes, heart disease, and osteoporosis. *Am J Clin Nutrition*. 2004; 39:326-327.

[9] Working Group of the Australian and New Zealand Bone and Mineral Society, Endocrine Society of Australia and Osteoporosis Australia. Vitamin D and adult bone health in Australia and New Zealand: a position paper statement. *Med J Aust* 2005;182:281-285.

[10] Cancer Chemoprevention and Cancer Treatment: is there a role for vitamin D, 1alpha, 25(OH)2-vitamin D3, or new analogs (deltanois)? Bethesda, MD, November 17-19, 2004. Sponsored by the National Cancer Institute, NIH, The Vitamin D Workshop, http://vitamined.ucr.edu/Cancer&CancerChemo.htm (accessed April 10, 2005).

[11] Webb AR, Kline L, Holick MF. Influence of season and latitude on the cutaneous synthesis of vitamin D3: exposure to winter sunlight in Boston and Edmonton will not promote vitamin D3 synthesis in the human skin. *J Clin Endorinol Metab* 1988; 67:373-378.

[12] Holick MF. Environment factors that influence the cutaneous production of vitamin D. *Am J Clin Nutr* 1995;61:6838S-645S.

[13] Alti T, Gullu S, Usal AR, Erdogen G. The prevalence of vitamin D levels in the elderly Turkish population. *Arch Gerontol Geriatr* 2005;40:53-60.

[14] Moore C, Murphy MM, Keast DR, Holick MF. Vitamin D intake in the United States. *J AM Diet Assoc* 2004;104:980-983.

[15] Hanley DA, Davison KS. Vitamin D insufficiency in North America. *J Nutr* 2005; 135:332-337.

[16] Chapuy MC, Preziosi P, Maamer M, et al. Prevalence of vitamin D insufficiency in an adult normal population. *Osteoporosis Int* 1997;7:439-443.

[17] Tangpricha V, Pearce EN, Chen TC, Holick MF. Vitamin D insufficiency among free-living healthy young adults. *Am J Med* 2002;112:659-662.

[18] Worstman J, Matsuoka LY, Chen TC, et al. Decreased bioavailability of vitamin D in obesity. *Am J Clin Nutr* 2000;2: 690-693. Erratum in : *Am J Clin Nutr* 2003;77:1342.

[19] Koutkia P, Lu Z, Chen TC, Holick MF. Treatment of vitamin D deficiency due to Crohn's disease with tanning bed ultraviolet B radiation. *Gastroeneterology* 2001; 121:1485-1488.

[20] Vestergaard P. Prevalence and pathogenesis of osteoporosis in patients with inflammatory bowel disease. *Minerva Med* 2004;95:469-480.

[21] Wortsman J, Matsuoka LY, Chen TC, et al. Decreased bioavailability of vitamin D in obesity. *Am J Clin Nutr* 2000;72:690-693.

[22] Holick MF. Photosynthesis of vitamin D in the skin: effect of environmental and life-style variables. *Fed Proc* 1987;46:1876-1882.

[23] Atli T, Gullu S, Usal AR, Erdogan G. The prevalence of vitamin D deficiency and effects of ultraviolet light on vitamin D levels in elderly Turkish population. *Arch Gerontol Geriatr* 2005;40:53-60.

[24] Holick MF. Sunlight and vitamin D for bone health and prevention of autoimmune diseases, cancers, and cardiovascular diseases. *Am J Clin Nutr* 2004;80:1678S-1688S.

[25] Cantorna MT, Zhu Y, Froicu M, Whittke A. Vitamin D status, 1-25-dihydroxyvitamin D3, and the immune system. *Am J Clin Nutr*

[26] DeLuca HF, Cantorna MT. Vitamin D: its role and uses in immunology. *FASEB J* 2001;15:2579-2585.

[27] Lyakh LA, Sanford M, Chekol S, et al. TGF beta and vitamin D3 utilize distinct pathways to suppress IL-12 production and modulate rapid differentiation of monocytes into CD83+ dendritic cells. *J Immunol* 2005;174:2061-2070.

[28] Drugarin D. The pattern of Th1 cytokine in autoimmune thyroditis. *Immunol Letts*, 2000; 71: 73-77.

[29] Smith EA, et al. Effects of long-term administration of vitamin D3 analogs to mice. *J Endocrinol Invest.* 1994; 17(6): 385-390.

[30] Zella JB, DeLuca HF. Vitamin D and autoimmune diabetes. *J Cell Biochem* 2003; 88:216-222.

[31] Embroy AF. Vitamin D supplementation in the fight against multiple sclerosis. *J Orthomolecular Med* 2004;19:27-38.

[32] Temper DI, Trent NH, Spencer DA, et al. Season of birth in multiple sclerosis. *Acta Neurol Scand* 1992;85:107-109.

[33] Willer Cj, Dyment DA, Sadovnick AD, et al. Timing of birth and risk of multiple sclerosis: population based study. *BMJ* 2005;330:120.

[34] Embroy AF, Snowdon LR, Vieth R. Vitamin D and seasonal fluctuations of gadolinium-enhancing magnetic resonance imaging lesions in multiple sclerosis. *Ann Neurol* 2000;48:271-271.

[35] Ericksen EF, Glenrup H. Vitamin D deficiency and aging: implications for general health and osteporosis. *Biogerontology* 2002;3:73-77.

[36] Holick MF. Vitamin D deficiency: what pain it is. *Mayo Clin Proc* 2003;78:1457-1459.

[37] Plotnikoff GA, Quigley JM. Prevalence of severe hypovitaminosis D in patients with persistent nonspecific musculoskeletal pain. *Mayo Clin Proc* 2003; 78:1463-1470.

[38] Plotnikoff GA, Quigley JM. Prevalence of severe hypovitaminosis D in patients with persistent nonspecific musculoskeletal pain. *Mayo Clin Proc* 2003; 78:1463-1470.

[39] Chiu K, et al. Hypovitaminosis D is associated with insulin resistance and beta cell function. *Am J Clin Nutrition.* 2004; 79: 820-825.

[40] Hypponen E, Laara E, Reunanen A, et al. Intake of vitamin D and risk of type I diabetes: a birth-cohort study. *Lancet* 2001; 358:1500-1503.

[41] Hypponen E. Micronutrients and risk of type I diabetes: vitamin D, vitamin E, and nicotinamide. *Nutr Rev* 2004; 62:340-347.

[42] Goldberg P, Fleming MC, Picard EH. Multiple sclerosis: decreased relapse rate through dietary supplementation with calcium, magnesium and vitamin D. *Med Hypothesis* 1986;21: 193-200.

[43] Embry AF. Vitamin D supplementation in the fight against multiple sclerosis. *J Orthomolecular Med* 2004; 19:27-38.

[44] Hayas CE, Cantorna MT, DeLuca HF. Vitamin D and multiple sclerosis. *Proc Soc Exp Biol Medi* 1997;216:21-27.

[45] Koziol JA. Feng AC. Seasonal variations in exacerbations and MRI parameters in relapsing remitting multiple sclerosis. *Neuroepidemiology* 2004; 23:217-223.

[46] Embroy AF, Snowdon LR, Vieth R. Vitamin D and seasonal fluctuations of gadolinium-enhancing magnetic resonance imaging lesions in multiple sclerosis. *Ann Neurol* 2000;48:271-272.

[47] Rajakumar K. Vitamin D, cod-liver oil, sunlight, and rickets: a historical perspective. *Pediatrics* 2003;112:e132-135.

[48] Bischoff-Ferrari HA, Conzelmann M, Dick W, et al. Effect of vitamin D on muscle strength and relevance in regard to osteoporosis prevention. *Z Rheumatol* 2003;62:518-521.

[49] Fuller KE. Low birth-weight infants: the continuing ethnic disparity and the interaction of biology and environment. *Ethn Dis* 2000;10:432-445.

[50] Specker B. Vitamin D requirements during pregnancy. *Am J Clin Nutr* 2004;80:1740S-1747S.

[51] Hypponens E, Lara E, Reunanen A, et al. Intake of vitamin D and risk of type I diabetes: a birth-cohort study. *Lancet* 2001;358:1500-1503.

[52] Pawley N, Bishop NJ. Prenatal and infant predictors of bone health: the influence of vitamin D. *Am J Clin Nutr* 2004;80:1748S-1751S.

[53] Grant W.B., Holick MF. Benefits and Requirements of Vitamin D for Optimal Health: A Review. *Alt Med Rev* 2005;10:94-111.

[54] Grant WB. An estimate of premature cancer mortality in the U.S. due to inadequate doses of solar ultraviolet-B radiation. *Cancer* 2002;94:1867-1875.

[55] Grant WB. Benefits of UVB exposure to reduce the risk of cancer – ecologic studies of cancer mortality rates. Proceedings of the CIE symposium '04; Light and Health: non-visual effects, 30 Sept.-2 Oct. 2004. Commision International de L, Eclairage, Vienna, Austria, 2004:174-177.

[56] Grant WB., Garland CF. A critical review of studies on vitamin D in relation to colorectal cancer. *Nutr Cancer* 2004;48:115-123.

[57] Baker SB, Worthley LI, The essentials of calcium, magnesium and phosphate metabolism: part I. Physiology Department of Critical Care Medicine, Flinders University of South Australia, Adelaide, South Australia. *Crit Care Resusc.* 2002 Dec;4(4):301-6.)

[58] Mazur A, et al. Magnesium and the inflammatory response: Potential physiopathological implications Equipe Stress Metabolique et Micronutriments, Unite de Nutrition Humaine UMR 1019, Centre de Recherche en Nutrition Humaine d'Auvergne, INRA, Theix, St. Genes Champanelle, France. Arch *Biochem Biophys.* 2006 Apr 19

[59] Carpenter TO et al "Effect of magnesium depletion on metabolism of 25-hydroxyvitamin D in rats"

[60] Cox SE et al; Vitamin A supplementation increases ratios of proinflammatory to anti-inflammatory cytokine responses in pregnancy and lactation. Department of Epidemiology and Population Health, London School of Hygiene and Tropical Medicine (LSHTM), London, UK.*Clin Exp Immunol.* 2006 Jun;144(3):392-400.

[61] Luo XM, "Retinoic acid exerts dual regulatory actions on the expression and nuclear localization of interferon regulatory factor-1" Department of Nutritional Sciences, 126-S Henderson Building, University Park, PA 16802, USA, *Exp Biol Med* (Maywood). 2006 May;231(5):619-31

[62] Wieringa FT et al; Reduced production of immunoregulatory cytokines in vitamin A- and zinc-deficient Indonesian infants. Department of Internal Medicine, University Hospital Nijmegen, The Netherlands --- *Eur J Clin Nutr.* 2004 Nov;58(11):1498-504.

[63] Chandra R and Sudhakaran L. Regulation of immune responses by Vitamin B6. *NY Acad Sci* 1990; 585:404-423.

[64] Leklem JE. Vitamin B6. In: Shils ME, Olson JA, Shike M, Ross AC, ed. *Modern Nutrition in Health and Disease.* 9th ed. Baltimore: Williams and Wilkins, 1999: 413-421.

[65] Leyland DM and Beynon RJ. The expression of glycogen phosphorylase in normal and dystrophic muscle. *Biochem J* 1991; 278:113-7.

[66] Okada M, Ishikawa K, Watanabe K. Effect of vitamin B6 deficiency on glycogen metabolism in the skeletal muscle, heart, and liver of rats. *J Nutr Sci Vitaminol* (Tokyo) 1991; 37:349-57.

[67] Revilla-Monsalve C et al, "Biotin supplementation reduces plasma triacylglycerol and VLDL in type 2 diabetic patients and in nondiabetic subjects with hypertriglyceridemia" *Biomed Pharmacother.* 2006 May;60(4):182-185. Epub 2006 Mar 31.

[68] L. C. Stene et al , Use of cod liver oil during pregnancy associated with lower risk of Type I diabetes in the offspring. *Diabetologia*, Volume 43, Number 9; September 2000

[69] Campan P et al; Pilot study on n-3 polyunsaturated fatty acids in the treatment of human experimental gingivitis.
Departement de Chirurgie Buccale, Faculte de Chirurgie Dentaire de Toulouse, France. *J Clin Periodontol.* 1997 Dec;24(12):907-13.

[70] Dayong Wu and Simin Nikbin Meydan ; " n-3 Polyunsaturated fatty acids and immune function."
Nutritional Immunology Laboratory, Jean Mayer USDA Human Nutrition Research Center on Aging at TUBS University,Boston, Proceedings of the Nutrition Society (1998), 57, 503-509

[71] Sergeeva M "Regulation of intracellular calcium levels by polyunsaturated fatty acids, arachidonic acid and docosahexaenoic acid, in astrocytes: possible involvement of phospholipase A2." *Reprod Nutr Dev.* 2005 Sep-Oct;45(5):633-46
Otto-von-Guericke-Universitat Magdeburg, Medizinische Fakultat, Institut fur Neurobiochemie, Leipziger Strasse 44, 39120 Magdeburg, Germany

9. TH-1 SUPPORT

[1] *Chung Kuo Yao Li Hsueh Pao* (1981 Sep) 2(3):200-4 (Published In Chinese) Chu DT Lepe-Zuniga J Wong WL LaPushin R Mavligit GM. Fractionated extract of Astragalus membranaceus, a Chinese medicinal herb, potentiates LAK cell cytotoxicity generated by a low dose of recombinantinterleukin-2.

[2] *Chung Hsi I Chieh Ho Tsa Chih* (1987 Jul) 7(7):403-4, 388 (Published InChinese) Geng CS [Advances in immuno-pharmacological studies on Astragalusmembranaceus].

[3] *Biol Response Mod* (1983) 2(3):227-37 Wang DY Yang WY [Effect of Astragalus polysaccharides on ribonucleic acid metabolism of spleen and liver cells of mice].

[4] *J Chung Kuo Yao Li Hsueh Pao* (1982 Sep) 3(3):204-7 (Published In Chinese) Wang DY Zhang W Xu GY [Protective effect of Astragalus polysaccharide on ribonucleases and theribonuclease inhibitor system].

[5] *Chung Kuo I Hsueh Ko Hsueh Yuan Hsueh Pao* (1983 Aug) 5(4):231-4 Chen LJ Shen ML Wang MY Zhai SK Liu MZ [Effect of Astragalus polysaccharides on phagocytic function in mice(author's transl)].

[6] *Chung Hsi I Chieh Ho Tsa Chih* (1984 Aug) 4(8):484-5 (Published In Chinese) Chang CY Hou YD Xu FM [Effects of Astragalus membranaceus on enhancement of mouse natural killer cell activity].

[7] Vrach Delo (1988 Jun) (6):51-4 Published In Russian Sun Y Hersh EM Lee SL McLaughlin M Loo TL Mavligit GM. Preliminary observations on the effects of the Chinese medicinal herbs Astragalus membranaceus and Ligustrum lucidum on lymphocyte blastogenic responses.

[8] *Chung Hsi I Chieh Ho Tsa Chih* (1986 Jan) 6(1):62-4 (Published In Chinese) He ZP Wang DZ Shi LY Wang ZQ Treating amenorrhea in vital energy-deficient patients with angelicasinensis-astragalus membranaceus menstruation-regulating decoction.

[9] *Chung Yao Tung Pao* (1986 Sep) 11(9):47-9 Ponomarenko AP [The effect of astragalus on the functional status of the liver in patients with chronic circulatory insufficiency].

[10] Chung Hsi I Chieh Ho Tsa Chih (1984 Oct) 4(10):615-7, 581 Skakun NP Blikhar EI Oleinik AN [Use of Astragalus dasyanthus in lesions of the liver in patients with pulmonary tuberculosis].

[11] Zhao, KS, Mancinia C, Doria G. Enhancement of the immune response in mice by Astragalus membranaceus extracts. Immunopharmacology 1990; 20: 225-233.

[12] Chang HM, But PPH eds. Pharmacology and applications of Chinese Materia Medica. Singapore: *World Scientific* 1987: p 1041-1046.

[13] Braunig, B., M. Dorn, E. Limburg, and E. Knick. 1992. Echinacea purpurea Radix For Strengthening the Immune Response in Flu-like Infections. *Zeitschrift fur Phytotherapie* 13:7-13 (In German; translated by Shanti Coble and Christopher Hobbs).

[14] Awang, D. V. C. and D. G. Kindack. 1991. Echinacea. Canadian Pharmaceutical Journal. 124(11):512-16.

[15] Schoneberger, D. 1992. The Influence of Immune-Stimulating Effects of Pressed Juice from Echinacea purpurea on the Course and Severity of Colds. *Forum Immunologie* 8:2-12. (In German, translated by Sigrid M. Klein).

[16] Melchart, D., K. Linde, F. Worku, R. Bauer, and H. Wagner. 1994. Immunomodulation with Echinacea - A Systematic Review of Controlled Clinical Trials. *Phytomedicine.* l(l):245-254.

[17] Braunig, B., M. Dorn, E. Limburg, and E. Knick. 1992. Echinacea purpurea Radix For Strengthening the Immune Response in Flu-like Infections. *Zeitschrift fur Phytotherapie* 13:7-13 (In German; translated by Shanti Coble and Christopher Hobbs).

[18] Bauer, R. and S. Foster. 1989. HPLC Analysis of Echinacea simulata and E. paradoxa roots. *Planta Medica* 55:637.

[19] Abe N, Ebina T, Ishida N. Interferon induction by glycyrrhizic acid. *Experientia* 1980; 36:304-305.20 Pompei R, et al. Antiviral activity of glycyrrhizic acid. Experientia 1980; 36:304.

[21] Csonka G, Tyrrell D. Treatment of herpes genitalis with carbonoxolone and cicloxolone creams. A double blinded placebo controlled trial. *Br J Ven Dis* 1984; 60:178-181.

[22] Hattori T, Ikematsu S, Kioto A, et al. Preliminary evidence for inhibitory effect of glycyrrhizin on HIV replication in patients with AIDS. *Antiviral Res* 1989; 11:255-261.

[23] Suzuki H, Ohta Y, Takino T, et al. Effects of glycyrrhizin on biochemical tests in patients with chronic hepatitis – double blind trial. *Asian Med J* 1984; 26:423-438.

[24] Mitscher L, Park Y, Clark D. Antimicrobial agents from higher plants. Antimicrobial isoflavonoids from Glycyrrhiza glabra. *J Natural Products* 1980; 43: 259-269.

[25] Kucera LS, Herrmann EC Jr. Antiviral substances in plants of the mint family (labiatae). I. Tannin of Melissa officinalis. *Proc Soc Exp Biol Med* 1967 Mar;124(3):865-9.

[26] Cohen RA, Kucera LS, Hermann EC JR. Antivrial activity of Mellisa officinalis (lemon balm) extract. *Proc Soc Exp Biol Med* 1964 Nov;117:431-4.

[27] Allahverdiyev A, Duran N, Ozguven M, Koltas S. Antiviral activity of the volatile oils of Melissa officinalis L. against Herpes simplex virus type-2. *Phytomedicine.* 2004 Nov;11(7-8):657-61.

[28] Dimitrova Z, Dimov B, Manolova N, Pancheva S, Ilieva D, Shishkov S. Antiherpes effect of Melissa officinalis L. extracts. *Acta Microbiol Bulg.* 1993;29:65-72.

[29] Kodama N, Murata Y, Nanba H. Administration of a polysaccharide from Grifola frondosa stimulates immune function of normal mice. *J Med Food.* 2004 Summer;7(2):141-5.

[30] Kodama N, Komuta K, Nanba H. Effect of Maitake (Grifola frondosa) D-Fraction on the activation of NK cells in cancer patients. *J Med Food.* 2003 Winter;6(4):371-7.

[31] Kodama N, Komuta K, Nanba H. Effect of Maitake (Grifola frondosa) D-Fraction on the activation of NK cells in cancer patients. *J Med Food.* 2003 Winter;6(4):371-7.32

[32] Seeram NP, Adams LS, Henning SM, Niu Y, Zhang Y, Nair MG, Heber D. In vitro antiproliferative, apoptotic and antioxidant activities of punicalagin, ellagic acid and a total pomegranate tannin extract are enhanced in combination with other polyphenols as found in pomegranate juice. *J Nutr Biochem.* 2005 Jun;16(6):360-7.

[33] Sudheesh S, Vijayalakshmi NR. Flavonoids from Punica granatum—potential antiperoxidative agents. *Fitoterapia.* 2005 Mar;76(2):181-6.

[34] Neurath AR, Strick N, Li YY, Debnath AK. Punica granatum (Pomegranate) juice provides an HIV-1 entry inhibitor and candidate topical microbicide. *BMC Infect Dis.* 2004 Oct 14;4(1):41.

[35] Zhang J, Zhan B, Yao X, Gao Y, Shong J. Antiviral activity of tannin from the pericarp of Punica granatum L. against genital Herpes virus in vitro. *Zhongguo Zhong Yao Za Zhi.* 1995 Sep;20(9):556-8, 576, inside backcover.

10. TH-2 SUPPORT

Kim HC, Healey JM. Effects of pine bark extract administered to immunosuppressed adult mice infected with Cryptosporidium parvum. *Am J Clin Med* 2001;29:469-75.

Cho KJ et al. Inhibition mechanisms of bioflavonoids extracted from the bark of Pinus maritime on the expression of proinflammatory cytokines. Ann NY Acad Sci. 2001;928:141-56.Rohdewald P. A review of the French maritime pine bark extract (Pycnogenol), a herbal medication with a diverse clinical pharmacology. *Int J Clin Pharmacol Ther.* 2002;40:158-6.

Dixon RA, Xie DY, Sharma SB. Proanthocyanidins--a final frontier in flavonoid research? *New Phytol.* 2005;165(1):9-28.

Cos P, De Bruyne T, Hermans N, Apers S, Berghe DV, Vlietinck AJ. Proanthocyanidins in health care: current and new trends. *Curr Med Chem.* 2004;11(10):1345-59.

Li WG et al. Anti-inflammatory effect and mechanism of proanthocyanidins from grape seeds. *Acta Pharmacol Sin* 2001; 22:1117-20.

Zhao M, Yang B, Wang J, Liu Y, Yu L, Jiang Y. Immunomodulatory and anticancer activities of flavonoids extracted from litchi (Litchi chinensis Sonn) pericarp. *Int Immunopharmacol.* 2007;7(2):162-6.

Sharma SD, Katiyar SK. Dietary grape-seed proanthocyanidin inhibition of ultraviolet B-induced immune suppression is associated with induction of IL-12. *Carcinogenesis.* 2006;27(1):95-102.

Lin LC, Kuo YC, Chou CJ. Immunomodulatory proanthocyanidins from Ecdysanthera utilis. *J Nat Prod.* 2002;5(4):505-8.

Klein C et al. From food to nutritional support to specific nutraceuticals: a journey across time in the treatment of disease. *J Gastroenterol.* 2000;35 Suppl 12:1-6.

Bagchi D, Bagchi M, Stohs S, Ray SD, Sen CK, Preuss HG. Cellular protection with proanthocyanidins derived from grape seeds. *Ann N Y Acad Sci.* 2002;957:260-70.

Li WG, Zhang XY, Wu YJ, Tian X. Anti-inflammatory effect and mechanism of proanthocyanidins from grape seeds. *Acta Pharmacol Sin.* 2001;22(12):1117-20.

Bagchi D, Bagchi M, Stohs SJ, Das DK, Ray SD, Kuszynski CA, Joshi SS, Pruess HG. Free radicals and grape seed proanthocyanidin extract: importance in human health and disease prevention. *Toxicology.* 200;148(2-3):187-97.

Zvetkova E et al. Aqueous extracts of Crinum latifolium (L.) and Camellia sinensis show immunomodulatory properties in human peripheral blood mononuclear cells. *Int Immunopharmacol.* 2001;12:2143-50.

Katiyar SK et al. Green tea polyphenols: DNA photodamage and photoimmunology. *J Photochem Photobiol B.* 2001;36:109-14.

Falchetti R et al. Effects of resveratrol on human immune cellfunction. *Life Sci* 2001; 70:81-96.

Feng WH, Wei HL, Liu GT. "Effect of Pycnogenol on the toxicity of heart, bone marrow and immune organs as induced by antitumor drugs." *Phytomedicine* 2002;9 :414-8.

11. PROTEIN POWDER

[1] Bach AC and Babyan VK. Medium-chain triglycerides: An update. *Am J Clin Nutr* 36,950-962, 1982.

[2] Seatib TB, et al. Thermic effect of medium-chain and long-chain triglycerides in man. *Am J Clin Nutr* 44, 630-634, 1986.

[3] Graf E. Antioxidant potential for ferulic acid. *Free Rad Biol Med* 13, 435-448, 1992.

[4] Scott BC, et al. Evaluation of the antioxidant actions of ferulic acid and catechins. *Free Rad Res Comms* 19, 241-253, 1993.

[5] Takemoto T, et al. Clinical trial of Hi-Z pills on gastrointestinal symptoms at 375 hospitals. *Shiyaku To Rinsho* 26, 2-27, 1977

[6] Sasagwa T, et al. Clinical studies on gamma-oryzanol in the treatment of gastro-enero neurosis. *Basic Pharmacol Ther* 4, 588-591,1980.

[7] Minakuchi C, et al. Clinical effects of gamma-oryzanol on gastric system complaints. *Shiyaka To Rhinsho* 25, 29-33,1976.

[8] Noda H et al. Biotin production by bifidobacteria. *J Nutr Sci Vitaminol* 40,181-188, 1994.

[9] Klimberg V, et al. Prophylactic glutamine protects the intestinal mucosa from radiation injury. *Cancer* July1;66(1):62-68, 1990.

[10] Noyar CM, et al. A double-blind placebo-controlled pilot study of glutamine therapy for abnormal intestinal permeability in patients with AIDS. *Am J Gastroenterol* 93(6), 972-975, 1998.

[11] Evans MA and Shronts EP. Intestinal fuels: glutamine, short-chain fatty acids, and dietary fiber. *J Amer Diet Assoc* 92, 1239-1246,1992.

[12] Shahani KM and Ayebo AD. Role f dietary lactobacilli in gastrointestinal microecology . *Am J Clin Nutr* 33, 2448-2457,1980.

[13] Shahani Km and Friend BA. Nutritional and therapeutic aspects of lactobacilli. *J Appl Nutr* 36, 125-152,1984.

[14] Barefoot SF et al. Detection and activity of lacticin B, a bacteriocin produced by Lactobacillus Acidophilus. *Appl Environ Microbiol* 45, 1808-1815, 1983.

[15] Tomomatsu H. Health effects of oligosaccharides. *Food Technol October*, 61-65,1994.

[16] Gibson GR, et al. Selective stimulation of bifidobacteria in the human colon by oligofructose and inulin. *Gastroenterology* 108, 975-982,1995.

[17] PDR for Herbal Medicines 1st Ed. *Medical Economics Co.* Montvale, New Jersey 1998.

[18] Ferrandiz ML, et al. Anti-inflammatory activity and inhibition of arachadonic acid metabolism by flavonoids. *Agents Action* 32,283-287,1991.

[19] Middelton E and Drzewieki G. Flavonoid inhibition of human basophil histamine release stimulated by various agents. *Biochem Pharmacol* 33, 3333-3338, 1984.

[20] Facino RM, et al. Free radicals scavenging action and anti-enzyme activities of procyanidines from Vitus vinifera: A mechanism for their capillary protective action. *Arzeim Forsch* 44, 592-601, 1994.

[21] Lindahl M, et al. Flavonoids as phosphaolipase A2 inhibitors: Importance of their structure for selective inhibition of group II phospholipase A2. *Inflammation* 21(3):347-356,1997.

[22] Nassauto G et al. Effects of silbinion on biliary lipid composition. Experimental and clinical study. *J Hepatol* 1991;12:290-295.

[23] Wagnar H. Antihepatotoxic flavonioids. In: CodyV, Middleton E, Harbourne JB, eds. Plant flavonoids in biology and medicine: biochemical, pharmacological, and structure-activity relationships. New York, NY: *Alan R Liss.* 1986:p545-558

[24] Adzet T. Polyphenolic compounds with biological activity and pharmacological activity. *Herbs Spices Medicinal Plants* 1986;1:167-184

[25] Hikino H, Kiso Y, Wagner H. Antihepatotoxic actions of flavanolignans from Silybum marianum fruits. *Plant Medica* 1984;50:248-250.

[26]Fiebrich F, Koch H. Siymarin, an inhibitor of prostaglandin synthetase. *Experentia* 1979;35:150-152.

[27] Feibrich F, Koch H. Silymarin an inbitor of lipoxygenase. *Experentia* 1979;35:148-150.

[28] Palasciano G, Protinacasa P, et al. The effect of silymarin on plasma levels of malonadialdehyde in patients receiving long-term treatment of psychotropic drugs. *Curr Ther Res* 1994;55:537-545.

[29] Sonnenbicher J, Goldberg M, Hane L, et al. Stimulatory effect of silibinin on the DNA synthesis in partially hepatectomized rat livers. Non-responsive in hepatoma and other malignant cel lines. *Biochem Pharm* 1986;35:538-541.

12. GUT HEALTH

[1] Sarker SA, Gyr K. Non-immunological defenses mechanisms of the gut. Gut 1992; 33:987-983.

[2] Balakrishnan V ,e t al. Deglycyrrhizinated liquorice in the treatment of chronic duodenal ulcer. J Assoc Phys Ind 1978:26; 811-814.

[3] Tewari S, Trembalowicz. Some experience with deglycyrrhizinated liquorice in the treatment of gastric and duodenal ulcers with special references to its spasmolytic effect. *Gut* 1968;9:48.

[4] Marle J, et al. Deglycrrhizinated Liquorice (DGL) and the renewal of rat stomach epithelium. *Eur J Pharm* 1981;72:219.

[5] Klimberg V, et al. Prophylactic glutamine protects the intestinal mucosa from radiation injury. *Cancer* July1;66(1):62-68, 1990.

[6] Noyar CM, et al. A double-blind placebo-controlled pilot study of glutamine therapy for abnormal intestinal permeability in patients with AIDS. *Am J Gastroenterol* 93(6), 972-975, 1998.

[7] Evans MA and Shronts EP. Intestinal fuels: glutamine, short-chain fatty acids, and dietary fiber. *J Amer Diet Assoc* 92, 1239-1246,1992.

[8] Parmar N Ghosh M. Gastric anti-ulcer activity of (+)-cyanidanol-3, a histdine decarboxylase inhibitor. *Eur J Pharmacol* 1981;69: 25-32.

[9] Wendt P, Reiman H, et al. The use of flavonoids as inhibitors of histidine decarboxylase in gastric diseases. Experimental and clinical studies. *Naunyn-Schmiedeberg's Arch Pharma* (Supplement) 1980;313:238.

[10] Beil W, Birkholz, Sewing KF. Effects of flavonoids on parietal cell acid secretion, gastric mucosal prostaglandin production and Helicobacter pylori growth. *Arzeneim Forsch* 1995;45:697-700.

[11] Kang Jy, et al. Effect of colloidal bismuth subcitrate on symptoms and gastric histology in non-ulcer dyspepsia. A double blind placebo controlled study. *Gut* 1990;31: 476-480.

[12] Marshall BJ, Valenzuela JE, McCallum RW. Bismuth subsalicylate suppression of Helicobacteria pylori in non-ulcer dyspepsia. A double blind placebo controlled trial. *Dig Dis Sci* 1993; 38:1674-1680.

[13] Graf E. Antioxidant potential for ferulic acid. *Free Rad Biol Med* 13, 435-448, 1992.

[14] Scott BC, et al. Evaluation of the antioxidant actions of ferulic acid and catechins. *Free Rad Res Comms* 19, 241-253, 1993.

[15] Takemoto T, et al. Clinical trial of Hi-Z pills on gastrointestinal symptoms at 375 hospitals. *Shiyaku To Rinsho* 26, 2-27, 1977

[16] Sasagwa T, et al. Clinical studies on gamma-oryzanol in the treatment of gastro-entero neurosis. *Basic Pharmacol Ther* 4, 588-591,1980.

[17] Minakuchi C, et al. Clinical effects of gamma-oryzanol on gastric system complaints. *Shiyaka To Rhinsho* 25, 29-33,1976.

[18] Zhou H, Jiao D. 312 cases of gastric and duodenal ulcer bleeding treated with 3 kinds of alcoholic extract rhubarb tablets. *Chung His I Chieh Tsa Chih* 1900; 10: 150-151, 131-132.

[19] Magiatis P, Melliou E, Skaltsounis AL, Chinou IB, Mitaku S. Chemical composition and antimicrobial activity of the essentia oils and Pistacia lentiscur var. chia. *Planta Med* 1999 Dec;65(8):749-52.

[20] Carson CF, Riley TV. Non-antibiotic therapies for infectious diseases. *Commun Dis Intell* 2003;27 Suppl:S143-6.

[21] Marone P, Bono L, Leone E, Bona S, Carretto E, Perversi L. Bactericidal activity of Pistacia lentiscus mastic gum against Helicobacter pylori. *J Chemother* 2001 Dec;13(6):611-4.

13. GUT INFECTIONS

[1] Amin AH, Subbaiah TV, Abbasi KM. Berberine sulfate: antimicrobial activity, bioassay, and mode of action. *Can J Microbiol* 1969; 15:1067-1076.

[2] Rabbani GH, Butler T, Knight J, et al. Randomized controlled trial of berberine sulfate therapy for diarrhea due to enterotoxigenic Escherichia coli and Vibrio cholerae. *J Inf Dis* 1987;155:979-984.

[3] Sack RB, Froehlich JL. Berberine inhibits intestinal secretory response of Vibrio cholerae and Escherichia coli enterotoxins. *Infect Immun* 1982;35:471-475.

[4] Sun D, Courtney HS, Beachey EH. Berberine sulfate blocks adherence of Streptococcus pyogenes to epithelial cells, fibronectin, and hexadecane. *Antimicrob Agents Chemother* 1988;32:1370-1374.

[5] Mahajan VM, Sharma A, Rattan A. Antimycotic activity of berberine sulphate: An alkaloid from an Indian medicinal herb. *Sabouraudia* 1982;20:79-81.

[6] Nakamoto K, Sadamori S, Hamada T. Effects of crude drugs and berberine hydrochloride on the activities of fungi. *J Prosthet Dent* 1990;64:691-694.

[7] Subbaiah TV, Amin AH. Effect of berberine sulphate on Entamoeba histolytica. *Nature* 1967;215:527-528

[8] Kaneda Y, Tanaka T, Saw T. Effects of berberine, a plant alkaloid, on the growth of anaerobic protozoa in axenic culture. *Tokai J Exp Clin Med* 1990;15:417-423.

[9] Ghosh AK, Bhattacharyya FK, Ghosh DK. Leishmania donovani: Amastigote inhibition and mode of action of berberine. *Exp Parasitol* 1985;60:404-413.

[10] Singhal KC. Anthelmintic activity of berberine hydrochloride against Syphacia obvelata in mice. *Indian J Exp Biol* 1976;14:345-347.

[11] Mohan M, Pant CR, Angra SK, Mahajan VM. Berberine in trachoma. *Indian J Ophthalmol* 1982;30:69-75.

[12] Sabir M, Mahajan VM, Mohapatra LN, Bhide NK. Experimental study of the antitrachoma action of berberine. *Indian J Med Res* 1976;64:1160-1167.

[13] Gudima SO, Memelova LV, Borodulin VB, et al. Kinetic analysis of interaction of human immunodeficiency virus reverse transcriptase with alkaloids. *Mol Biol* (Mosk) 1994;28:1308-1314.

[14] Kaneda Y, Torii M, Tanaka T, Aikawa M. In vitro effects of berberine sulphate on the growth and structure of Entamoeba histolytica, Giardia lamblia and Trichomonas vaginalis. *Ann Trop Med Parasitol* 1991;85:417-425.

[15] Kumazawa Y, Itagaki A, Fukumoto M, et al. Activation of peritoneal macrophages by berberine alkaloids in terms of induction of cytostatic activity. *Int J Immunopharmacol* 1984;6:587-592.

[16] Huang CG, Chu ZL, Yang ZM. Effects of berberine on synthesis of platelet TXA2 and plasma PGI2 in rabbits. *Chung Kuo Yao Li Hsueh Pao* 1991;12:526-528.

[17] Fleming, Thomas ed. *PDR for Herbal Medicines 1st ed.* Medical Economics Company, Montvale, NJ, 1998.

[18] Moore, Michael. *Medicinal Plants of the Desert and Canyon West.* Museum of New Mexico Press, Santa Fe, NM, 1989.

[19] Kay, M.A. *Healing with Plants in the American and Mexican West.* University of Arizona Press, Tucson, AZ, 1996.

[20] Arcila-Lozano CC, Loarca-Pina G, Lecona-Uribe S, Gonzalez de Mejia E. Oregano: properties, composition and biological activity. *Arch Latinoam Nutr.* 2004 Mar;54(1):100-11.

[21] Force M, Sparks WS, Ronzio RA. Inhibition of enteric parasites by emulsified oil of oregano in vivo. *Phytother Res.* 2000 May;14(3):213-4.

[22] Walter BM, Bilkei G. Immunostimulatory effect of dieatary oregano etheric oils on lymphocytes from growth-retarded, low-weight growing-finishing pigs and productivity. *Tijdschr Diergeneeskd.* 2004 Mar 15;129(6):178-81.

14. PHASE I AND II LIVER DETOXIFICATION

[1] Heafield MT, et al. Xenobiotic metabolism in Alzheimer's disease. *Neurology.* 1990;40:1095-1098.

[2] Steventon GB, et al. Xenobiotic metabolism in Parkinson's disease. *Neurology.* 1989;39:883-887.

[3] Perlmutter D. Parkinson's diseases – new perspectives. *Townsend Lett.* Jan 1997:48-50.

[4] Magil MK, et al. A multiple chemical sensitivity syndrome. *Am Acad Fam Phys.* www.http://www.aafp.org/afp/980901ap/magil.html.

[5] Meyer, et al. Genetic polymorphisms of drug metabolism. *Prog Liver Dis.* 1990; 9:307-323.

[6] Iarbovici D. Single blood test might predict drugs' effects on patients. *J NIH Res.* 1997;9:34-35

[7] Lee WM. Drug induced hepatoxicity. *N Engl J Med.* 1995;333:1118-1127.

[8] Ridgen S. Entero-hepatic resuscitation program for CFIDS. *The CFIDS Chronicle. Spring* 1995:46-49.

[9] Ridgen S, et al. Evaluation of the effect of modified entero-hepatic resuscitation program in chronic fatigue syndrome patients. *J Adv Med.* 1998;11(4):247-262.

[10] McKinnon RA, et al. Possible role of cytochromes P450 in lupus erythematosus and related disorders. *Lupus.* 1994;3:473-478.

[11] Faber K. The dandelion Taraxacum officinale. *Pharmaize* 1958;13:423-436.

[12] Susnik F. Present state of knowledge of the medicinal plant Taraxacum officinale. Weber. *Med Razgledi* 1982;21:323-328.

[13] Bohm K. Choleretic action of some medicinal plants. *Arzneimittel Forsch* 1959;9: 376-378.

[14] Nassauto G et al. Effects of silbinion on biliary lipid composition. Experimental and clinical study. *J Hepatol* 1991;12:290-295.

[15] Wagnar H. Antihepatotoxic flavonioids. In: CodyV, Middleton E, Harbourne JB, eds. Plant flavonoids in biology and medicine: biochemical, pharmacological, and structure-activity relationships. New York, NY: *Alan R Liss.* 1986:p545-558

[16] Adzet T. Polyphenolic compounds with biological activity and pharmacological activity. *Herbs Spices Medicinal Plants* 1986;1:167-184

[17] Hikino H, Kiso Y, Wagner H. Antihepatotoxic actions of flavanolignans from Silybum marianum fruits. *Plant Medica* 1984;50:248-250.

[18] Fiebrich F, Koch H. Siymarin, an inhibitor of prostaglandin synthetase. *Experentia* 1979;35:150-152.

[19] Feibrich F, Koch H. Silymarin an inbitor of lipoxygenase. *Experentia* 1979;35:148-150.

[20] Palasciano G, Protinacasa P, et al. The effect of silymarin on plasma levels of malonadialdehyde in patients receiving long-term treatment of psychotropic drugs. *Curr Ther Res* 1994;55:537-545.

[21] Sonnenbicher J, Goldberg M, Hane L, et al. Stimulatory effect of silibinin on the DNA synthesis in partially hepatectomized rat livers. Non-responsive in hepatoma and other malignant cell lines. *Biochem Pharm* 1986;35:538-541.

[22] Darnis F, Orcel L, de Saint-Maur PP, Mamaou P. Use of a titrated extract of Centella asiatica in chronic hepatic disorders. *Sem Hosp Paris* 1979;55:1749-1750.

[23] El Zawahry MD, Kahil AM, El Banna MH. Madecassol. A new therapy for hepatic fibrosis. *Bull Soc Int Chir* (Belgium) 1975;34:296-297.

[24] Belcaro GV, Grimaldi R, Guidi G. Improvement of capillary permeability in patients with venous hypertension after treatment with TTFCA. *Angiology* 1990; 41(7):533-540.

[25] Pointel JP, Boccalon H, Cloarec M, et al. Titrated extract of Centella asiatca (TECA) in the treatment of venous insufficiency of the lower limbs. *Angiology* 1987;38(11):46-50.

[26] Hikino H, Kiso Y, Sandah S, Shoji J. Antihepatotoxic actions of ginesenosides form Panax ginseng roots. *Planta Medica* 1985;52: 62-64.

[27] Yammato M, Uemura T, Nakama S, et al. Serum HDL-cholesterol-increasing and fatty liver-improving action of Panax ginseng in high cholesterol diet-feed rats with clinical effects on hyperlipidemia in man. *Am J Chin Med* 1983;11:96-101.

[28] Bombardelli E, Cirstoni A, Lietta A. The effect of acute and chronic (Panax) ginseng saponins treatment on adrenal function; biochemical and pharmacological. Proceedings 3rd International Ginseng Symposium.Seoul: *Korean Research Institute.* 1980: p 9-16.

[29] Oura H, Hiai S, Seno H. Synthesis and characterization of nuclear RNA induced b Radix ginseng extract in rat liver. *Chem Pharm Bull* 1971;19:1598-1605.

[30] Oura H, Hiai S, Nabatini S, Nakagawa H, et al. Effect of ginseng o endoplasmic reticulum and ribosome. *Planta Medica* 1975;28:76-88.

[31] Johnston CJ, Meyer CG, Srilakshmi JC. Vitamin C elevates red blood cell glutathione levels in healthy adults. *Am J Clin Nutr* 1993; 58: 103-105.

[32] Jain A, Buist NR, Keenaaway NG, et al. Effect of ascorbate or N-acetlycysteine treatments in patient with hereditary glutathione synthetase deficiency. *J Pediatr* 1994; 124: 229-233.

[33] Skvortsova RI, Pzniakovski VM, Agarkova IA. Role of vitamin factor in preventing phenol poisoning. *Vopr Pitan* 1981; 2: 32-35.

15. METHYLATION

[1] Brattstoerm L, et al. Plasma homocysteine in women on oral oestrogen-containing contraceptives and in men with oestrogen-treated prostatic carcinoma. *Scand J Clin Lab Invest.* 52, 1982:283-287.

[2] Smithells RW, et al. Possible prevention of neural-tube defects by periconceptional vitamin supplementation. *Lancet,* Feb 16, 1980:339-342. Butterworth CE, et al. Folate deficiency and cervical dysplasia. *JAMA.* 1992; 267:528-533.

[3] Lindenbaum J, et al. Neuropsychiatric disorders caused by cobalamin deficiency in the absence of anemia or macrocytosis. *N Eng J Med.* 1988;318:1720-1728.

[4] Allen RH, et al. Serum beatine, N,N-dimethlyglycine and N-methylglycine levels in patients with cobalamin deficiency and related inborn errors of metabolism. *Metab.* 1993;42(11):1448-1460.

[5] Zingh JM, Jones PA. Genetic and epigenetic aspects of DNA methylation on genome expression, evolution, mutation and carcinogenesis. *Carcinogenesis.* 1997; 18(5):869-882.

[6] Smythies JR. The role of the one-carbon cycle in neuropsychatric disease. *Biol Psychiatry.* 1984;19(5):755-758.

[7] Finkelstein JD. Homocysteine: a history in progress. *Nutr Rev.* 2000;58(7):193-204.

[8] Krumdieck CL, Prince CW. Mechanisms of homocysteine toxicity on connective tissues: implications of morbidity of aging. *J Nutr.* 2000;130:365S-368S.

16. GALLBLADDER/BILE

[1] Faber K. The dandelion Taraxacum officinale. *Pharmaize* 1958;13:423-436.

[2] Susnik F. Present state of knowledge of the medicinal plant Taraxacum officinale. Weber. *Med Razgledi* 1982;21:323-328.

[3] Bohm K. Choleretic action of some medicinal plants. *Arzneimittel Forsch* 1959;9:376-378.

[4] Nassauto G et al. Effects of silbinion on biliary lipid composition. Experimental and clinical study. *J Hepatol* 1991;12:290-295.

[5] Wagnar H. Antihepatotoxic flavonoids. In: CodyV, Middleton E, Harbourne JB, eds. Plant flavonoids in biology and medicine: biochemical, pharmacological, and structure-activity relationships. New York, NY: *Alan R Liss.* 1986:p545-558

[6] Adzet T. Polyphenolic compounds with biological activity and pharmacological activity. *Herbs Spices Medicinal Plants* 1986;1:167-184

[7] Hikino H, Kiso Y, Wagner H. Antihepatotoxic actions of flavanolignans from Silybum marianum fruits. *Plant Medica* 1984;50:248-250.

[8]Fiebrich F, Koch H. Siymarin, an inhibitor of prostaglandin synthetase. *Experentia* 1979;35:150-152.

[9] Feibrich F, Koch H. Silymarin an inbitor of lipoxygenase. *Experentia* 1979;35:148-150.

[10] Palasciano G, Protinacasa P, et al. The effect of silymarin on plasma levels of malonadialdehyde in patients receiving long-term treatment of psychotropic drugs. *Curr Ther Res* 1994;55:537-545.

[11] Sonnenbicher J, Goldberg M, Hane L, et al. Stimulatory effect of silibinin on the DNA synthesis in partially hepatectomized rat livers. Non-responsive in hepatoma and other malignant cel lines. *Biochem Pharm* 1986;35:538-541.

[12] Gujral S. Bhumra H. Swaroop M. Effects of ginger (zingebar officinale Roscoe) oleoresin on serum and hepatic cholesterol levels in cholesterol fed rats. *Nutr Rep Intl* 1978;17:183-189.

[13] Giri J, Sakthi Devi TK, Meerarani S. Effect of ginger on serum cholesterol levels. *Ind J Nutr Diet* 1984;21:433-436.

[14] Srinivasan K, Sambaiah K. The effect of spices on cholesterol 7 alpha-hydroxylase activity and the serum and hepatic cholesterol levels in rat. *Int J Vitam Nutr Res* 1991;61:364-369.

[15] Tushilin SA, Drieling DA, Narodetskaja RV, Lukash LK. The treatment of patients with gallstones by lecithin. *Am J Gastroenerol* 1976:65:231.

[16] Hannin I, Ansell GB. Lecithin. Technological, biological, and therapeutic aspects. New York, NY:*Plenum Press*.1987.

[17] Jenkins SA. Vitamin C and gallstone formation: a preliminary report. *Experientia* 1977;33:1616-1617.

17. THYROID HORMONE SYNTHESIS

[1] Panda S, Kar A. Gugulu (Commiphora mukul) induces triiodothyronine production: possible involvement in lipid peroxidation. *Life Sciences.* 1999;65(12):137-141

[2] Singh R, Mohammad AN, Ghosh S. Hypolipidemic and antioxidant effects of Commiphora mukul as an adjunct to dietary therapy in patients with hypercholesterolemia. *Cardiovascular Drugs Therapy.* 1994;8:659-664.

[3] Olivieri O, Gerelli D, Stanzial AM, et al. Selenium, zinc and thyroid hormones in healthy subjects: low T3/T4 ratio in the elderly is related to low selenium status. *Biol Trace Elem Res* 1996;51:31-41.

[4] Olivieri O, Girelli D, Azzini M, et al. Low selenium status in the elderly influences thyroid hormones. *Clin Sci* 1995;89:637-642.

[5] Kralik A, Eder K, Kirchgessner M. Influence of zinc and selenium deficiency on parameters relating to thyroid hormone metabolism. *Horm Metab Res* 1996;28:223-226.

[6] Calomme M, Vanderpas J, Francois B, et al. Effects of selenium supplementation on thyroid hormone metabolism in phenylketunuria subjects on the phenylalanine restricted diet. *Biol Trac Elem Res* 1995; 47:349-353.

[7] Lehmann C, Egerer K, Weber M et al. Effects of selenium administration on various laboratory parameters of patients at risk for sepsis syndrome. *Med Klin* 1997;92:14-16.

[8] Kauf E, Dawczynski H, Jahreis G, et al. Sodium selenite therapy and thyroid-hormone status in cystic fibrosis and congenial hypothyroidism. *Bio Trac Elem Res* 1994;40:247-253.

[9] Olivieri O, Girelli D, Azzini M, et al. Low selenium status in the elderly influences thyroid hormones. *Clin Sci* 1995;89:637-642.

[10] Zhu Z, Kumura M, Itokawa Y. Iodothyronine deiodinase activity in methionine-deficient rats fed selenium-deficient or selenium-sufficent diets. *Biol Trac Elem Res.* 1995;48(2):197-213.

[11] Fujimoto S, Indo Y, Higahi A, et al. Conversion of thryoxine into tri-idothyronine in zinc deficient rat liver. *J Pediatr Gastroenterol Nutr* 1986;5:799-805.

[12] Nishiyama S, Futagoishi-Suginohara Y, Matsukura M. Zinc supplementation alter thyroid hormone metabolism in disabled patients with zinc deficiency. *J Am Coll Nutr* 1994;13:62-67.

[13] Fujimoto S, Indo Y, Higashi, et al. Conversion of thyroxine into tri-idothryoinine in zinc deficient rat liver. *J Pediatr Gastroenterol Nutr* 1986;5:799-805.

[14] Licastro F, et al. Zinc effects the metabolism of thyroid hormones in children with Down's syndrome:normalization of thyroid stimulating hormone and of reversal of triiodothyronin plasmic levels of dietary zinc supplementation. *Int J Neruosci* 1992;65(1-4):259-268.

[15] Napolitano G, Palka G, Lio S, et al. Is zinc deficiency a cause of subclinical hypothyroidism in Down's syndrome? *Ann Genet* 1990;33(1):9-15.

[16] Sustrova M, Strbak V. Thyroid function and plasma immunoglobulins in subjects with Down's syndrome (DS) during ontogenesis and zinc therapy. *J Endocrinol Invest* 1994;17(6):385-390.

[17] Osius N, Karmaus W, Kruse H, Witten J. Exposure to polychlorinated biphenyls and levels of thyroid hormones in children. *Environ Heath Prespect* 1999;107:843-9.

[18] Pavia JM, Paier B, Noll M, Hagmuller K, Zaninovich A. Evidence suggesting that cadmium induces a non-thyroidal illness syndrome in rat. *J Endocrinol* 1997;154:113-7.

[19] Gupta p, Kar A. Cadmium induced thyroid dysfunction in chicken: hepatic type I iodothyronine 5'-monodeiodinase activity and role of lipid peroxidation. *Comp Biochem Physiol C Pharmacol Toxicol Endocrinol.* 1999;123:39-44.

[20] Gutupa P, Kar A.Role of ascorbic acid in cadmium induced thyroid dysfunction and lipid peroxidation. *J Apple Toxicol* 1998;18:317-20.

[21] Brucker –DF. Effects of environmental synthetic chemicals on thyroid function. *Thyroid* 1998;8:827-56.

[22] Barreg aL, Lindstedt G, Schultz A, Sallsten G. Endorine function in mercury exposed chloralkali workers. *Occup Environ Med* 1994;51:536-540.

[23] Johnston CJ, Meyer CG, Srilakshim JC. Vitamin C elevated red blood cell glutathione in healthy adults. *Am J Clin Nutr* 1993;58:103-105.

[24] Jain A, Buist NR, Kennaaway NG, et al. Effect of ascorbate or N-acetlysyteine treatment in patient with hereditary glutathione synthase deficiency. *J Pediatr* 1994;124:229-233.

18. THYROID FUNCTION

[1] Panda S, Kar A. Withania somnifera and Bauhinia purpurea in the regulation of circulating thyroid hormone concentrations in female mice. *J Ethnopharmacol.* 1999;65(12):137-141.

[2] Panda S, Kar A. Changes in thyroid hormone concentrations after administration of ashwaganda root extract to adult mice. *J Pharm Pharmacol.* 1998;50:1065-1058.

[3] Osius N, Karmaus W, Kruse H, Witten J. Exposure to polychlorinated biphenyls and levels of thyroid hormones in children. *Environ Heath Prespect* 1999;107:843-9.

[4] Pavia JM, Paier B, Noll M, Hagmuller K, Zaninovich A. Evidence suggesting that cadmium induces a non-thyroidal illness syndrome in rat. *J Endocrinol* 1997;154:113-7.

[5] Gupta p, Kar A. Cadmium induced thyroid dysfunction in chicken: hepatic type I iodothyronine 5'-monodeiodinase activity and role of lipid peroxidation. *Comp Biochem Physiol C Pharmacol Toxicol Endocrinol.* 1999;123:39-44.

[6] Gutupa P, Kar A.Role of ascorbic acid in cadmium induced thyroid dysfunction and lipid peroxidation. *J Apple Toxicol* 1998; 18:317-20.

[7] Brucker –DF. Effects of environmental synthetic chemicals on thyroid function. *Thyroid* 1998;8:827-56.

[8] Barreg AL, Lindstedt G, Schultz A, Sallsten G. Endocrine function in mercury exposed chloralkali workers. *Occup Environ Med* 1994;51:536-540.

[9] Eleskka M, et al. Withania somnifera, a plant with a great therapeutical future. *Rev Med Chir Soc Med Nat Iasi.* 1989;93:349-350.

[10] Grandhi A, et al. A comparative pharmacological investigation of Ashwagandha and Ginseng. *J Ethnopharmacol.* 1994;44:131-135.

[11] Lu Z, Gu Y, Rooney SA. Transcriptional regulation of the lung fatty acid synthase gene by glucocorticoid, thyroid hormone and transforming growth factor-beta 1. *Biochem Biophys Acta.* 2001;1532;213-212.

[12] Zhang J, Lazar MA. The mechanism of action of thyroid hormones. *Ann Rev Physiol* 2000;62:439-466.

[13] Contorna MT. Vitamin D and autoimmunity: is vitamin D status an environmental factor affecting autoimmune disease prevalence? *PSEBM*. 2000;223:230-233.

[14] Olivieri O, Gerelli D, Stanzial AM, et al. Selenium, zinc and thyroid hormones in healthy subjects: low T3/T4 ratio in the elderly is related to low selenium status. *Biol Trace Elem Res* 1996;51:31-41.

[15] Olivieri O, Girelli D, Azzini M, et al. Low selenium status in the elderly influences thyroid hormones. *Clin Sci* 1995;89:637-642.

[16] Kralik A, Eder K, Kirchgessner M. Influence of zinc and selenium deficiency on parameters relating to thyroid hormone metabolism. *Horm Metab Res* 1996;28:223-226.

[17] Calomme M, Vanderpas J, Francois B, et al. Effects of selenium supplementation on thyroid hormone metabolism in phenylketunuria subjects on the phenylalanine restricted diet. *Biol Trac Elem Res* 1995; 47:349-353.

[18] Lehmann C, Egerer K, Weber M et al. Effects of selenium administration on various laboratory parameters of patients at risk for sepsis syndrome. *Med Klin* 1997;92:14-16.

[19] Kauf E, Dawczynski H, Jahreis G, et al. Sodium selenite therapy and thyroid-hormone status in cystic fibrosis and congenial hypothyroidism. *Bio Trac Elem Res* 1994;40:247-253.

[20] Olivieri O, Girelli D, Azzini M, et al. Low selenium status in the elderly influences thyroid hormones. *Clin Sci* 1995;89:637-642.

[21] Zhu Z, Kumura M, Itokawa Y. Iodothyronine deiodinase activity in methionine-deficient rats fed selenium-deficient or selenium-sufficent diets. *Biol Trac Elem Res*. 1995;48(2):197-213.

[22] Fujimoto S, Indo Y, Higahi A, et al. Conversion of thryoxine into tri-idothyronine in zinc deficient rat liver. *J Pediatr Gastroenterol Nutr* 1986;5:799-805.

[23] Nishiyama S, Futagoishi-Suginohara Y, Matsukura M. Zinc supplementation alter thyroid hormone metabolism in disabled patients with zinc deficiency. *J Am Coll Nutr* 1994;13:62-67.

[24] Fujimoto S, Indo Y, Higashi, et al. Conversion of thyroxine into tri-idothryoinine in zinc deficient rat liver. *J Pediatr Gastroenterol Nutr* 1986;5:799-805.

[25] Licastro F, et al. Zinc effects the metabolism of thyroid hormones in children with Down's syndrome:normalization of thyroid stimulating hormone and of reversal of triiodothyronin plasmic levels of dietary zinc supplementation. *Int J Neruosci* 1992;65(1-4):259-268.

[26] Napolitano G, Palka G, Lio S, et al. Is zinc deficiency a cause of subclinical hypothyroidism in Down's syndrome? *Ann Genet* 1990;33(1):9-15.

[27] Sustrova M, Strbak V. Thyroid function and plasma immunoglobulins in subjects with Down's syndrome (DS) during ontogenesis and zinc therapy. *J Endocrinol Invest* 1994;17(6):385-390.

19. THYROID-PITUITARY AXIS
N/A

20. HYPOPHYSEAL-GONADAL AXIS

[1] Vicktorov D, Kaloyanov , et al. Clinical Investegations on Tribestan in males with disorders in sexual function. *MBI* 1982.

[2] Kourmanov F, Bozedijieva M, et al. Clinical trial on Tribestan, *Exp Med* 1982.

[3] Kerr JB, Krester, Cyclic variation of Serotli cell lipid content throughout the spermatogenic cycle in rat, *J Reprod Fertil* 1975.

[4] Leboland C, Clermont P, Definition of the state of the cycle of the seminiferous epithelium in the rat. *Annals of New York Acad Sci* 548-573,1952.

[5] Mancini R, Seiguer A, et al. Effect of gonadotrophins of the recovery of spermatogenesis in hypophysectomized patients. *J Clin Endocrinol Metab* 467-478, 1969.

[6] Tomova M, et al. Steroid Saponin and Steroidsapogenine VI. Furstanol bisglykosis aus Tribulus terrestris L, *Plant Medica* 188-191, 1978.

[7] Cicero AF, et al. Hexanic Maca extract improves rat sexual performance more effectively than methonolic and chloroformic Maca extracts. *Andrologia* 34(3), 177-9, 2002.

[8] Balick MJ, et al. Maca: from traditional food crop to energy and libido stimulant. *Altern Ther Health Med* 8(2), 96-8, 2002.

[9] Gonzales GF, et al. Effect of Lepidium meyeni (maca) roots on spermatogenesis of male rats. *Asian J Androl* 3(3), 231-3, 2001.

[10] Balick MJ, Lee R. Maca: from traditional food crop to energy and libido stimulant. *Altern Ther Health Med* 8(2), 96-82, 2002.

[11] Fahim MS. Effect of Pannax Ginseng on testosterone level on prostate in male rats. *Arch Androl* 8(4):261-3, 1982.

[12] Yamamato M, et al. Stimulatory effect of Panax Ginseng principles on DNA and protein synthesis in rat testes. *Arzneimittelforschung*, 27(7), 1404-5, 1977.

[13] Shibata S, Tanaka J, Shoji, and Saito H. Chemistry and pharmacology of Panax. *Economic and Medicinal Plant Research,* 1; 217-284, 1985.

[14] Kim C, et al. Influence of ginseng on mating behavior in male rats, *Am J Chinese Med,* 4;163-8, 1976.

[15] Netter et al. Effect of zinc administration on plasma testosterone, dihydrotestosterone and sperm count. *Arch Androl,* 69-73,1985.

[16] Taikara H, et al. Zinc sulphate therapy for infertile males with or without Varicocelectomy, *Urology,* 638-41, 1987.

[17] Tikkiwal M, et al. Effect of zinc administration on seminal zinc and fertility of oligospermic males, *Ind J Physiol Pharmacol, 30-4, 1987.*

21. PROGESTERONE METABOLISM

[1] Amann W. Removing an ostipation using Agnolyt. *Ther Gegnew* 1965;104:1263-1265.

[2] Weiss RF. Herbal Medicine. Beaconsfield, England:*Beaconsfield Publishers Ltd.,* 1988.

[3] Losh EG, Kayser E. Diagnosis and treatment of dyshormonal menstrual periods in the general practice. *Gybacol Praxis* 1990;14:489-495.

[4] Propping D, Katzorke T. Treatment of corpus luteum insufficiency. *Zetis Allgemeinmedizin* 1987;63:932-933.

[5] Milewicz A, Gejdel, et al. Vitex angus castus extract in the treatment of luteal phase defects due to hyperprolactinemia: results of a randomized placebo-controlled double blind study. *Arzneim-Forsch Drug Res* 1993;43:752-756.

[6] Muhlenstedt D, Wutke W, Schneider HPG. Short luteal phase and prolactin. *Fertil Steril* 1977;373-374.

[7] Propping D, Katzorke T. Treatment of corpus luteum insufficiency. *Zetis Allgemeinmedizin* 1987;63:932-933.

[8] Dittmar FW Bohnert KJ, et al. Premenstrual syndrome: treatment with phytopharmaceutical. *TW Gynakol* 1992;5:60-68.

[9] Lauritzen CH, Reuter HD, Repeges R, et al. Treatment of premenstrual tension type syndrome with Vitex agnus castus: controlled doulble-blind study versus pyridoxine. *Phytomed* 1997;4:183-189.

[10] Bleier W. Phytotherapy in irregular mentstrual cycles or bleeding periods and other gynecological disorders of endocrine origin. *Zentralblatt Gyekal* 1959;81:701-709.

[11] Weiss RF. Herbal Medicine. Beaconsfield, England:Beaconsfield Publishers Ltd., 1988.

[12] Grieve M. A Modern Herbal. *New York, NY: Dover Publications,*1984.

[13] Kurdo K, Takagi K. Physiologically active substances in Capsella bursa-patoris. *Nature* 220(168):707-708,1968.

[14] Shipcohliev T. Uterogenic actions of extracts from a group of medicinal plants. *Vet Med Nauki* 1981; 18(4):94-98.

22. ESTROGEN METABOLISM

[1] Adlercreutz H, Mazur W. Phyto-oestrogens and Western diseases. *Ann Med* 1997;29:95-120.

[2] Price KR, Fenwick GR. Naturally occurring oestrogens in foods – a review. *Food Addit Contam* 1985;2:73-106.

[3] Hirano T, Fukuoka K, Oka K, et al. Antiproliferative activity of mammalian lignan derivatives against the human breast carcinoma cell line, ZR-75-1. *Cancer Invest* 1990;8:595-602.

[4] Hartman PE, Shenkel DM. Antimutagens and anticarcinogens: a survey of putative interceptor molecules. *Environ Mol Mutagen* 1990;15;145-182.

[5] Hirano T, Gotoh M, Ika K. Natural flavinoids and lignans are potent cyto-static agents against human leukemic HL-60 cells. *Life Sci* 1994;55:1061-1069.

[6] MacRae WD, Hudson JB, Towers GH, The antiviral action of lignans. *Plant Med* 1989;55:531-535.

[7] Wu ES, Loch JT 3rd, Toder BH, et al. Flavones. 3. Synthesis , biological activities, and conformational analysis of isoflavone derivatives and related compounds. *J Med Chem* 1992;18:3519-3525.

[8] Jha HC, Recklinghausen G, Zilkah F. Inhibition of in vitro microsomal lipid peroxidation by isoflavonoids. *Biochem Pharmacol* 1985;34:1367-1369.

[9] Wei H, Wei L, Frenkel K, et al. Inhibition of tumor promoter-induced hydrogen peroxide formation in vitro and in vivo by genistein. *Nutr Cancer* 1993;20:1-12.

[10] Wagner JD, Cefalu WT, Anthony MS, et al. Dietary soy protein and estrogen replacement therapy improve cardiovascular risk factors and decrease aortic cholesteryl ester content in ovariectomized cynomolgu monkeys. *Metabolism* 1997;46:698-705.

[11] Bradlow HL Sepkovic DW, Telang NT, et al. Multifunctional aspects of the action of indole-3-carbinol as an anti tumor agent. *Ann NY Academy Sci* 1997;28-29:111-116.

[12] Michnovicz JJ, Bradlow HL. Altered estrogen metabolism and excretion in humans following consumption of indole-3-carbinol. *Nutr Cancer* 1991;16(1):59-66.

[13] Michnovicz JJ, Adlercreutz H, Bradlow HL. Changes in levels of urinary estrogen metabolites after oral indole-3-carbinol treatments in humans. *J Natl Cancer Inst* 1997;89(10):718-23.

[14] Wong GY, Bradlow L, Sepkovic D, et al. Dose-ranging study of indole-3-carbinol for breast cancer prevention. *J Cell Biochem Suppl* 1997;28-29:111-16.

[15] Yuan F, Chen DZ, Liu K, et al. Anti-esrogenic activities of indole-3-carbinol in cervical cells: implications for prevention of cervical cancer. *Anticancer Res* 1999;19(3A)1673-80.

[16] Michnovicz JJ, Bradlow HL. Induction of estradiol metabolism by dietary indole-3-carbinol in humans. *J Natl Cancer Inst* 1990;82;947-949.

[17] Telang NT, Katdare M, Bradlow HL, et al. Inhibition of proliferation and modulation of estradiol metabolism: novel mechanisms for breast cancer prevention by the phytochemical indole-3-carbinol. *Proc Soc Exp Bio Med* 1997;216:246-252.

[18] Tully DB, Allgood VE, Cidlowski JA. Modulation of steroid receptor-mediated gene expression by vitamin B6. *FASEB J* 1994;8(3):343-49.

[19] Brucker A. Essay on the phytotherapy of hormonal disorders in women. *Med Welt* 1960;44:231-2333.

[20] Warnecke G. Influencing menopausal symptoms with a phytoherapeutic agent. *Med Welt* 1985;36:871-874.

[21] Stoll W. Phytopharmacon influences atrophic vaginal epithelium. Double-blind-study – Cimicifuga vs. estrogenic substances. *Therapeuticum* 1987;1:23-31.

[22] Lieberman S. A review of the effectivness of Cimicifuga racemoasa for the symptoms of menopause. *J Women's Health.* 7(5):525-529,1998.

[23] Miksicek RJ. Commonly occurring plant flavoniods have estrogenic activity. *Molecular Pharmacology* 1993;44:37-43.

[24] Duker EM, et al. Effects of extracts from Cimicifuga racemosa on gonadotropin release in menopausal women and ovariectomized rats. *Planta Medica* 1991;57:420-424.

[25] Hirata JD, et al. Does dong quai have estrogenic effects in postmenopausal women? A double-blind placebo-controlled trial. *Fertil Steril* 68(6):981-986,1997.

[26] Ozaki Y. Antiinflammatory effect of tetramethylpyraziane and ferulic acid. *Chem Pharm Bull* 1992;40(4):954-956.

[27] Bensky D, et al. *Chinese Herbal Medicine Materica Medica*, Seattle, WA:East-land Press, 1986.

[28] Sherman JA. *The Complete Botanical Prescriber.* Portland OR: John Sherman, 1993.

[29] Hikino H. Recent research on Oriental medicinal plants. *Econ Med Plant Res* 1985;1:53-85.

[30] Thastrup O, Fjaland B, Lemmich J. Coronary vasodilatory, spasmolytic and cAMP-phosphodiesterase inhibitory properties of dihydropyranocoumarins and dihydrofuranocoumarins. *Acta Pharmacol et Toxical* 1983;52:246-53.

[31] Yamada H, Kiyohara H, Cyong JC, et al. Studies on polysachharides from Angelica. *Plant Medica* 1984;48:163-167.

[32] Yager JD, Liehr JG. Molecular mechanisms of estrogen carcinogenesis. *Annu Rev Pharmacol Toxicol* 1996;36:203-32.

[33] Buttterworth M, Lau SS, Monks TJ. 17 Beta-estradiol metabolism by hamster hepatic microsomes. Implications fo the catechol-O-methyl transferase-mediated detoxification of catechol estrogens. *Drug Metab Dispos* 1996;24(4):588-94.

23. TESTOSTERONE METABOLISM

[1] Nankin HR, Calkin JM. Decreased bioavailable testosterone in aging and normal impotent men. *J Clin Endocrinol Metab* 1986:63:1418-1420.

[2] Gray A Berlin JA, McKinley JB, Longcope C. An examination of research design effects on the association of testosterone and male aging: results of meta-analysis. *J Clin Epidemiol* 1991;44:671-684.

[3] Simon D, Presiosi P, Barret-Conner E, Roger M, Saint M, Nahoul K, et al. The influence of aging on plasma sex hormones in men: the Telecom Study. *Am J Epidemiol* 1982; 135:783-791.

[4] Deslypere JP, Vermeulen A. Leydig cell function in normal men: effects of age, life-style, residence, diet and activity. *J Clin Endocrinol Metab* 1984; 59:995-962.

[5] Vermeulen A, Desylpere JP. Testicular endocrine function in the aging male. *Maruritas* 1985; 7:273-279.

[6] Nankin HR, Calkin JM. Decreased bioavailable testosterone in aging and normal impotent men. *J Clin Endocrinol Metab* 1986:63:1418-1420.

[7] Kellis JT and Vickery LE. Inhibition of human estrogen synthetase (aromatase) by Flavones. *Science* 225, 1032-1024.

[8] Campbell DR and Kruzer MS. Flavonoid inhibition of aromatase enzyme activity in human preadipocytes. *J of Steroid Biochem and Mol Bio* 46, 381-388, 1993.

[9] Le Bail JC, et al. Aromatase and 17-beta-hydroxysteroid dehydrogenase inhibition by flavonids, *Cancer Letters* 133, 101-106, 1998.

[10] Pauget C, et al. Synthesis and aromatase inhibitory activity of flavones. *Pharm Res,* 19(3), 286-91, 2002.

[11] Vinh TK, et al. Evaluation of 7-hydroxy-flavones as inhibitors of oestrone and oestradiol biosynthesis. *J Enzyme Inhib* 16(5), 417-24, 2001.

[12] Jeong HJ, et al. Inhibition of aromatase by flavonoids. *Arch Pharm Res* 22(3), 309-312,1997.

[13] Saarinen N, et al. No evidence for the in vivo activity of aromatase-inhibitory flavonoids. *J Steroid Biochem* 78(3), 231-9, 2001.

[14] Hertog, Mg, et al. Dietary antioxidant flavonoids and risks of coronary heart disease: The Zutphen Elderly Study. *Lancet* 342, 1007-1011.

[15] Chaumdry PS, et al. Inhibition of human lens aldose reductast by flavonids, sulindac, and indomethicin. *Biochem Phamacol* 32, 1995-1998, 1983.

[16] Yoshimoto T, et al. Flavonoids: Potent inhibitors of arachidonate 5-lipoxygenase. *Biochem Biophys Res Common* 11, 612-618, 1983.

[17] Ferrandiz ML and Alcaraz MJ. Anti-inflammatory activity and inhibition of arachidonic acid metabolism by flavonoids. *Agents Action* 32, 283-287, 1991.

[18] Middleton E and Drzewieki G, Flavonoid inhibition of human basophil histamine release. *Int Arch Allergy Appl Immunol* 77, 155-157, 1985.

[19] Kaul T, Middleton E, and Ogra P. Antiviral effects of flavonoids on human viruses. *J Med Virol* 15, 71-79, 1985.

[20] Mukhtar H, et al. Tea compounds: Antimutagenic and anticarcinogenic effects. *Prev Med* 21, 351-360, 1992.

[21] Larroca LM, et al. Growth-inhibitory effect of quercetin and presence of type II estrogen binding sites in primary human transitional cell carcinomas. *J Urol* 152, 1029-1033, 1994.

[22] Wang ZY, et al. Protection against polycyclic aromatic hydrocarbon-induced skin tumor initiation in mice by green tea polyphenols. *Carinogenesis* 10, 411—415, 1989.

24. SEROTONIN

[1] Sarzi Puttini P, Caruso I. Primary fibromylagia syndrome and 5-hydroxy-L-tryptophan: a 90-day open study. *J Int Med Res*1992;20(2):182-9.

[2] De Benedittis G, Massei R. Serotonin precursors in chronic primary headache. A double-blind cross-over study with L-5-hydroxytryptophan vs. placebo. *Journal of Neurosurgical Sciences* 1985;29(3):239–48.

[3] Rahman MK, Nagatsu T, Sakurai T, Hori S, Abe M, Matsuda M. Effect of pyridoxal phosphate deficiency on aromatic L-amino acid decarboxylase activity with L-DOPA and L-5-hydroxytryptophan as substrates in rats. *Jpn. J. Pharmacol.* 1982;32(5):803-11.

[4] Birdsall TC."5-Hydroxytryptophan: a clinically-effective serotonin precursor. *Alternative medicine review : a journal of clinical therapeutic* 1998;3(4):271-80.

[5] Bouchard S, Roberge AG. Biochemical properties and kinetic parameters of dihydroxyphenylalanine--5-hydroxytryptophan decarboxylase in brain, liver, and adrenals of cat. *Can. J. Bioche* 1979; 57(7):1014-8.

[6] Meryer S. Use of neurotransmitter precursors for treatment of depression. *Alter Med Rev* 2000;5(1):64-71.

[7] Turner EH, Loftis JM, Blackwell AD. Serotonin a la carte: supplementation with the serotonin precursor 5-hydroxytryptophan. *Pharmacol. Ther* 2006;109 (3):325-38.

[8] Bruni O, Ferri R, Miano S, Verrillo E. L-5-Hydroxytryptophan treatment of sleep terrors in children 2004;163(7):402-7.

[9] Randløv C, J. Mehlsen, CF, Thomsen, C. Hedman, H, von Fircks and K. Winther. The efficacy of St. John's Wort in patients with minor depressive symptoms or dysthymia - a double-blind placebo-controlled study" *Phytomedicine.* 2006; 13(4): 215–221.

[10] Woelk H, et al. Comparison of St John's wort and imipramine for treating depression: randomised controlled trial. *Br Med J* 2000; 321:536-9.

[11] Schrader E, et al. Equivalence of St John's wort extract (Ze 117) and fluoxetine: a randomised, controlled study in mild-moderate depression. *Int Clin Psychopharmacology* 2000;15:61-68.

[12] Laakmann G, Schule C, Baghai T, Kieser M. St. John's wort in mild to moderate depression: the relevance of hyperforin for the clinical efficacy. *Pharmacopsychiatry* 1998;31 (Suppl 1):54-9.

[13] Harrer G, Schmidt U, Kuhn U, Biller A. Comparison of equivalence between the St. John's wort extract LoHyp-57 and fluoxetine. *Arzneimittelforschung* 1999;49 (4):289-96

[14] Philipp M, Kohnen R, Hiller KO. Hypericum extract versus imipramine or placebo in patients with moderate depression: randomised multicentre study of treatment for eight weeks. *Br Med J* 1999;319 (7224):1534-8.

[15] Lecrubier et al. "Efficacy of St. John's wort extract WS 5570 in major depression: a double-blind, placebo-controlled trial." *Am J Psychiatry.* 2002;159(8):1361-6.

[16] Nahrstedt A, Butterweck V. Biologically active and other chemical constituents of the herb of Hypericum perforatum L. *Pharmacopsychiatry* 1997;30 (Suppl 2):129-34.

[17] Chatterjee SS, Bhattacharya SK, Wonnemann M, Erdelmeier C.Antidepressant activity of hypericum perforatum and hyperforin: the neglected possibility. *Pharmacopsychiatry* 1988;31 (Suppl 1):7-15.

[18] Bressa GM. S-Adenosyl-L-methionine (SAMe) as antidepressant: meta-analysis of clinical studies. *Acta Neurol Scand* 1994;89:7-14.

[19] Bressa GM. S-Adenosyl-L-methionine (SAMe) as antidepressant: meta-analysis of clinical studies. *Acta Neurol Scand* 1994;89:7-14.

[20] Curcio M, Catto E, Stramentinoli G, Algeri S. Effect of S-adenosyl-L-methionine on serotonin metabolism in rat brain. *Prog Neuropsychopharmacol Biol Psychiatry* 1978;2:65-71.

[21] Fonlupt P, Barailler J, Roche M, Cronenberger L, Pacheco H. Effets de la S-adénosylméthionine et de la S-adénosylhomocystéine sur la synthèse, in vivo, de la noradrénaline et de la sérotonine dans différentes parties du cerveau de rat. *C R Seances Acad Sci D* 1979; 288: 283-6.

[22] Bottiglieri T, Laundy M, Martin R, Carney MWP, Nissenbaum H, Toone BK, et al. S-Adenosylmethionine influences monoamine metabolism. *Lancet* 1984;ii:224.

[23] Baldessarini R. Neuropharmacology of [SAMe]. *Am J Med* 1987;83 (suppl 5A):95-103.

[24] B. Kagan et al,"Oral [SAMe] in depression: a... double-blind, placebo controlled trial. *Am J Psychiat* 1990;147:591-95.

[25] E. Reynolds et al. Methylation and mood." *Lancet II* 1984:196-98.

25. DOPAMINE

[1] Tharakan B, Dhanasekaran M, Mize-Berge J, Manyam BV. Anti-parkinson botanical Mucuna pruriens prevents levodopa induced plasmid and genomic DNA damage. *Phytother Res* 2007;11{Epub ahead of print}

[2] Mizra L and Wagner H. Extraction of bioactive principles from Mucuna pruriens seeds. *Indian J Biochem Biophys* 2007;44(1):56-60.

[3] Katzenschlager R, Evans A, Manson A, et al. Mucuna pruriens in Parkinson's disease: a double blind clinical and pharmacological study. *J Neurol Neurosrug Psychiatry* 2004; 75(12);1672-7.

[4] Manyam BV, Dhanasekaran M, Hare TA. Neuroprotective effects of the antiparkinson drug Mucuna pruriens. *Phytother Res* 2004;18(9):706-12.

[5] Singhal B, Lalkaka J, Sankhia C. Epidemiology and treatment of Parkinson's disease in India. *Parkinsonism Relat Disord* 2003;9 Suppl 2:S105-9.

[6] Mayam BV & Sanchez-Ramos JR. Traditional and complimentary therapies for Parkinson's disease. *Adv Neurol* 1999;80:565-74.

[7] Sebelli H, Fink P, Fawcett J. Tom C. Sustained antidepressant effect of PEA replacement. *J Neuropsychiatry Clin Neurosci* 1996;8(2): 168-71.

[8] Guang-Xi Z, Hiroshi S, et al. Decreased B-phenylethylamine in CSF in Parkinson's Disease. *J Neurol Neurosurg Psychiatry* 1997;63:754-758.

[9] Michell S, Lewis G, et al. *Biomarkers of Parkinson's disease.* 2004;127(8):1693-1705.

[10] Karoum F, Wolf M, Mosniam AD. Effects of the administration of amphetmaine eithier alone or in combination with resperine or cocaine, or regional brain beta-phenetylamine and dopamine release. *Am J Ther* 1997;4(9/10):333-342.

[11] Kausage A. Decrease beta-phenletylamine in urin of children with attention deficit hyperactivity disorder and autistic disorder. *No To Hattatsu* 2002; 34(3):243-8.

[12] McGuire S, Sortwell C, et al. Dietary supplementation with blueberry extract improves survival of transplanted dopamine neurons. *Nutritional Neuroscience* 2006;9:251-258.

[13] Crews F, Nixon K, et al. BHT blocks NF-kappa B activation and ethanol-induced brain damage. *Alcohol Clin Exp Res* 2006;30(11):1938-49.

[14] Ahukitt-Hale B, Carey AN, et al. Beneficial effects of fruit extracts on neuronal function and behavior in a rodent model of accelerated aging. *Neurobiol Aging* 2006:10:1187-94.

[15] Lau FC, Shukitt Hale B, Joseph JA. The beneficial effects of fruit polyphenols on brain aging. *Neurobiol Aging* 2005;26(1):128-32.

[16] Russell AL, McCarty MF. DL-phenylalanine markedly potentiates opiate analgesia - an example of nutrient/pharmaceutical up-regulation of the endogenous analgesia system. *Med Hypotheses.* 2000;55(4):283-8.

[17] Beckmann H, Athen D, Olteanu M, Zimmer R. DL-phenylalanine versus imipramine: a double-blind controlled study. *Arch Psychiatr Nervenkr.* 1979;227(1):49-58.

[18] Wood DR, Reimherr FW, Wender PH. Treatment of attention deficit disorder with DL-phenylalanine. *Psychiatry Res.* 1985;16(1):21-6.

[19] Borison RL, Maple PJ, Havdala HS, Diamond BI. Metabolism of an amino acid with antidepressant properties. *Res Commun Chem Pathol Pharmacol.* 1978;21(2):363-6.

[20] Ehrenpreis S. Analgesic properties of enkephalinase inhibitors: animal and human studies. *Prog Clin Biol Res*;192:363-70.

[21] Janssen PA, Leysen JE, Megens AA, Awouters FH. Does phenylethylamine act as an endogenous amphetamine in some patients? *Int J Neuropsychopharmcol* 1999; 2(3):229-240

22 Anderson PJ, Rogers QR, Morris JG. Cats require more dietary phenylalanine or tyrosine for melanin deposition in hair than for maximal growth. *J Nutr.* 2002;132(7):2037-42.

23 Harmer CJ, McTavish SF, Clark L, Goodwin GM, Cowen PJ. Tyrosine depletion attenuates dopamine function in healthy volunteers. *Psychopharmacology* (Berl). 2001;154(1):105-11.

24 Rasmussen DD, Ishizuka B, Quigley ME, Yen SS. Effects of tyrosine and tryptophan ingestion on plasma catecholamine and 3,4-dihydroxyphenylacetic acid concentrations. *J Clin Endocrinol Metab.* 1983;57(4):760-3.

25 Meyers S. Use of neurotransmitter precursors for treatment of depression. *Altern Med Rev.* 2000 5(1):64-71.

26 Young SN. Behavioral effects of dietary neurotransmitter precursors: basic and clinical aspects. *Neurosci Biobehav Rev.* 1996;20(2):313-23.

27 Montgomery AJ, McTavish SF, Cowen PJ, Grasby PM. Reduction of brain dopamine concentration with dietary tyrosine plus phenylalanine depletion: an [11C]raclopride PET study. *Am J Psychiatry.* 2003;160(10):1887-9.

28 Guilarate TR. Effects of vitamin B-6 nutrition on the levels of dopamine, dopamine metabolites, dopa decarboxylase activity, and GABA in the developing rat corpus striatum. *Neurochemical Research* 1989;14:571-578.

29 Tang F, Wei LL. Vitamin B-6 deficiency prolongs the time course of evoked dopamine release from rat striatum. *J Nutr* 2004; 134:3350-3354.

30 Guilarte, T. R., Wagner, H. N., Jr & Frost, J. J. Effects of perinatal vitamin B6 deficiency on dopaminergic neurochemistry. *J. Neurochem* 1987;48:432-439.

31 Guilarte, T. R.Effect of vitamin B-6 nutrition on the levels of dopamine, dopamine metabolites, dopa decarboxylase activity, tyrosine, and GABA in the developing rat corpus striatum. *Neurochem. Res* 1989;14:571-578.

32 Bayoumi, R. A., Kirwan, J. R. & Smith, W. R.. Some effects of dietary vitamin B6 deficiency and 4-deoxypyridoxine on -aminobutyric acid metabolism in rat brain. *J. Neurochem* 1972;19:569-576.

33 Weber C. & Ernesrt ME. Antioxidants, supplements, and Parkinson's disease. *Ann Pharmacother.* 2006 May;40(5):935-8.

34 Benton D. Selenium intake, mood and other aspects of psychological functioning. *Nutr Neurosci.* 2002;5(6):363-74.

35 Grimble RF. The effects of sulfur amino acid intake on immune function in humans. *J Nutr.* 2006 ;136(6 Suppl):1660S-1665S.

CHAPTER REFERENCES

CHAPTER ONE
[1] Facts About Thyroid Disease, 2005. American Academy of Clinical Endocrinologists: http://www.aace.com/public/awareness/tam/2005/pdfs/thyroid_disease_fact_sheet.pdf.
[2] Eastwood GI, Braverman LE, White EM, Vander Salm TJ. Reversal of lower esophageal sphincter hypotension and esophageal aperistalsis after treatment for hypothyroidism. *J Clin Gastroenterol* 1982;4:307-310.
[3] Valenti S, Guido R, Fazzuoli, et al. Decreased steroidogenesis and camp production in vitro by leydig cells isolated from rats made hypothyroid during adulthood. *Int J Androl* 1997; 20:279-286.
[4] Purandare A, Godil M, Ahnn SH, et al. Effect of hypothyroidism and its treatment on the IGF system in infants and children. *J Pediatr Endocrinol Metab* 2003;16: 35-42.
[5] Purandare A, Godil M, Ahnn SH, et al. Effect of hypothyroidism and its treatment on the IGF system in infants and children. *J Pediatr Endocrinol Metab* 2003;16: 35-42.
[6] Muller MJ, Burger AC, Ferrannini E, et al. Glucoregulatory function of thyroid hormones: role of pancreatic hormones. *Am J Physio* 1989;256: E101-E110.
[7] Oge A, Sozmen E, Karaoglue AO. Effect of thyroid function on LDL oxidation in hypothyroidism and hyperthyroidism. *Endocr Res* 2004;30: 481-489.
[8] Boado RJ, Romeo HE, Chuluvan HE. et al. Evidence suggesting that the sympathetic nervous system mediates thyroidal depression in turpentine-induced nonthyroidal illness syndrome. *Neuroendocrinology* 1991;53:360-364.
[9] Kitmura S, Jinno N, Suzuki T, et al. Thyroid hormone-like and estrogenic activity of hydroxylated PCBs in cell culture. *Toxicology* 30, 377-387.
[10] Lin SY, Wang YY, Lin PH, et al. Lower serum thyroxine levels are associated with metabolic syndrome in Chinese population. *Metabolism* 2005;54: 1525-1528.
[11] Saha B & Maity C. (2002). Alteration of serum enzymes in primary hypothyroidism. *Clin Chem Lab Med* 40, 609-611.
[12] Purandare A, Godil M, Ahnn SH, et al. Effect of hypothyroidism and its treatment on the IGF system in infants and children. *J Pediatr Endocrinol Metab* 2003;16: 35-42.
[13] Mani S. Signaling mechanisms in progesterone-neurotransmitter interactions. *J Mol Endocrinol* 2003;30(2):127-37.
[14] Hampl R, Kancheva R, Hill M, et al. Interpretation of sex-hormone-binding globulin levels in thyroid disorders. *Thyroid* 2003; 13,:755-760.
[15] Oge A, Sozmen E, Karaoglue AO. Effect of thyroid function on LDL oxidation in hypothyroidism and hyperthyroidism. *Endocr Res* 2004;30: 481-489.

CHAPTER TWO
[16] American Autoimmune Related Diseases Association, Inc.
[17] ACTA Bio Medica 2003;74;9-33. *Update on polyendocrine systems (APS).*
[18] ACTA Bio Medica 2003;74;9-33. *Update on polyendocrine systems (APS).*

[19] Bailleres. Autoimmunity and hypothyroidism. *Clin Endocrin Metab.* 1988 Aug;2(3):591-617.

[20] Ness-Abramof R, Nabriski DA, Braverman LE, Shilo L, Weiss E, Reshef T, Shapiro MS, Shenkman L. Prevalence and evaluation of B12 deficiency in patients with autoimmune thyroid disease. *Am J Med Sci* 2006 Sep;332(3):119-22.

[21] Elfström P, Montgomery SM, Kämpe O, Ekbom A, Ludvigsson JF. Risk of thyroid disease in individuals with celiac disease. *J Clin Endocrinol Metab* 2008 Oct;93(10):3915-21. Epub 2008 Jul 8.

[22] Risk factors for and prevalence of thyroid disorders in a cross-sectional study among healthy female relatives of patients with autoimmune thyroid disease. *Clin Endocrinol* (Oxf) 2003 Sep;59(3):396-401.

[23] High iodine intake is a risk factor of post-partum thyroiditis: result of a survey from Shenyang, China. J *Endocrinol Invest* 2005 nov;38(10):876-81.

[24] Thyroid. 2004 Jul;14(7):510-20.

[25] Thyroid-related autoantibodies and celiac disease: a role for a gluten-free diet? *J Clin Gastroenterol* 2002 Sep;35(3):245-8.

[26] Prevalence of thyroid disorders in untreated adult celiac disease patients and effect of gluten withdrawal: an Italian multicenter study. *Am J Gastroenterol* 2001 Mar;96(3):751-7.

[27] Prevalence of coeliac disease in patients with thyroid autoimmunity. *Horm Res* 1999;51(3):124-7.

[28] Celiac disease in North Italian patients with autoimmune thyroid diseases. *Autoimmunity* 2008 Feb;41(1):116-21.

[29] Celiac disease in Dutch patients with Hashimoto's thyroiditis and vice versa. *World J Gastroenterol* 2007 Mar 21;13(11):1715-22.

[30] The presence of the antigliadin antibodies in autoimmune thyroid diseases. *Hepatogastroenterology* 2003 Dec;50 Suppl 2:cclxxix-cclxxx.

[31] *Physiol Res.* 2003;52(1):79-88.

[32] Clinical and sub-clinical autoimmune thyroid disease in adult celiac disease *Dig Dis Sci* 2001 Dec;46(12):2631-5.

[33] Surks M, Sievert R. Drugs and thyroid function. *NEJM* 1995; 333(25):1688.

[34] Weetman A. Grave's Disease. *NEJM* 2000; 343(17):1236.

[35] American Thyroid Association

[36] Bailleres. Autoimmunity and hypothyroidism. *Clin Endocrin Metab* 1988 Aug;2(3):591-617.

[37] Evolution of thyroid autoimmunity during iodine prophylaxis--the Sri Lankan experience. *Eur J Endocrinol* 2003 Aug;149(2):103-10.

[38] High prevalence of thyroid dysfunction and autoimmune thyroiditis in adolescents after elimination of iodine deficiency in the Eastern Black Sea Region of Turkey. *Thyroid* 2006 Dec;16(12):1265-71.

[39] Effect of iodine intake on thyroid diseases in China Effect of iodine intake on thyroid diseases in China. *N Engl J Med* 2006 Jun 29;354(26):2783-93.

[40] Why measure thyroglobulin autoantibodies rather than thyroid peroxidase autoantibodies? *Thyroid* 2004 Jul;14(7):510-20.

[41] Autoimmune thyroid disorders and celiac disease. *Eur J Endocrinol* 1994 Feb;130(2):137-40.

[42] The presence of the antigliadin antibodies in autoimmune thyroid diseases. *Hepatogastroenterology* 2003 Dec;50 Suppl 2:cclxxix-cclxxx.

[43] Autoimmune thyroid diseases and coeliac disease. *Eur J Gastroenterol Hepatol* 1999 Aug;11(8):939-40.

[44] Risk factors for and prevalence of thyroid disorders in a cross-sectional study among healthy female relatives of patients with autoimmune thyroid disease. *Clin Endocrinol* (Oxf) 2003 Sep;59(3):396-401.

[45] Clinical and sub-clinical autoimmune thyroid disease in adult celiac disease *Dig Dis Sci*. 2001 Dec;46(12):2631-5.

[46] IgA and IgG antigliadin, IgA anti-tissue transglutaminase and antiendomysial antibodies in patients with autoimmune thyroid diseases and their relationship to thyroidal replacement therapy. *Physiol Res* 2003;52(1):79-88.

[47] The American Journal of Gastroenterology Genetic Background of Celiac Disease and Its Clinical Implications Victorien M. Wolters, M.D.; Cisca Wijmenga, Ph.D., *Am J Gastroenterol* 2008;103(1):190-195.)

[48] Celiac disease in North Italian patients with autoimmune thyroid disease. *Autoimmunity* 2008;4(1):116-21.

[49] Celiac disease in Dutch patients with Hashimoto's thyroiditis and vice versa. *World J Gastroenterol* 2007 Mar 21;13(11):1715-22.

[50] Thyroid-related autoantibodies and celiac disease: a role for a gluten-free diet? *J Clin Gastroenterol* 2002 Sep;35(3):245-8.

[51] Amino N, Hidaka Y, Takano T, et al. Possible Induction of Graves' disease in painless thyroiditis by gonasotropin-releasing hormone analogues. *Thyroid* 2003;13(8):815-8.

[52] Ishii K, Hayashi A, Tamaoka A, et al. A case of Hashimoto's encephalopathy with a relapsing course related to the menstrual cycle. *Rinsho Shinkeigaku*1993;33(9):995-7.

[53] Risk of subclinical hypothyroidism in pregnant women with asymptomatic autoimmune thyroid disorders. *J Clin Endocrinol Metab* 1994;79(1):197-204.

[54] Guan HX, Li CY, LI FS, et al. Thyroid function and thyroid autoimmunity at the late pregnancy: data from 664 pregnant women. *Zhanghua Fu Chan Ke Za Zhi* 2006;41(8):529-32.

[55] Massoudi MS, Meilahn EN, Orchard TJ, et al. Prevalence of thyroid antibodies among healthy middle-aged women. Findings from the thyroid study in healthy women. *Ann Epidemiol* 1995:5(3):229-33.

[56] Sozen I, Arici A. Hyperinsulinism and its interaction with hyperandrogenism in polycystic ovary syndrome. *Obest Bynecol Surv* 2000;55:321-328.

[57] Nestler J. Insulin resistance effects on sex hormones and ovulation in the polycystic ovary syndrome. In:Reaven G, Laws A, eds. *Contemporary Endocrinology: Insulin Resistance*. Totowa NJ: Humana Press; 1999.347-365.

[58] Wu XK, et al. Ovarian-adrenal cross-talk in polycystic ovary syndrome: evidence of wedge. *Euro J Endocrinol* 2000;143:383-388.

[59] Inflammatory markers, insulin resistance and carotid intima-media thickness in North-Indian type 2 diabetic subjects. *J Assoc Physicians India* 2007 Oct; 55:693-9.

[60] Autoimmune thyroid disorders and celiac disease. *Eur J Endocrinol* 1994 Feb;130(2):137-40.

[61] Lisa A Houghton and Reinhold Vieth. The case against ergocalciferol (vitamin D2) as a vitamin supplement. From the School of Nutrition and Dietetics, Acadia University, Wolfville, Canada (LAH); the Department of Nutritional Sciences, University of Toronto, Toronto, Canada (RV); and the Mount Sinai Hospital, Toronto, Canada (RV).

[62] Drugarin D. The pattern of Th1 cytokine in autoimmune thyroditis. *Immunol Letts* 2000; 71: 73-77.

[63] Smith EA, et al. Effects of long-term administration of vitamin D3 analogs to mice. *J Endocrinol Invest* 1994; 17(6): 385-390.

[64] Holick MF. Sunlight and vitamin D for bone health and prevention of autoimmune diseases, cancers, and cardiovascular diseases. *Am J Clin Nutr* 2004;80:1678S-1688S.

[65] DeLuca HF, Cantorna MT. Vitamin D: its role and uses in immunology. *FASEB J* 2001;15:2579-2585.

[66] Cantorna MT, Zhu Y, Froicu M, Whittke A. Vitamin D status, 1-25-di-hydroxyvitamin D3, and the immune system. *Am J Clin Nutr* 2004;80:1717S-1720S.

[67] Drugarin D. The pattern of Th1 cytokine in autoimmune thyroditis. *Immunol Letts* 2000; 71: 73-77.

[68] Smith EA, et al. Effects of long-term administration of vitamin D3 analogs to mice. *J Endocrinol Invest* 1994; 17(6): 385-390.

[69] Koutkia P, Lu Z, Chen TC, Holick MF. Treatment of vitamin D deficiency due to Crohn's disease with tanning bed ultraviolet B radiation. *Gastroeneterology* 2001; 121:1485-1488.

[70] Vestergaard P. Prevalence and pathogenesis of osteoporosis in patients with in-flammatory bowel disease. *Minerva Med* 2004;95:469-480.

[71] Wortsman J, Matsuoka LY, Chen TC, et al. Decreased bioavailability of vitamin D in obesity. *Am J Clin Nutr* 2000;72:690-693.

[72] Holick MF. Photosynthesis of vitamin D in the skin: effect of environmental and life-style variables. *Fed Proc* 1987;46:1876-1882.

[73] Atli T, Gullu S, Usal AR, Erdogan G. The prevalence of vitamin D deficiency and effects of ultraviolet light on vitamin D levels in elderly Turkish population. *Arch Gerontol Geriatr* 2005;40:53-60.

[74] Jacob CM, Pastorino AC, Fahl K, Carneiro-Sampaio M, Monteiro RC. Autoimmunity in IgA Deficiency: revisiting the role of IgA as a silent house-keeper. *J Clin Immunol* 2008 May;28Suppl 1:S56-61. Epub 2008 Jan 17.

[75] Tlaskalová-Hogenová H, Stopánková R, Tucková L, Farré MA, Funda DP, Verdú EF, Sinkora J, Hudcovic T, Reháková Z, Cukrowska B, Kozáková H, Prokesová L. Autoimmunity, immunodeficiency and mucosal infections: chronic intes-tinal inflammation as a sensitive indicator of immunoregulatory defects in re-sponse to normal luminal microflora. *Folia Microbiol (Praha)* 1998;43(5):545-50.

[76] Girschick HJ, Guilherme L, Inman RD, Latsch K, Rihl M, Sherer Y, Shoenfeld Y, Zeidler H, Arienti S, Doria A. Bacterial triggers and autoimmune rheumatic diseases. *Clin Exp Rheumatol* 2008 Jan-Feb;26(1 Suppl 48):S12-7.

[77] Paroli M, Schiaffella E, Di Rosa F, Barnaba V. Persisting viruses and autoimmu-nity. *J Neuroimmunol* 2000 Jul 24;107(2):201-4.

[78] Husman TM. Clusters of autoimmune diseases in microbial exposure in mois-ture damaged buildings. *Journal of Allergy and Clinical Immunology* 2004 Feb;113(2;1): S59.

[79] Molina V, Shoenfeld Y. Infection, vaccines and other environmental triggers of autoimmunity. *Autoimmunity* 2005 May;38(3):235-45.

[80] Langer P, Kocan A, Tajtaková M, Petrík J, Chovancová J, Drobná B, Jursa S, Rádiková Z, Koska J, Ksinantová L, Hucková M, Imrich R, Wimmerová S, Gasperíková D, Shishiba Y, Trnovec T, Seböková E, Klimes I. Fish from indus-trially polluted freshwater as the main source of organochlorinated pollutants and increased frequency of thyroid disorders and dysglycemia. *Chemosphere* 2007 Apr;67(9):S379-85. Epub 2007 Jan 11.

[81] Langer P, Tajtáková M, Fodor G, Kocan A, Bohov P, Michálek J, Kreze A. Increased thyroid volume and prevalence of thyroid disorders in an area heavily polluted by polychlorinated biphenyls. *Eur J Endocrinol* 1998 Oct;139(4):402-9.

[82] Rádiková Z, Tajtáková M, Kocan A, Trnovec T, Seböková E, Klimes I, Langer P. Possible effects of environmental nitrates and toxic organochlorines on human thyroid in highly polluted areas in Slovakia. *Thyroid* 2008 Mar;18(3):353-62.

[83] Langer P, Kocan A, Tajtakova M, Petrik J, Chovancova J, Drobna B, Jursa S, Pavuk M, Trnovec T, Seböková E, Klimes I. Human thyroid in the population

exposed to high environmental pollution by organochlorinated pollutants for several decades. *Endocr Regul* 2005 Jan;39(1):13-20.

[84] ACTA Bio Medica 2003;74;9-33. *Update on polyendocrine systems (APS).*

[85] Queiroz MS. [Type 1 diabetes and autoimmune polyendocrine syndromes]. *Arq Bras Endocrinol Metabol* 2008 Mar;52(2):198-204. Portuguese.

[86] Blanchin S, Coffin C, Viader F, Ruf J, Carayon P, Potier F, Portier E, Comby E, Allouche S, Ollivier Y, Reznik Y, Ballet JJ. Anti-thyroperoxidase antibodies from patients with Hashimoto's encephalopathy bind to cerebellar astrocytes. *J Neuroimmunol* 2007 Dec;192(1-2):13-20. Epub 2007 Oct 26.

CHAPTER THREE

[87] Ozawa M, Sato K, Han DC, et al. Effects of tumor necrosis factor-alpha/cachetin on thyroid hormone metabolism in mice. *Endocrinology* 1998;123:1461-1467.

[88] Rittig MG. Smooth and rough lipopolysaccharides phenotypes of Brucella induce different intracellular trafficking and cytokine/chemokine release in human monocytes. *Journal of Leukocyte Biology* 2004;5(4):196-200.

[89] Hermus RM, Sweep CG, van der Meer MJ, et al. Continuous infusion of interleukin-1Beta induces a non-thyroidal illness syndrome in rat. *Endocrinology* 1992;131:2139-2146.

[90] Lyson K, McCann SM. The effect of interleukin-6 on pituitary hormone release in vivo and vitro. *Neuroendocrinology* 1991;54:262-266.

[91] Mechanisms of disease: the role of intestinal barrier function in the pathogenesis of gastrointestinal autoimmune diseases. *Nat Clin Pract Gastroenterol Hepatol* 2005 Sep;2(9):416-22. Review.

[92] The proinflammatory cytokines IL-2, IL-15 and IL-21 modulate the repertoire of mature human natural killer cell receptors. *Arthritis Res Ther* 2007;9(6):R125. PMID: 18053164.

[93] Effective collaboration between IL-4 and IL-21 on B cell activation. *Immunobiology* 2008;213(7):545-55. Epub 2008 Feb 20.

[94] B cells are involved in the modulation of pathogenic gut immune response in food-allergic enteropathy. *Clin Exp Immunol* 2008 Nov;154(2):153-61. Epub 2008 Sep 5.

[95] Effect of acute hyperglycaemia and/or hyperinsulinaemia on proinflammatory gene expression, cytokine production and neutrophil function in humans. *Diabet Med* 2008 Feb;25(2):157-64.

[96] Exposure to the fish parasite Anisakis causes allergic airway hyperreactivity and dermatitis. *J Allergy Clin Immunol* 2006 May;117(5):1098-105.

[97] Myeloid Dendritic Cells of Patients With Chronic HCV Infection Induce Proliferation of Regulatory T Lymphocytes. *Gastroenterology* 2008 Aug 7.

[98] Autoantibodies to the translational suppressors T cell intracytoplasmic antigen 1 and T cell intracytoplasmic antigen 1-related protein in patients with rheumatic diseases: increased prevalence in systemic lupus erythematosus and systemic sclerosis and correlation with clinical features. *Arthritis Rheum* 2008 May;58(5):1226-36.

[99] Whipworm: DDW 2004: Abstract 580, presented May 18, 2004; abstract 644, presented May 18, 2004.

[100] American Autoimmune Related Diseases Association, Inc. http://www.aarda.org/mission_statement.php

[101] American Autoimmune Related Diseases Association, Inc. http://www.aarda.org/mission_statement.php

[102] Mechanisms of disease: the role of intestinal barrier function in the pathogenesis of gastrointestinal autoimmune diseases. *Nat Clin Pract Gastroenterol Hepatol* 2005 Sep;2(9):416-22. Review.

[103] The cytokine hypothesis of depression: inflammation, oxidative & nitrosative stress (IO&NS) and leaky gut as new targets for adjunctive treatments in depression. *Neuro Endocrinol Lett* 2008 Jun;29(3):287-91. Review.

[104] Sex-specific programming of offspring emotionality after stress early in pregnancy. *J Neurosci* 2008 Sep 3;28(36):9055-65.

[105] Activation of the maternal immune system alters cerebellar development in the offspring. *Brain Behav Immun* 2008 Aug 9.

[106] Preliminary evidence for a modulation of fetal dopaminergic development by maternal immune activation during pregnancy. *Neuroscience* 2008 Jun 23;154(2):701-9. Epub 2008 Apr 25.

[107] Maternal infection leads to abnormal gene regulation and brain atrophy in mouse offspring: implications for genesis of neurodevelopmental disorders. *Schizophr Res* 2008 Feb;99(1-3):56-70. Epub 2008 Jan 9.

[108] Maternal autoimmune diseases, asthma and allergies, and childhood autism spectrum disorders: a case-control study. *Arch Pediatr Adolesc* Med. 2005 Feb;159(2):151-7.

[109] Maternal health in pregnancy and intellectual disability in the offspring: a population-based study. *Ann Epidemiol* 2006 Jun;16(6):448-54. Epub 2005 Sep 22.

[110] A shift in the Th(1)/Th(2) ratio accompanies the clinical remission of systemic lupus erythematosus in patients with end-stage renal disease. *Nephrol Dial Transplant* 2002 Oct;17(10):1790-4.

[111] Lu B, Moser AH, Shigenaga JK, Feingold KR, Grunfeld C. Type II nuclear hormone receptors, coactivator, and target gene repression in adipose tissue in acute-phase response. *J Lipid Res* 2006;47 (10):2179-90.

[112] Kimura H and Caturegli P. Chemokine orchestration of autoimmune thyroiditis. *Thyroid* 2007;47(10):1005-11.

[113] Yamazaki K, Suzuki K, Yamada E, et al. Suppression of iodide uptake and thyroid hormone synthesis with stimulation of the type I interferon system by double-stranded ribonucleic acid in cultured human thyroid follicles. *Endocrinology* 2007;148(7):3226-35.

[114] Kwakkel J, Wiersinga WM, Boelen A. Interleukin-1 beta modulates endogenous thyroid hormone receptors alpha gene transcription in liver cells. *J Endocrinol* 2007:194(2):257-65.

[115] Implementation of a regulatory gene network to simulate the TH1/2 differentiation in an agent-based model of hypersensitivity reactions. *Bioinformatics* 2008 Jun 1;24(11):1374-80. Epub 2008 Apr 14.

[116] Th1-like dominance in high-risk first-degree relatives of type I diabetic patients. *Diabetologia* 2000 Jun;43(6):742-9.

[117] Cytokine-modulated regulation of helper T cell populations. *J Theor Biol* 2000 Oct 21;206(4):539-60.

[118] Measurement of intracellular interferon-gamma and interleukin-4 in whole blood T lymphocytes from patients with systemic lupus erythematosus. *Immunol Lett* 2000 Nov 1;74(3):207-10.

[119] IL-10, TGF-beta, IL-2, IL-12, and IFN-gamma cytokine gene polymorphisms in asthma. *J Asthma* 2008 Nov;45(9):790-4.

[120] American Autoimmune Related Diseases Association, Inc. http://www.aarda.org/mission_statement.php

[121] Manifestations of chronic disease during pregnancy. *JAMA* 2005 Dec 7;294(21):2751-7. Review.

[122] Risk of subclinical hypothyroidism in pregnant women with asymptomatic autoimmune thyroid disorders. *J Clin Endocrinol Metab* 1994;79(1):197-204.

[123] Guan HX, Li CY, LI FS, et al. Thyroid function and thyroid autoimmunityat the late pregnancy: data from 664 pregnant women. *Zhanghua Fu Chan Ke Za Zhi* 2006;41(8):529-32.

[124] Extradigestive manifestations of Helicobacter pylori gastric infection. *Gut* 1999 Jul;45 Suppl 1:I9-I12. Review.

[125] Screening frequency for celiac disease and autoimmune thyroiditis in children and adolescents with type 1 diabetes mellitus - data from a German/Austrian multicentre survey. *Pediatr Diabetes* 2008 Aug 18.

[126] Coeliac disease in Dutch patients with Hashimoto's thyroiditis and vice versa. *World J Gastroenterol* 2007 Mar 21;13(11):1715-22.

[127] Holick MF. Sunlight and vitamin D for bone health and prevention of autoimmune diseases, cancers, and cardiovascular diseases. *Am J Clin Nutr* 2004;80:1678S-1688S.

[128] Cantorna MT, Zhu Y, Froicu M, Whittke A. Vitamin D status, 1-25-dihydroxyvitamin D3, and the immune system. *Am J Clin Nutr* 2004;80:1717S-1720S.

[129] DeLuca HF, Cantorna MT. Vitamin D: Its role and uses in immunology. *FASEB J* 2001;15:2579-2585.

[130] Adequate level of vitamin D is essential for maintaining good health. *Postepy Hig Med Dosw* (Online). 2008 Oct 9;62:502-10. Polish.

[131] Vitamin D receptor gene polymorphisms are associated with risk of Hashimoto's thyroiditis in Chinese patients in Taiwan. *J Clin Lab Anal* 2006;20(3):109-12.

[132] Association of vitamin D receptor gene 3'-variants with Hashimoto's thyroiditis in the Croatian population. *Int J Immunogenet* 2008 Apr;35(2):125-31. Epub 2008 Feb 11.

[133] Vitamin D receptor gene polymorphisms are associated with risk of Hashimoto's thyroiditis in Chinese patients in Taiwan. *J Clin Lab Anal* 2006;20(3):109-12.

[134] Association of vitamin D receptor gene polymorphism with susceptibility to Graves' disease in Eastern Croatian population: case-control study. *Croat Med J* 2005 Aug;46(4):639-46.

[135] Vitamin D receptor gene polymorphisms in Hashimoto's thyroiditis. *Thyroid* 2001 Jun;11(6):607-8. No abstract available.

[136] Vitamin D receptor initiation codon polymorphism in Japanese patients with Graves' disease. *Thyroid* 2000 Jun;10(6):475-80.

[137] Vitamin D 1alpha-hydroxylase (CYP1alpha) polymorphism in Graves' disease, Hashimoto's thyroiditis and type 1 diabetes mellitus. *Eur J Endocrinol* 2002 Jun;146(6):777-81.

[138] Fidelus RK. Glutathione and lymphocyte activation: a function of aging and auto-immune disease. *Immunology* 1987;61:503-508.

[139] Droge W, et al. Functions of glutathione and glutathione disulfide in immunology and immunopathology. *FASEB J* 1994;8:1131-1138.

[140] Kinscheref R, et al. Effect of glutathione depletion and oral N-acetyl-cysteine treatment on CD4+ and CD8+ cells. *FASEB J* 1994;8:448-451.

[141] Wu D, et al. In vitro glutathione supplementation enhances interleukin-2 production and mitogenic response of peripheral blood mononuclear cells from young and old subjects. *J Nutr* 1994;124:655-663.

[142] Witschi A, et al. The systemic availability of oral glutathione. *Euro J Clin Pharmacol* 1992; 43:667-669.

[143] See references for TH-1 stimulators in Nutritional Compounds chapter.

[144] The effect of Echinacea purpurea, Astragalus membranaceus and Glycyrrhiza glabra on CD69 expression and immune cell activation in humans. *Phytother Res* 2006 Aug;20(8):687-95.

[145] The effect of Echinacea purpurea, Astragalus membranaceus and Glycyrrhiza glabra on CD69 expression and immune cell activation in humans. *Phytother Res* 2006 Aug;20(8):687-95. PMID: 16807880.

[146] The effect of Echinacea purpurea, Astragalus membranaceus and Glycyrrhiza glabra on CD69 expression and immune cell activation in humans. *Phytother Res* 2006 Aug;20(8):687-95. PMID: 16807880.

[147] Czop, Joyce K., "The Role of Beta.-Glucan Receptors on Blood and Tissue Leukocytes in Phagocytosis and Metabolic Activation". *Pathology and Immunopathology Research* 1986; 5:286-296.

[148] Kodman N, Komuta K, Nanba H. Effect of Maitake (Grifola frondosa) D-Fraction on the activation of NK cells in cancer patients. *Journal of Medicinal Food* 2003;6(4):371-377.

[149] The effect of Echinacea purpurea, Astragalus membranaceus and Glycyrrhiza glabra on CD69 expression and immune cell activation in humans. *Phytother Res* 2006 Aug;20(8):687-95.

[150] Allahverdiyea A, Duran N, Ozguven M, Koltas S. Antiviral activity of the volatile oils of Melissa officalis L. against Herpes simplex virus type-2. *Phytomedicine* 2004;11:657-671.

[151] See references for TH-2 stimulators in Nutritional Compounds chapter.

[152] Horrigan LA, Kelly JP, Connor TJ. Immunomodulatory effects of caffeine: friend or foe? *Pharmacol Ther* 2006;113(3):877-892.

[153] A review of complementary and alternative approaches to immunomodulation. *Nutr Clin Pract* 2008 Feb;23(1):49-62. Review.

[154] Li WG. Anti-inflammatory effect and mechanism of proanthocyanidins from grape seeds. *Acta Pharmacol Sin* 2001;22:1117-1120.

[155] Cho KJ. Inhibition of mechanisms of bioflavonoids extracted from the bark of Pinus maritime on the expression of proinflammatory cytokines. *Ann NY Acad Aci* 2001;928:141-156.

[156] Evidence of effectiveness of herbal antiinflammatory drugs in the treatment of painful osteoarthritis and chronic low back pain. Phytother Res. 2007 Jul;21(7):675-83. Review.

[157] Nevestani T, Shariatzadeh N, Gharav iA, Kalayi A, Khalaji N. Physiologic dose of lycopene suppressed oxidative stress and enhances serum levels of immunoglobulin M in patients with Type 2 diabetes mellitus: a possible role in the prevention of long-term complications. *J Endocrinol Invest* 2007;30(10):833-838.

[158] A review of complementary and alternative approaches to immunomodulation. *Nutr Clin Pract* 2008 Feb;23(1):49-62.

[159] Rohdewald P. A review of Frenc maritime pine bark extract (Pycnogenol), a herbal medication with a diverse clinical pharmacology. *Int J Clin Pharmacol Ther* 2002;40:158-160

[160] Effect of specific colostral antibodies and selected lactobacilli on the adhesion of Helicobacter pylori on AGS cells and the Helicobacter-induced IL-8 production. *Scand J Immunol* 2008 Sep;68(3):280-6.

[161] Effects of probiotic bacteria and their genomic DNA on TH1/TH2-cytokine production by peripheral blood mononuclear cells (PBMCs) of healthy and allergic subjects. *Immunobiology* 2008;213(8):677-92. Epub 2008 Apr 2.

[162] Probiotics and immunology: separating the wheat from the chaff. *Trends Immunol* 2008 Oct 4.

[163] Effect of specific colostral antibodies and selected lactobacilli on the adhesion of Helicobacter pylori on AGS cells and the Helicobacter-induced IL-8 production. *Scand J Immunol* 2008 Sep;68(3):280-6.

[164] A review of complementary and alternative approaches to immunomodulation. *Nutr Clin Pract* 2008 Feb;23(1):49-62.

[165] Retinoic acid production by intestinal dendritic cells and its role in T-cell trafficking. *Semin Immunol* 2008 Oct 10.

166 Retinoic acid promotes mouse splenic B cell surface IgG expression and maturation stimulated by CD40 and IL-4. Cell *Immunol* 2007 Sep;249(1):37-45. Epub 2007 Dec 20.

167 A short-term dietary supplementation with high doses of vitamin E increases NK cell cytolytic activity in advanced colorectal cancer patients. *Cancer Immunol Immunother* 2007 Jul;56(7):973-84. Epub 2006 Dec 2.

168 Effect of vitamin E supplementation on lymphocyte distribution in gut-associated lymphoid tissues obtained from weaned piglets. *J Vet Med A Physiol Pathol Clin Med* 2006 Sep;53(7):327-33.

169 Immune Components of Bovine Colostrum and Milk. *J Anim Sci* 2008 Oct 24.

170 Effect of specific colostral antibodies and selected lactobacilli on the adhesion of Helicobacter pylori on AGS cells and the Helicobacter-induced IL-8 production. *Scand J Immunol* 2008 Sep;68(3):280-6.

171 Serum IgG, blood profiles, growth and survival in goat kids supplemented with artificial colostrum on the first day of life. *Trop Anim Health Prod* 2008 Feb;40(2):141-5.

172 Immunomodulatory effects of bovine colostrum in human peripheral blood mononuclear cells. *New Microbiol* 2007 Oct;30(4):447-54.

173 Exosomes with immune modulatory features are present in human breast milk. *J Immunol* 2007 Aug 1;179(3):1969-78.

174 A review of complementary and alternative approaches to immunomodulation. *Nutr Clin Pract* 2008 Feb;23(1):49-62.

175 Boswellic acids: A leukotriene inhibitor also effective through topical application in inflammatory disorders. *Phytomedicine* 2008 Jun;15(6-7):400-7. Epub 2008 Jan 28.

176 A review of complementary and alternative approaches to immunomodulation. *Nutr Clin Pract* 2008 Feb;23(1):49-62.

177 Evidence of effectiveness of herbal antiinflammatory drugs in the treatment of painful osteoarthritis and chronic low back pain. *Phytother Res* 2007 Jul;21(7):675-83.

178 Pure compound from Boswellia serrata extract exhibits anti-inflammatory property in human PBMCs and mouse macrophages through inhibition of TNFalpha, IL-1beta, NO and MAP kinases. *Int Immunopharmacol* 2007 Apr;7(4):473-82. Epub 2007 Jan 8.

179 A review of complementary and alternative approaches to immunomodultion. *Nutr Clin Pract* 2008 Feb;23(1):49-62.

180 Curcumin-induced inhibition of cellular reactive oxygen species generation: novel therapeutic implications. *J Biosci* 2003 Dec;28(6):715-21.

181 Effect of curcumin and capsaicin on arachidonic acid metabolism and lysosomal enzyme secretion by rat peritoneal macrophages. *Lipids* 1997 Nov;32(11):1173-80.

182 *Clin Microbiol Infect* 2001 Mar;7(3):138-43.

CHAPTER FOUR

183 American Association of Clinical Endocrinologists

184 Hermus RM, Sweep CG, van der Meer MJ, et al. Continuous infusion of interleukin-1Beta induces a non-thyroidal illness syndrome in rat. *Endocinrology* 1992;131:2139-2146.

185 Rettori V, Jurcovicova J,McCAann SM. Central action of interleukin-1 in altering the release of TSH, growth hormone, and prolactin in the male rat. *J Neurosci Res* 1987;18:179-183.

186 Bartalena L, Grasso L, Brogioni S, et L. Interleukin-6 on pituitary-thyroid-axis in the rat. *Eur J Endcrinol* 1994;131:302-306.

[187] Lyson K, McCann SM. The effect of interleukin-6 on pituitary hormone release in vivo and vitro. *Neuroendocrinology* 1991;54:262-266.

[188] Ozawa M, Sato K, Han DC, et al. Effects of tumor necrosis factor-alpha/cachetin on thyroid hormone metabolism in mice. *Endocrinology* 1998;123:1461-1467.

[189] Rettori V, Milenkovic L, Beutler BA, et al. Hypothalamus action of cachectin to alter pituitary hormone release. *Brain Res Bull* 1989;23:471-475.

[190] Tsigos C, Chrousos GP. Hypothalamic-pituitary-adrenal axis, neuroendocrine factors and stress. *J Psychosom Res* 2002 Oct;53(4):865-71.

[191] Krysiak R, Okopień B, Szkróbka W, Herman ZS. [Thyroid disorders in pregnancy and after delivery] [Article in Polish] *Przegl Lek* 2007;64(3):159-64.

[192] LoPresti, JS and Nicoloff JT. Thyroid response to critical illness. *Endocrinology of Critical Disease* Human Press. Totowa. NJ. 1997. Pp 157-173.

[193] Strakis CA, Chrousos GP. Neuroendocrinology and Pathophysiology of the Stress System, *Ann NY Acad Sci* Vol. 771, pp 1-18, 1995.

[194] Corrsmite EP, Heyligenberg R, Endert E, et al. Acute effects of interferon-alpah-administration on thyroid hormone metabolism in healthy men. *J Clin Endcorin Metab* 1995:80:3140-3144.

[195] Van der Poll T, Romijn JA, Wiersinga WM, et al. Tumor necrosis factor: a putative mediator of the sick euthyroid syndrome in man. *J Clin Endocrinol Metab* 1990;71:1567-1572.

[196] Stouthared JM, Van der Poll T, Endert E., et al. Effects of acute and chronic interleukin-6 administration on thyroid hormone metabolism in human. *J Clin Endocrinol Metab* 1994;79:1342-1346.

[197] Bisschop PH, Toorians AW, Endert E, Wiersinga WM, Gooren LJ, Fliers E. The effects of sex-steroid administration on the pituitary-thyroid axis in transsexuals. *Eur J Endocrinol* 2006 Jul;155(1):11-6.

[198] Sarkis MI, Sievert R. Drugs and thyroid function. *NEJM* 1995;333(25): 168801694.

[199] Knopp RH, Bergelin RO, Wahl PW, Walden CE, Chapman MB. Chemical alterations in pregnancy and oral contraceptive use. *Obstet Gynecol* 5;66:682-90, 1985.

[200] Steingold KA, Matt DW, DeZiegler D, Sealey JE, Fratkin M, Rezinkov S. Comparison of transdermal to oral estradiol administration on hormonal and hepatic parameters in women with premature ovarian failure. *J Clin Endocrinol Metab* 1991:73:275-80.

[201] Geola FL, Frumar AM, Tataryn IV, et al. Biological effects of various doses of conjugated equine estrogens in postmenopausal women. *J Clin Endocrinol Metab* 1980;51:620-5.

[202] Ben-Rafael Z, Mastroianni L, Strauss JF, Flickinger GL, Arendasch-Durand B. Changes in Thyroid function tests and sex hormone binding globulin associated with treatment of gonadotropin. *Fertil Steril* 1987:48;318-320.

[203] Williams GR, Neuberger JM, Ranklin JA, Sheppard MC. Thyroid hormone receptor expression in the "sick euthyroid syndrome." *Lancet* 1989;2(8678-8679):1477-1481.

[204] Reidel W, Layka H, Neeck G. Secretory pattern of GH, TSH, Thyroid hormones, ACTH, cortisol, FSH, and LH in patients with fibromyalgia syndrome following systemic injection of the relevant hypothalamic-releasing hormones. *J Rheumatol* 1998;57 (Suppl 2):81-87.

[205] Limpach A, Dalton M, Mules R, Gadson P. Homocysteine inhibits retinoic acid synthesis: a mechanism for homocysteine-induced congenital defects. *Experimental Cell Res* 2000;260:166-174.

[206] Mandell AJ. Non-equilibrium behavior of some brain enzyme and receptor systems. *Annu Rev Pharmacol Toxicol* 1984;24:237-274.

[207] Block ER, Edwards D. Effect of plasma membrane fluidity on serotonin transport by endothelial cells. *Am J Physiol* 1987;253(5,Pt 1):C672-678.

[208] Storlien LH, Kriketos AD, Calvert GB, Bauer LA, Jenkins AB. Fatty acids, triglycerides and syndromes of insulin resistance. *Prostaglandins Leukot Essent Fatty Acids* 1997;57(4-5):379-385.

[209] Shamberger RJ. Erythrocyte Fatty Acid Studies in Patients. *J Advance Med* 1997;10(3):195-205.

[210] Simopoulos AP. Omega-3 fatty acids in health and disease and in growth and development. *Am J Clin Nutr* 1991;54(3):438-463.

[211] Storlien LH, et al. Fatty acids, triglycerides and syndromes of insulin resistance. *Prostaglandin Leukot Essent Fatty Acids* 1997;57(4-5):379-385.

[212] Brenner R. Nutrition and hormonal factors influencing desaturation of essential fatty acids. *Prog Lipid Res* 1982;20;41-48.

[213] See references for nutritional compounds for thyroid metabolism in Nutritional Compounds chapter.

[214] Zhang J, Lazar MA. The mechanism of action of thyroid hormones. *Ann Rev Physiol* 2000;62:439-466.

[215] Zhang J, Lazar MA. The mechanisms of action of thyroid hormones. *Ann Rev Physiol* 2000;62:439-466.

[216] Jacques H, Deshais Y, Sovoie L. Relationship between dietary tyrosine and plasma cholesterol in the rat. *Can J Physiol Pharmacol* 1988;23(1-2):17-30.

[217] Stewart RM, Hemli S, Daniels GH, Kolodny Eh. Maloof F. The pituitary-thyroid axis in adults with phenylketonuria. *J Clin Endocrinol Metab* 1976;42(6):1179-1181.

[218] Rasmussen DD, Ishizuka B, Quigley ME, Yen SS. Effects of tyrosine and tryptophan ingestion on plasma catecholamine and 3,4-dihydroxyphenylacetic acid concentrations. *J Clin Endocrinol Metab* 1983;57(4):760-3.

[219] Carralho DV, Ferriera ACF, Coelho SM, et al. Thyroid peroxidase activity in inhibited by amino acids. *Brazilian Journal of Medical and Biological Research* 2000;33:335-361.

[220] Rocotta R, Ramierz A, Velesco D. Metabolic effects of chronic infusions of epinephrine and norepinphrine in rats. *Am J Physio Endocrinol Metab* 1986;250(5):E518-E522.

[221] Masimi-Repiso AM, Coleoni AH. Effects of epinephrine and 5-hydroxytrptamine on in vivo thyroid iodine organification. *Acta Endocrinol (Copenh)* 1981;97(2):207-12.

CHAPTER FIVE

[222] Venkat Narayan KM, Boyle JP, Thompson TJ, Sorensen SW, Williamson DF. Lifetime risk for diabetes mellitus in the United States. *Journal of the American Medical Association* 2003;290(14):1884-1890.

[223] Liu S, Willett WC. Dietary glycemic load and atherothrombotic risk. *Curr Atheroscler Rep* 2002;4(6):454-461.

[224] Scott, H, et al. *Scan J Gastroenterol* 1980, 15:81.

[225] Kamada H, et al. Influence of hyperglycemia on oxidative stress and matrix metalloproteinase-9 activation after focal cerebral ischemia/reperfusion in rats. *Stroke* 2007;38:1044-1049.

[226] Fuenmayor NM, et al. Relations between fasting serum insulin, glucose, and dehydroepiandrosterone-sulfate concentrations in obese patients with hypertension: short term effects of antihypertensive drugs. *J Card Pharm* 1997;30:523-527.

[227] Nestler JE, Clore JN, Blackard WG. Dehydroepiandrosterone: the missing link between hyperinsulinemia and atherosclerosis. *FASEB* 1992 1992;9;3073-3074.

228 Wu XK, et al. Ovarian-adrenal cross-talk in polycystic ovary syndrome: evidence of wedge reCategory. *Euro J Endocrinol* 2000;143:383-388.
229 Fuenmayor NM, et al. Relations between fasting serum insulin, glucose, and de-hydroepiandrosterone-sulfate concentrations in obese patients with hypertension: short term effects of antihypertensive drugs. *J Card Pharm* 1997;30:523-527.
230 Nestler JE, Clore JN, Blackard WG. Dehydroepiandrosterone: the missing link between hyperinsulinemia and atherosclerosis. *FASEB* 1992;9:3073-3074.
231 Storlien LH, et al. Fatty acids, triglycerides and syndromes of insulin resistance. *Prostaglandin Leukot Essent Fatty Acids* 1997;57(4-5):379-385.
232 Brenner R. Nutrition and hormonal factors influencing desaturation of essential fatty acids. *Prog Lipid Res* 1982;20;41-48.
233 Inflammatory markers, insulin resistance and carotid intima-media thickness in North-Indian type 2 diabetic subjects. *J Assoc Physicians India* 2007 Oct; 55:693-9.
234 Hermus RM, Sweep CG, van der Meer MJ, et al. Continuous infusion of inter-leukin-1 Beta induces a non-thyroidal illness syndrome in rat. *Endocrinology* 1992;131:2139-2146.
235 Rettori V, Jurcovicova J, McCaann SM. Central action of interleukin-1 in altering the release of TSH, growth hormone, and prolactin in male rat. *J Neurosci Res* 1987;18:179-183.
236 Bartalena L, Grasso L, Brogioni S, et al. Interleukin-6 on pituitary-thyroid-axis in the rat. *Eur J Endocrinol* 1994;131:302-306.
237 Lyson K, McCann SM. The effect of interleukin-6 on pituitary hormone release in vivo and vitro. *Neuroendocrinology* 1991;54:262-266.
238 Ozawa M, Sato K, Han DC, et al. Effects of tumor necrosis factor-alpha/cachetin on thyroid hormone metabolism in mice. *Endocrinology* 1998;123:1461-1467.
239 Rettori V, Milenkovic L, Beutler BA, et al. Hypothalamus action of cachetin to alter pituitary hormone release. *Brain Res Bull* 1989;23:471-475.
240 Wu XK, et al. Ovarian-adrenal cross-talk in polycystic ovary syndrome: evidence of wedge reCategory. *Euro J Endocrinol* 2000;143:383-388.
241 Grimm JJ. Interaction of physical activity and diet: implications for insulin-glucose dynamics. *Public Health Nutr* 1999;2:363-368.
242 Moore MA, et al. Implications of the hyperinsulinemia-diabetes-cancer link for preventative effors. *Eur J Cancer Prev* 1998;7:89-107.
243 Despres JP, et al. Hyperinsulinemia as an independent risk factor of ischemic heart disease. *N Eng J Med* 1996;334:952-957.
244 Tiihonen M, Partinen M. Narvanen S. The severity of obstructive sleep apnea is associated with insulin resistance. *J Sleep Res* 1993;2:56-61.
245 Arthur LS, Selvakumar R, Seshardir MS. Hyperinsulinemia in polycystic ovary disease. *J Reprod Med* 1999;44:783-787.
246 Benzi L, et al. Intracellular hyperinsulinemia: a metabolic characteristic of obesity with and without type II diabetes: intracellular insulin in obesity and type II diabetes. *Diabetes Res Clin Pract* 1999;46:231-237.
247 Stoll BA. Essential fatty acids, insulin resistance and breast cancer risk. *Nutr Cancer* 1998;31:72-77.
248 Muller MJ, Burger AC, Ferrannini E, et al. Glucoregulatory function of thyroid hormones: role of pancreatic hormones. *Am J Physio* 1989;256: E101-E110.
249 Chris D. Meletis, Nieske Zabriskie. Supporting Gastrointestinal Health with Nutritional Therapy. *Alternative and Complementary Therapies* June 1, 2008, 14(3): 132-138. doi:10.1089/act.2008.14305.

[250] Gut microbiota and lipopolysaccharide content of the diet influence development of regulatory T cells: studies in germ-free mice. *BMC Immunol* 2008 Nov 6;9(1):65.PMID: 18990206

[251] The gut immune system and type 1 diabetes. *Ann NY Acad Sci* 2002 Apr;958:39-46.

[252] The "perfect storm" for type 1 diabetes: the complex interplay between intestinal microbiota, gut permeability, and mucosal immunity. *Diabetes* 2008 Oct;57(10):2555-62.

[253] The gut immune system and type 1 diabetes. *Ann NY Acad Sci* 2002 Apr;958:39-46.

[254] The "perfect storm" for type 1 diabetes: the complex interplay between intestinal microbiota, gut permeability, and mucosal immunity. *Diabetes* 2008 Oct;57(10):2555-62.

[255] Chronic fatigue syndrome: inflammation, immune function, and neuroendocrine interactions. *Curr Rheumatol Rep 2007* Dec;9(6):482-7.

[256] Atrophic body gastritis in patients with autoimmune thyroid disease: an underdiagnosed association. *Arch Intern Med* 1999 Aug 9-23;159(15):1726-30.

[257] Atrophic body gastritis in patients with autoimmune thyroid disease: an underdiagnosed association. *Arch Intern Med* 1999 Aug 9-23;159(15):1726-30.

[258] Possible chronic thyroiditis revealed by [18F]-FDG-PET/CT scan in a euthyroid patient with recurrent gallbladder carcinoma. *Thyroid* 2007 Nov;17(11):1157-8.

[259] Is bile flow reduced in patients with hypothyroidism? *Surgery* 2003 Mar;133(3):288-93.

[260] Coordinate regulation of gallbladder motor function in the gut-liver axis. *Hepatology* 2008 Jun;47(6):2112-26.

[261] Schmidt, Michael A. 1995. *Tired of Being Tired: Overcoming Chronic Fatigue & Low Energy.* Frog Books, pages 97-98.

[262] *Clin Microbiol Infect* 2001 Mar;7(3):138-43.

[263] Van der Poll T, Endert E, Coyle SM, Agosti JM, Lowry SF. Neutralization of TNF does not influence endotoxin induced changes in thyroid hormone metabolism in humans. *Am J Physiol* 1999;276:357-62.

[264] Van der Poll T, Van Zee KJ, Endert E, et al. Interleukin-1 receptor blockade does not effect endotoxin-induced changes in plasma thyroid hormone and thyrotropin concentrations in man. *J Clin Endocrinol Metab* 1995;80(4):1341-6.

[265] Boelen A, Kwakkel J, Platvoet-ter Shicporst M, et al. Interleukin-18, a proinflammatory cytokine, contributes to the pathogenesis of non-thyroidal illness mainly via the central part of the hypothalamus-pituitary-thyroid axis. *European Journal of Endocrinology* 151(4):497-502.

[266] Beigneux AP, Moser AH, Shingenga JK, et al. Sick euthyroid syndrome is associated with decreased TR expression and DNA binding in mouse liver. *Am J Physiol Endocrin Metab* 2003;284(1):E228-36

[267] Wynsome, Dr. Rebecca, N. D. Eighty percent of immune and hormonal stress comes from my gut?! *PCC Sound Consumer* Nov. 2002.

[268] Prevalence of celiac disease in patients with autoimmune thyroiditis. *Minerva Endocrinol* 2007 Dec;32(4):239-43.

[269] Celiac disease and autoimmune thyroid disease. *Clin Med Res* 2007 Oct;5(3):184-92. Review.

[270] Hays, Marguerite T. *Endocrine Research* 1988 June;14(2,3):203-224.

[271] Potent anti-microbial activity of traditional Chinese medicine herbs against Candida species. *Mycoses* 2008 Jan;51(1):30-4.

[272] Antibacterial activity of a Chinese herbal medicine, Gosyuyu (Wu-Chu-Yu), against Helicobacter pylori. *Nippon Rinsho* 2005 Nov;63 Suppl 11:592-9. Japanese.

273 LoPresti, JS and Nicoloff, JT. Thyroid response to critical illness. *Endocrinology of Critical Disease* Humana Press. Totowa. NJ. 1997. pp 157-173.

274 Strakis, CA and Chrousos, GP. Neuroendocrinology and Pathophysiology of the Stress System, *Ann NY Acad Sci* Vol. 771, pp. 1-18,1995.

275 Stockigt, JR. and Baverman. Update on the Sick Euthyroid Syndrome. *Diseases of the Thyroid* Humana Press, Totowa, NJ, 1997, pp. 49-68.

276 LoPresti, JS and Nicoloff, JT. Thyroid response to critical illness. *Endocrinology of Critical Disease* Humana Press. Totowa. NJ. 1997. pp 157-173.

277 Strakis, CA and Chrousos, GP. Neuroendocrinology and Pathophysiology of the Stress System, *Ann NY Acad Sci* Vol. 771, pp. 1-18,1995.

278 Stockigt, JR. and Baverman. Update on the Sick Euthyroid Syndrome. *Diseases of the Thyroid* Humana Press, Totowa, NJ, 1997, pp. 49-68.

279 Stockigt, JR. and Braverman. Update on the Sick Euthyroid Syndrome. Diseases of the Thyroid Humana Press, Totowa, NJ, 1997, pp. 49-68.

280 Atrophic body gastritis in patients with autoimmune thyroid disease: an under-diagnosed association. *Arch Intern Med* 1999 Aug 9-23;159(15):1726-30.

281 Coordinate regulation of gallbladder motor function in the gut-liver axis. *Hepatology* 2008 Jun;47(6):2112-26.

282 Influence of stressors on normal intestinal microbiota, intestinal morphology, and susceptibility to Salmonella enteritidis colonization in broilers. *Poult Sci* 2008 Sep;87(9):1734-41.

283 Guhad, FA, et al. Salivary IgA as a marker of social stress in rats. *Neurosci Lett* 216(2). 137-140, 1996.

284 Cunningham-Rundies, C., et al. *Proc Nat Acada Sci USA* 1978;75:3387.

285 Scott, H., et al. Scan. J. *Gastroenterol* 1980;15:81.

286 Association between hypothyroidism and small intestinal bacterial overgrowth. *J Clin Endocrinol Metab* 2007 Nov;92(11):4180-4. Epub 2007 Aug 14.

CHAPTER SEVEN

287 Thyroid disorders and diabetes mellitus. *Minerva Med* 2008 Jun;99(3):263-7.

288 Reversible subclinical hypothyroidism in the presence of adrenal insufficiency. *Endocr Pract* 2006 Sep-Oct;12(5):572.

289 Chronic fatigue syndrome. A brief review of functional disturbances and poten-tial therapy. *J Sports Med Phys Fitness* 2005 Sep;45(3):381-92.

290 Facts About Thyroid Disease, 2005. American Academy of Clinical Endocrinologists: http://www.aace.com/public/awareness/tam/2005/pdfs/thy-roid_disease_fact_sheet.pdf.

291 Reversible subclinical hypothyroidism in the presence of adrenal insufficiency. *Endocr Pract* 2006 Sep-Oct;12(5):572.

292 Van Der Pomp G., et al. Elevated basal cortisol levels and attenuated ACTH and cortisol responses to a behavioral challenge in women with metastatic breast cancer. *Psychoneuroendocrinology* 1996 21(4):361-374.

293 Sapolsky RM. Kre LC. McEwens BS. 1986. The Neuroendocrinology of stress and aging: the glucocorticoid cascade hypothesis. *Endocr Rev* 7:284-301.

294 Meaney MJ. Aitken DH. Van Berkel C, Bhatnager S, Sapolsky RM. Effect of neonatal handling of age-related impairment associated with hippocampus. *Science* 239:766-768.

295 LoPresti, JS and Nicoloff, JT. Thyroid response to critical illness. *Endocrinology of Critical Disease.* Human Press. Totowa, NJ. 1997, pp.157-173.

296 Strakis, CA and Chrousos, GP. Neuroendocrinology and Pathophysiology of the Stress System, *Ann NY Acad Sci* Vol. 771, pp.1-18, 1995.

297 Stockigt, JR. and Braverman. Update on the Sick Euthyroid Syndrome. *Diseases of the Thyroid* Humana Press, Totowa, NJ, 1997, pp. 49-68.

[298] Guhad, FA, et al. Salivary IgA as a marker of social stress in rats. *Neurosci Lett* 1996;216(2):137-140.

[299] Cunningham-Rundies, C., et al. *Proc Nat Acada. Sci USA* 1978;75:3387.

[300] Scott, H., et al. Scan. J. *Gastroenterol* 1980;15:81.

[301] Reversible subclinical hypothyroidism in the presence of adrenal insufficiency. *Endocr Pract* 2006 Sep-Oct;12(5):572.

[302] Gastrointestinal symptoms are associated with hypothalamic-pituitary-adrenal axis suppression in healthy individuals. *Scand J Gastroenterol* 2007 Nov;42(11):1294-301.

[303] Active and inactive thyroid hormone levels in elective and acute surgery. *Acta Chir Scand* 1979;145(2):77-82.

[304] Decreased levels of dehydroepiandrosterone sulphate in severe critical illness: a sign of exhausted adrenal reserve? *Crit Care* 2002 Oct;6(5):434-8. Epub 2002 Jul 9.

[305] Chronic stress, hormone profiles and estrus intensity in dairy cattle. *Horm Behav* 2008 Mar;53(3):493-501. Epub 2007 Dec 23.

[306] The HPA axis in HIV-1 infection. *J Acquir Immune Defic Syndr* 2002 Oct 1;31 Suppl 2:S89-93.

[307] Stress as a risk factor in the pathogenesis of rheumatoid arthritis. *Neuroimmunomodulation* 2006;13(5-6):277-82. Epub 2007 Aug 6.

[308] Impact of platinum group metals on the environment: a toxicological, genotoxic and analytical chemistry study. *J Environ Sci Health A Tox Hazard Subst Environ Eng* 2006;41(3):397-414.

[309] Impact of platinum group metals on the environment: a toxicological, genotoxic and analytical chemistry study. *J Environ Sci Health A Tox Hazard Subst Environ Eng* 2006;41(3):397-414.

[310] Addison's disease due to Histoplasma duboisii infection of the adrenal glands. *Saudi Med J* 2008 Jun;29(6):904-6.

[311] The effects of the fungicide methyl thiophanate on adrenal gland morphophysiology of the lizard, Podarcis sicula. Arch Environ *Contam Toxicol* 2007 Aug;53(2):241-8. Epub 2007 Jun 2.

[312] Adrenal toxicology: a strategy for assessment of functional toxicity to the adrenal cortex and steroidogenesis. *J Appl Toxicol* 2007 Mar-Apr;27(2):103-15.

[313] The stress response in critical illness. *New Horiz* 1994 Nov;2(4):426-31.

[314] The overtraining syndrome in athletes: a stress-related disorder. *J Endocrinol Invest* 2004 Jun;27(6):603-12.

[315] The impact of a 17-day training period for an international championship on mucosal immune parameters in top-level basketball players and staff members. *Eur J Oral Sci* 2008 Oct;116(5):431-7.

[316] Overview of gut immunology. *Adv Exp Med Biol* 2008;635:1-14.

[317] The adrenal cortex and life. *Mol Cell Endocrinol* 2008 Sep 17.

[318] Exercise and circulating cortisol levels: the intensity threshold effect. *J Endocrinol Invest* 2008 Jul;31(7):587-91.

[319] Effects of maternal prenatal stress on offspring development: a commentary. *Arch Womens Ment Health* 2008; Oct 31.

[320] Prenatal exposure to maternal depression, neonatal methylation of human glucocorticoid receptor gene (NR3C1) and infant cortisol stress responses. *Epigenetics* 2008 Mar-Apr;3(2):97-106.

[321] The long-term behavioural consequences of prenatal stress. *Neurosci Biobehav Rev* 2008 Aug;32(6):1073-86. Epub 2008 Mar 18.

CHAPTER NINE

[322] Bernal J, et al. Thyroid hormones and brain development. *Eur J Endocrinol* 1995;133:390-398.

[323] Flavin RSL, et al. Regulation of microglial development: A novel role for thyroid hormones. *The Journal of Neuroscience* 2001;21(6):2028-2038.

[324] Legrand J. *J Physiol Paris* 1983;78:603-652.

[325] Porterfield SP, et al. *Endocr Rev* 1993;14:94-106.

[326] Calza L, et al. Thyroid hormone-induced plasticity in the adult rat brain. *Brain Res Bull* 1997;44(4):549-57.

[327] Strawen JR, Ekhator NN. Pituitary-thyroid state correlates with central dopaminergic and serotonergic activity in healthy humans. *Neuropsychobiology* 2004; 49(2):84-7.

[328] Tiovonen M, Tuomainen P, Mannisto PT. Effects of hypothalamic paraventricular nucleus lesion on cold-stimulated TSH responses to 5-HT in male rats. *Acta Physiol Scan* 1990;139(1):233-40.

[329] Soldin OP and Aschner M. Effects of manganese on thyroid hormone homeostasis: potential links. *Neurotoxicology* 2007; 28(5):951-6.

[330] Electrical responses of cultured thyroid cells to serotonin. *J Endocrinol* 1985;107(3):397-401.

[331] Maayan ML, Sellitto RV, Volpert EM. Dopamine and L-dopa: inhibition of thyrotropin-stimulated thyroidal thyroxine release. *Endocrinology* 1986;118(2): 632-6.

[332] Foord SM, Peters JM, Dieguez C, et al. Thyrotropin regulates thyrotroph responsiveness to dopamine in vitro. *Endocrinology* 1986; 118(4):1319-26.

[333] Garbutt JC, Loosen PT, Glenn M. Lack of effect of dopamine receptor blockade on the TSH response to TRH in borderline personality disorder. *Psychiatry Res* 1987; 21(4): 307-11.

[334] Cooper DS, Klibanski A, Ridgway EC. Dopaminergic modulation of TSH and its subunits: in vitro studies. *Clinical Endocrinol* (Oxf) 1983;18(3):265-75.

[335] Strawen JR, Ekhator NN. Pituitary-thyroid state correlates with central dopaminergic and serotonergic activity in healthy humans. *Neuropsychobiology* 2004; 49(2):84-7.

[336] Oh-Nishi, Saji M, Furudate SI, Suzuki N. Dopamine D(2)-like receptor function is converted from excitatory to inhibitory by thyroxine in the developmental hippocampus. *J Neuroendocrinol* 2005;17(12):836-45.

[337] Peterson AL, Gilman TL, Banks ML, Sprague JE. Hypothyroidism alters striatal dopamine release medidated by 3,4 methylendioxymethamphteamine (MDMA ecstasy). *Synapse* 2006;59(5):317-9.

[338] Sidneva LN and Adamskaia EI. The relationship between changes in the concentration of catecholamines in the hypothalamus and the level of thyroid hormones in the body. *Probl Endokrinol* (Mosk) 1975;21(6):84-8

[339] Peterson AL, Gilman TL, Banks ML, Sprague JE. Hypothyroidism alters striatal dopamine release medidated by 3,4 methylendioxymethamphteamine (MDMA ecstasy). *Synapse* 2006;59(5):317-9.

[340] Garcia-Moreno JM, Chacon-Pena J. Hypothyroidism and Parkinson's disease and the issue of diagnostic confusion. *Mov Disord* 2003 Sep;18(9):1058-9.

CHAPTER TEN
[341] Tiovonen M, Tuomainen P, Mannisto PT. Effects of hypothalamic paraventricular nucleus lesion on cold-stimulated TSH responses to 5-HT in male rats. *Acta Physiol Scan* 1990;139(1):233-40.

[342] Soldin OP and Aschner M. Effects of manganese on thyroid hormone homeostasis: potential links. *Neurotoxicology* 2007; 28(5):951-6.

[343] Electrical responses of cultured thyroid cells to serotonin. *J Endocrinol* 1985;107(3):397-401.

344 Sapronov NS, Fedotova YO. The effect of L-tryptophan on conditioned reflex learning and behavior in rats with experimental pathology of the thyroid gland. *Neurosci Behav Physiol* 2002 May-Jun;32(3):237-41.

345 Foltyn W, Nowakowska-Zajdel E, Danikiewicz A, Brodziak A. [Hypothalamic-pituitary-thyroid axis in depression] [Article in Polish] *Psychiatr Pol* 2002;36(2):281-92.

346 Maayan ML, Sellitto RV, Volpert EM. Dopamine and L-dopa: inhibition of thyrotropin-stimulated thyroidal thyroxine release. *Endocrinology* 1986;118(2): 632-6.

347 Foord SM, Peters JM, Dieguez C, et al. Thyrotropin regulates thyrotroph responsiveness to dopamine in vitro. *Endcrinology* 1986; 118(4):1319-26.

348 Garbutt JC, Loosen PT, Glenn M. Lack of effect of dopamine receptor blockade on the TSH response to TRH in borderline personality disorder. *Psychiatry Res* 1987; 21(4): 307-11.

349 Cooper DS, Klibanski A, Ridgway EC. Dopaminergic modulation of TSH and its subunits: in vitro studies. *Clinical Endocrinol (Oxf)* 1983;18(3):265-75.

350 Hermus RM, Sweep CG, van der Meer MJ, et al. Continuous infusion of interleukin-1Beta induces a non-thyroidal illness syndrome in rat. *Endocrinology* 1992;131:2139-2146.

351 Rettori V, Jurcovicova J,McCAann SM. Central action of interleukin-1 in altering the release of TSH, growth hormone, and prolactin in the male rat. *J Neurosci Res* 1987;18:179-183.

352 Bartalena L, Grasso L, Brogioni S, et L. Interleukin-6 on pituitary-thyroid-axis in the rat. Eur J Endcrinol. 1994;131:302-306.

353 Lyson K, McCann SM. The effect of interleukin-6 on pituitary hormone release in vivo and vitro. *Neuroendocrinology1991*;54:262-266

354 Ozawa M, Sato K, Han DC, et al. Effects of tumor necrosis factor-alpha/cachetin on thyroid hormone metabolism in mice. *Endocrinology* 1998;123:1461-1467.

355 Rettori V, Milenkovic L, Beutler BA, et al. Hypothalamus action of cachectin to alter pituitary hormone release. *Brain Res Bull* 1989;23:471-475.

356 Drucker D, Josse R. Inappropriate TSH secretion with abnormal thyrotroph sensitivity to dopamine. *Clin Invest Med* 1985;8(2):117-20.

357 Marchesi C, Chiodera P, De Risio C. et al. Dopaminergic control of TSH secretion in endogenous depression. *Psychiatry Res* 1988;25(3):277-82.

358 Dieguez C, Peters JR, Page MD, et al. Thyroid function in patients with hyperprolactinemia: relationship to dopaminergic inhibition of TSH release. *Clin Endocrinol (Oxf)* 1986;25(4):435-40.

359 Patients with primary hypothyroidism presenting with prolactinomas. *Am J Med* 1987;83(4):765-9.

360 Hermus RM, Sweep CG, van der Meer MJ, et al. Continuous infusion of interleukin-1 Beta induces a non-thyroidal illness syndrome in rat. *Endoncrinology* 1992;131:2139-2146.

361 Rettori V, Jurcovicova J, McCaann SM. Central action of interleukin-1 in altering the release of TSH, growth hormone, and prolactin in male rat. *J Neurosci Res* 1987;18:179-183.

362 Bartalena L, Grasso L, Brogioni S, et al. Interleukin-6 on pituitary-thyroid-axis in the rat. *Eur J Endcrinol 1994*;131:302-306.

363 Lyson K, McCann SM. The effect of interleukin-6 on pituitary hormone release in vivo and vitro. *Neuroendocrinology* 1991;54:262-266.

364 Ozawa M, Sato K, Han DC, et al. Effects of tumor necrosis factor-alpha/cachetin on thyroid hormone metabolism in mice. *Endocrinology* 1998;123:1461-1467.

[365] Rettori V, Milenkovic L, Beutler BA, et al. Hypothalamus action of cachetin to alter pituitary hormone release. *Brain Res Bull* 1989;23:471-475.

[366] High iodine intake is a risk factor of post-partum thyroiditis: result of a survey from Shenyang, China. *J Endocrinol Invest* 2005 Nov;38(10):876-81.

[367] Pedersen IB, Knudsen N, Jørgensen T, Perrild H, Ovesen L, Laurberg P. Thyroid peroxidase and thyroglobulin autoantibodies in a large survey of populations with mild and moderate iodine deficiency. *Clin Endocrinol (Oxf)* 2003 Jan;58(1):36-42.

[368] *Thyroid* 2004 Jul;14(7):510-20.

[369] Mani S. Signaling mechanisms in progesterone-neurotransmitter interactions. *J Mol Endocrinol* 2003;30(2):127-37.

[370] Olivieri O, Girelli D, Azzini M, et al. Low selenium status in the elderly influences thyroid hormones. *Clin Sci* 1995;89:637-642.

[371] Kralik A, Eder K, Kirchgessner M. Influence of zinc and selenium deficiency on parameters relating to thyroid hormone metabolism. *Horm Metab Res* 1996;28:223-226.

[372] Calomme M, Vanderpas J, Francois B, et al. Effects of selenium supplementation on thyroid hormone metabolism in phenylketunuria subjects on the phenylalanine restricted diet. *Biol Trac Elem Res* 1995; 47:349-353.

[373] Lehmann C, Egerer K, Weber M et al. Effects of selenium administration on various laboratory parameters of patients at risk for sepsis syndrome. *Med Klin* 1997;92:14-16.

[374] Kauf E, Dawczynski H, Jahreis G, et al. Sodium selenite therapy and thyroid-hormone status in cystic fibrosis and congenial hypothyroidism. *Bio Trac Elem Res* 1994;40:247-253.

[375] Olivieri O, Gerelli D, Stanzial AM, et al. Selenium, zinc and thyroid hormones in healthy subjects: low T3/T4 ratio in the elderly is related to low selenium status. *Biol Trace Elem Res* 1996;51:31-41.

[376] Olivieri O, Girelli D, Azzini M, et al. Low selenium status in the elderly influences thyroid hormones. *Clin Sci* 1995;89:637-642.

[377] Kralik A, Eder K, Kirchgessner M. Influence of zinc and selenium deficiency on parameters relating to thyroid hormone metabolism. *Horm Metab Res* 1996;28:223-226.

[378] Calomme M, Vanderpas J, Francois B, et al. Effects of selenium supplementation on thyroid hormone metabolism in phenylketunuria subjects on the phenylalanine restricted diet. *Biol Trac Elem Res* 1995; 47:349-353.

[379] Lehmann C, Egerer K, Weber M, et al. Effects of selenium administration on various laboratory parameters of patients at risk for sepsis syndrome. *Med Klin* 1997;92:14-16.

[380] Kauf E, Dawczynski H, Jahreis G, et al. Sodium selenite therapy and thyroid-hormone status in cystic fibrosis and congenial hypothyroidism. *Bio Trac Elem Res* 1994;40:247-253.

[381] Zhu Z, Kumura M, Itokawa Y. Iodothyronine deiodinase activity in methionine-deficient rats fed selenium-deficient or selenium-sufficient diets. *Biol Trac Elem Res* 1995;48(2):197-213.

[382] Fujimoto S, Indo Y, Higahi A, et al. Conversion of thryoxine into tri-idothyronine in zinc deficient rat liver. *J Pediatr Gastroenterol Nutr* 1986;5:799-805.

[383] Nishiyama S, Futagoishi-Suginohara Y, Matsukura M. Zinc supplementation alter thyroid hormone metabolism in disabled patients with zinc deficiency. *J Am Coll Nutr* 1994;13:62-67.

[384] Licastro F, et al. Zinc effects the metabolism of thyroid hormones in children with Down's syndrome:normalization of thyroid stimulating hormone and of reversal of triiodothyronin plasmic levels of dietary zinc supplementation. *Int J Neruosci* 1992;65(1-4):259-268.

385 LoPresti, JS and Nicoloff, JT. Thyroid response to critical illness. *Endocrinology of Critical Disease*. Human Press. Totowa. NJ. 1997. pp 157-173.

386 Strakis, CA and Chrousos, GP. Neuroendocrinology and Pathophysiology of the Stress System, *Ann NY Acad Sci* Vol. 771, pp. 1-18,1995.

387 Stockigt, JR, Braverman, LE, ed. Update on the Sick Euthyroid Syndrome. *Diseases of the Thyroid*. Humana Press, Totowa, NJ, 1997, pp. 49-68.

388 Ongphiphadhanakul B, Fang SL, Tang KT, et al. Tumor necrosis factor-alpha decreased thyrotropin-induced 5'deiodinase activity in FRTL-5 thyroid cells. *Eur J Endocrinol* 1994;130:502-507.

389 Pekary AE, Berg L, Santini F, et al. Cytokines modulate type I iodthyronine deiodinase mRNA levels and enzyme activity in FRTL 5 rat thyroid cells. *Mol Cell Endocrinol* 1994:101:R31-R35.

390 Yu J, Koenig RJ. Regulation of hepatocyte thryoxine 5'deiodinase by T3 and nuclear receptor coactivators as a model of sick euthyroid syndrome. *J Biol Chem* 2000;275:38296-38301.

391 Molnar I, Balazs C, Szegedi G, et al. Inhibition of type 2.5 deiodinase by tumor necrosis factor alpha, interleukin-6 and interferon gamma in human thyroid tissue. *Immunol Lett* 2002;80:3-7.

392 Nagaya T, Fujieda M, Otsuka G, et al. A potential role o activated NF-KB in pathogenesis of euthyroid sick syndrome. *J Clin Invest* 2000:106:393-402.

393 LoPresti, JS and Nicoloff, JT. Thyroid response to critical illness. *Endocrinology of Critical Disease*. Human Press. Totowa. NJ. 1997. pp 157-173.

394 Strakis, CA and Chrousos, GP. Neuroendocrinology and Pathophysiology of the Stress System, *Ann NY Acad Sci* Vol. 771, pp. 1-18,1995.

395 Stockigt, JR, Braverman, LE, ed. Update on the Sick Euthyroid Syndrome. *Diseases of the Thyroid*. Humana Press, Totowa, NJ, 1997, pp. 49-68.

396 Corrsmite EP, Heyligenberg R, Endert E, et al. Acute effects of interferon-alpha-administration on thyroid hormone metabolism in healthy men. *J Clin Endcorin Metab* 1995:80:3140-3144.

397 Van der Poll T, Romijn JA, Wiersinga WM, et al. Tuor necrosis factor: a putative mediator of the sick euthyroid syndrome in man. *J Clin Endocrinol Metab* 1990;71:1567-1572.

398 Stouthared JM, Van der Poll T, Endert E. et al. Effects of acute and chronic interleukin-6 administration on thyroid hormone metabolism in human. *J Clin Endocrinol Metab* 1994;79:1342-1346.

399 Strawen JR, Ekhator NN. Pituitary-thyroid state correlates with central dopaminergic and serotonergic activity in healthy humans. *Neuropsychobiology* 2004; 49(2):84-7.

400 Strawen JR, Ekhator NN. Pituitary-thyroid state correlates with central dopaminergic and serotonergic activity in healthy humans. *Neuropsychobiology* 2004; 49(2):84-7.

401 Bisschop PH, Toorians AW, Endert E, Wiersinga WM, Gooren LJ, Fliers E. The effects of sex-steroid administration on the pituitary-thyroid axis in transsexuals. *Eur J Endocrinol* 2006 Jul;155(1):11-6.

402 Knopp RH, Bergelin RO, Wahl PW, Walden CE, Chapman MB. Chemical alterations in pregnancy and oral contraceptive use. *Obstet Gynecol* 1985;5;66:682-90.

403 Steingold KA, Matt DW, DeZiegler D, Sealey JE, Fratkin M, Rezinkov S. Comparison of transdermal to oral estradiol administration on hormonal and hepatic parameters in women with premature ovarian failure. *J Clin Endocrinol Metab* 1991:73:275-80.

404 Geola FL, Frumar AM, Tataryn IV, et al. Biological effects of various doses of conjugated equine estrogens in postmenopausal women. *J Clin Endocrinol Metab* 1980;51:620-5.

405 Ben-Rafael Z, Mastroianni L, Strauss JF, Flickinger GL, Arendasch-Durand B. Changes in Thyroid function tests and sex hormone binding globulin associated with treatment of gonadotropin. *Fertil Steril* 1987;48;318-320.

406 Sarkis MI & Sievert R. Drugs and thyroid function. *NEJM* 1995;333(25): 168801694.

407 Deysigg R, Weissel M. Ingestion of androgenic-anabolic steroids induces mild thyroidal impairment in male body builders. *J Clin Endocrinol Metab* 1993;76:1069-71.

408 Malarkey WB, Strauss RH, Leizman DJ, et al. Endocrine effects in female weight lifters who self-administer testosterone and anabolic steroids. *Am J Obstet Gynecol* 1991;165:1385-90.

409 Graham RL, Gambrell RD Jr. Changes in thyroid function tests during danazol therapy. *Obstet Gynecol* 1980;55:395-7.

410 Lu B, Moser AH, Shigenga JK, Feingold KR, Grunfeld C. Type II nuclear hormone receptors, coactivator, and target gene repression in adipose tissue in acute-phase response. *J Lipid Res* 2006;47 (10):2179-90.

411 Kimura H and Caturegli P. Chemokine orchestration of autoimmune thyroiditis. *Thyroid* 2007;47(10):1005-11.

412 Yamazaki K, Suzuki K, Yamada E, et al. Suppression of iodide uptake and thyroid hormone synthesis with stimulation of the type I interferon system by double-stranded ribonucleic acid in cultured human thyroid follicles. *Endocrinology* 2007;148(7):3226-35.

413 Kwakkel J, Wiersinga WM, Boelen A. Interleukin-1 beta modulates endogenous thyroid hormone receptors alpha gene transcription in liver cells. *J Endocrinol* 2007:194(2):257-65.

414 Williams GR, Neuberger JM, Ranklin JA, Sheppard MC. Thyroid hormone receptor expression in the "sick euthyroid syndrome." *Lancet* 1989;2(8678-8679):1477-1481.

415 Reidel W, Layka H, Neeck G. Secretory pattern of GH, TSH, Thyroid hormones, ACTH, cortisol, FSH, and LH in patients with fibromyalgia syndrome following systemic injection of the relevant hypothalamic-releasing hormones. *J Rheumatol* 1998;57 (Suppl 2):81-87.

416 Sterling K. Thyroid hormone action at the cell level. *N Engl J Med* 300(3):117-122.

417 Zhang J, Lazar MA. The mechanisms of action of thyroid hormones. *Ann Rev Physiol* 2000;62:439-466.

418 Limpach A, Dalton M, Mules R, Gadson P. Homocysteine inhibits retinoic acid synthesis: a mechanism for homocysteine-induced congenitial defects. *Experimental Cell Res* 2000;260:166-174.

INDEX

lactoluse/mannitol test, 129, 130
L-arginine, 80, 162, 171, 195, 226
L-carnitine, 145, 146, 170, 195
LDL cholesterol, 13, 193
leaky gut
  about, 123
  adrenal stress and, 130–131667
  autoimmune disease triggers and, 47
  defined, 239
  dysglycemia and, 104
  gluten intolerance and, 29, 31
  mercury and, 62
  Repair Stage of colon health program, 129
lecithin (phosphatidylcholine), 84, 128, 162, 222
lemon balm, 54, 209
lemon juice, 109, 110
Lepidium mayenil, 162, 227
Levothyroid, 91
Levothyroixine, 91
Levoxyl, 91
L-glutamine, 129
L-glutathione, 84, 161
licorice, 54, 146, 153, 201–202, 209
lime juice, 109, 110
lipase, 12
lipid markers, 14
lipid peroxidation, 195, 203
lipopolysaccharides (LPS), 122
liposomal creams
  for adrenal balancing, 200
  for adrenal dysfunction, 143
  for adrenal exhaustion, 200–201
  for neurotransmitter deficiency, 171
  nutritional support for thyroid under-conversion, 82
liver
  conversion of T4 hormones, 3, 4, 10
  detoxification, 15, 83, 84, 161, 203, 218–221
  estrogen metabolism, 14
  excess hormones and, 157, 159
  glucose utilization, 193
  homocysteine and, 18
  hypothyroidism and, 11–12, 13
long pepper fruit, 126
low-carbohydrate diet for dysglycemia, 102–103, 104–107
low thyroid function, see hypothyroidism
luteinizing hormone (LH), 158, 228
lycopene, 55

macronutrients in protein powder, 211
macrophages, 44, 239
magnesium
  for adrenal dysfunction alarm and resistance, 143–145
  alarm reaction nutritional support, 143
  estrogen metabolism and, 162, 231

CPSIA information can be obtained at www.ICGtesting.com
Printed in the USA
BVOW070046230513

321430BV00002B/108/P